Atlas of Pulmonary Pathology

PATHCO P.C.
R. M. Kotz, D.O.   L. W. Icle, D.O.
3126 - 44th
Des Moines, Iowa 50310
(515) 255-7526

Current Histopathology

Consultant Editor
Professor G. Austin Gresham, TD, ScD, MD, FRC Path.
Professor of Morbid Anatomy and Histology, University of Cambridge

Volume Three

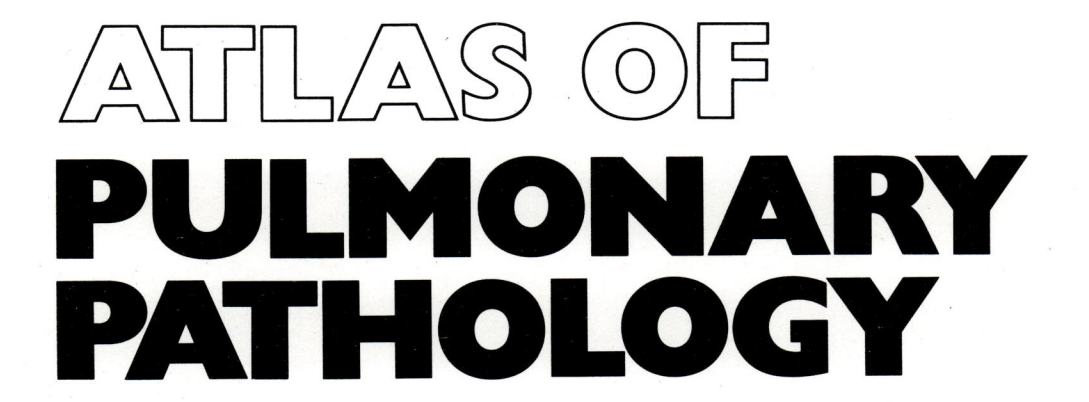

ATLAS OF PULMONARY PATHOLOGY

BY A. R. GIBBS
Department of Pathology,
The Welsh National School of Medicine, Cardiff, Wales

AND R. M. E. SEAL
Department of Pathology,
Llandough Hospital, Glamorgan, Wales

with a chapter by **J. G. Leopold,**
Welsh National School of Medicine

J. B. Lippincott Company
PHILADELPHIA AND TORONTO

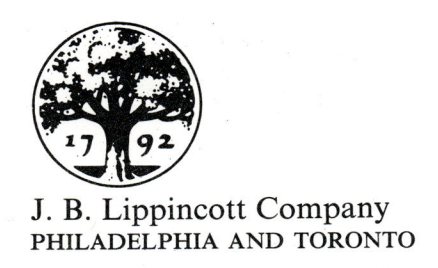

Published and distributed in North America by
J. B. Lippincott Company

Published in Great Britain by
MTP Press Limited
Falcon House
Cable Street
Lancaster, England

Copyright © 1982 A. R. Gibbs and R. M. E. Seal

All rights reserved. No part of this publication may be reproduced, stored in a retrieval system, or transmitted in any form or by any means, electronic, mechanical, photocopying, recording or otherwise, without prior permission from the publishers.

ISBN 0-397-58283-8

LCCN 81-86053

Printed in Great Britain

Contents

	Consultant editor's note	7
	Introduction	9
1	Congenital disorders	11
2	Chronic bronchitis and emphysema by Dr J. G. Leopold	15
3	Bronchiectasis	25
4	Pneumonias	27
5	Interstitial pneumonias	39
6	Tuberculosis	47
7	Non-tuberculous granulomatous conditions	53
8	Asthma and related conditions	59
9	Systemic diseases affecting the lung	63
10	Pathology of the pulmonary vasculature	69
11	Pulmonary angiitides	75
12	Diseases of uncertain aetiology	79
13	Occupational lung disorders – I. coal and silica	83
14	Occupational lung disorders – II. silicate pneumoconioses	91
15	Occupational lung disorders – III. metals, fumes and organic materials	99
16	Lung carcinomas	103
17	Carcinoid and salivary-gland type tumours	111
18	Mixed tumours	115
19	Primary lymphoproliferative conditions	119
20	Miscellaneous rare pulmonary tumours	123
21	Pleural tumours	127
	Index	131

Current Histopathology Series

Already published in this series:
Volume 1   Atlas of Lymph Node Pathology
Volume 2   Atlas of Renal Pathology

Other volumes currently scheduled in this series include the following titles:

Atlas of Breast Pathology

Atlas of Cytology

Atlas of Gastro-intestinal Pathology

Atlas of Gynaecological Pathology

Atlas of Joint and Connective Tissue Pathology

Atlas of Liver Pathology

Atlas of Male Reproductive System Pathology

Atlas of Muscle Pathology

Atlas of Neuropathology

Atlas of Oral Pathology

Atlas of Skin Pathology

Atlas of Toxicology

Consultant Editor's Note

At the present time books on morbid anatomy and histology can be divided into two broad groups: extensive textbooks often written primarily for students and monographs on research topics.

This takes no account of the fact that the vast majority of pathologists are involved in an essentially practical field of general Diagnostic Pathology, providing an important service to their clinical colleagues. Many of these pathologists are expected to cover a broad range of disciplines and even those who remain solely within the field of histopathology usually have single and sole responsibility within the hospital for all this work. They may often have no chance for direct discussion on problem cases with colleagues in the same department. In the field of histopathology, no less than in other medical fields, there have been extensive and recent advances, not only in new histochemical techniques but also in the type of specimen provided by new surgical procedures.

There is a great need for the provision of appropriate information for this group. This need has been defined in the following terms.

1. It should be aimed at the general clinical pathologist or histopathologist with existing practical training, but should also have value for the trainee pathologist.
2. It should concentrate on the practical aspects of histopathology taking account of the new techniques which should be within the compass of the worker in a unit with reasonable facilities.
3. New types of material e.g. those derived from endoscopic biopsy should be covered fully.
4. There should be an adequate number of illustrations on each subject to demonsterate the variation in appearance that is encountered.
5. Colour illustrations should be used wherever they aid recognition.

The present concept stemmed from this defirition but it was immediately realized that these aims could only be achieved within the compass of a series, of which this volume is one. Since histopathology is, by its very nature, systematized, the individual volumes deal with one system or where this appears more appropriate with a single organ.

This is the third volume of the *Current Histopathology* series. It provides a modern account of pulmonary disease illustrated by photographs of macroscopic and microscopic material. Once more the aim is to provide ready access to a developing field of histopathology. Modern ideas of aetiology and modern classifications are clearly presented.

G. Austin Gresham
Cambridge

Dedication

To Gillian, Geoffrey and Edward.

Introduction

The field of pulmonary medicine is evolving rapidly and the role of the pathologist always changing. Statements formerly accepted as fact are being challenged; new concepts and classifications are being put forward and new entities established. This has left a very considerable number of pathologists and clinicians confused and ignorant about severe pulmonary conditions. In this volume we have attempted to bring some order to this chaos and to provide the information necessary for a reasonable comprehension of these disorders. At first sight it might seem that we have overemphasised and discussed more fully certain disorders over more common ones but it is the authors' experience that problems particularly arise for example, in relation to occupational lung disease, interstitial pneumonias, asthmatic disorders, angiitides, lymphoproliferative disorders and the classification of lung tumours. The weight and balance of this volume therefore reflects this. We hope that we have provided in this volume the majority of the information and guidance necessary to approach particular diagnostic problems and reach satisfactory conclusions. It is only by careful and accurate interpretation of lung material that correct diagnosis will be established and appropriate treatment instituted.

Acknowledgements

We wish to express our gratitude to Dr J. G. Leopold for his comments on several chapters in this book. We thank Professor E. D. Williams for his advice on Chapter 17, Dr. J. C. Wagner for advice on Chapters 13, 14 and 21 and Dr Jones Williams for advice on Chapter 7.

We are grateful to many of our colleagues in Wales for use of their material: Dr W. Beasley, Dr T. Dauncey, Dr D. M. D. Evans, Dr R. W. Fortt, Dr J. Gough, Dr B. Knight, Dr G. Melville Jones, Dr T. Parry, Dr D. B. Richards, Dr A. L. Wells and Dr Geraint Williams. We have also made extensive use of the late Professor Jethro Gough's pulmonary collection housed in the Welsh National School of Medicine.

We also wish to express our appreciation of our colleagues outside Wales: Professor Bryan Corrin (The Brompton Hospital), Dr J. C. Briggs (Bristol), Dr K. W. Chan (Hong Kong), Professor Gee (Leeds), Dr A. Morley (Newcastle-Upon-Tyne) and Dr N. Sannerkin (Bristol).

We wish to thank our clinical colleagues, particularly Dr A. Cockcroft, Dr J. Edwards and Dr J. Lyons, for providing useful information.

A publication such as this is heavily dependent on skilful contributions from Departments of Medical Illustration. Special thanks are due to Mr D. Llewellyn for producing the plates and several of the macroscopic illustrations and also to Mr P. Langham and Mr R. Boothby.

We express appreciation to Mr W. Sullivan, Mr C. Lediard and the staff of the pathology laboratories of the University Hospital of Wales and Llandough Hospital.

Our thanks are due to Miss J. Stitfall and Mrs V. Hamilton for typing the manuscript.

Specific acknowledgements

Professor K. M. Laurence and the Editor of *Journal of Clinical Pathology* – Chapter 1 Figures 8, 9 and 10
Mr P. Cartwright – Chapter 4 Figure 14 (right)
Dr J. C. Wagner – Chapter 4 Figure 27
Professor B. Corrin – Chapter 5 Figure 4
Dr W. Jones Williams – Chapter 7 Figure 3 (right)
Dr Nej Sannerkin – Chapter 8 Figure 5 (right)
Dr A. Morley – Chapter 8 Figures 9, 10 and 11
Professor B. Corrin – Chapter 10 Figure 6
Dr J. C. Wagner – Chapter 14 Figure 13
Professor B. Corrin and Dr J. Abrahams – Chapter 15 Figure 3 (right)
Dr Nej Sannerkin – Chapter 18 Figure 5
Professor B. Corrin – Chapter 20 Figures 7 and 8
Dr J. C. Wagner – Chapter 21 Figure 12
Professor C. A. Wagenvoort and the Editor of *Chest* – Chapter 10 Plate
Dr R. W. Furtt and Dr D. Pollock – Chapter 12 Figure 7

Congenital Disorders

Minor anomalies of the lung are not uncommon; severe malformations resulting in impaired pulmonary function are rare. They may co-exist with anomalies of other organs.

Pulmonary Abnormalities

Primary Agenesis, Aplasia and Hypoplasia are rare anomalies. The causative factors must have been operative between the 24th day and 24th week of intrauterine life.

Agenesis is unilateral or bilateral complete absence of pulmonary tissue. Unilateral agenesis is compatible with long life[1], although many cases die of respiratory-tract infections or concomitant malformations of other organs. *Aplasia* refers to suppression of development of all but a rudimentary bronchus; in *hypoplasia* the bronchus is malformed and terminates in a fleshy mass of incompletely differentiated tissue.

Secondary Hypoplasia results from interference of the capacity of the thoracic cage in early fetal life, e.g. by diaphragmatic hernia (Figure 1.1), cardiomegaly, abdominal masses, etc. The number of bronchial branches and amount of alveolar tissue is usually reduced.

Bronchopulmonary Abnormalities

Minor Abnormalities of Lobation are not uncommon and are of no functional significance. Most common is the *azygos lobe*, which occurs in 1% of the population[1], where a fold of pleura enclosing the azygos vein separates the right upper lobe into two portions. The most common supernumerary lobe is the left middle lobe[2]. An *'infracardiac'* lobe occurs when a fissure separates the medial basal segment from the remainder of the right lower lobe.

Sequestrated Lobe is a mass of pulmonary tissue which does not communicate with the bronchial tree and is supplied by an aberrant systemic artery. It may be described as: *intralobar*, when the mass is within the visceral pleura; *extralobar*, when it is outside the visceral pleura but still attached to the lungs; or *completely sequestrated*, when the mass is entirely independent of the lungs.

Intralobar sequestrations are three to four times more frequent than the extralobar type. The intralobar type exhibits no propensity for either side but the extralobar variety occurs on the left side in 80% of cases. The latter is often associated with a diaphragmatic hernia or a pulmonary arteriovenous fistula.

The sequestrated lobe is usually well demarcated, grey or dark red, firm and fleshy (Figure 1.2). In town dwellers the sequestrated segment stands out as non-pigmented. Solitary or multiple cysts may be evident (Figure 1.3). Histologically, bronchi, bronchioles, lymphoid tissue and thick atherosclerotic arteries are present (Figures 1.2 and 1.3). There is usually considerable fibrosis and there may or may not be alveoli. Venous drainage from extralobar sequestration is to the azygos system and from intralobar sequestration to the pulmonary venous system.

Most *Abnormalities of the Bronchial Tree* are of no clinical significance. There are two major categories[3]: (1) a normal branch may arise in an abnormal position (displaced bronchus); (2) supernumerary branches may be present. The most common supernumerary branch arises from the lateral side of the right main bronchus or lower part of the right side of the trachea to connect with the right upper lobe.

Other common anomalies include a bifurcate pattern to the division of the right upper lobe bronchus (normally trifurcate) and a trifurcate pattern to the left upper lobe bronchus (normally bifurcate).

Congenital Bronchiectasis is much rarer than the acquired disease. Due to abnormal development of the bronchial tree, the lung reveals dilated tubular bronchi which extend almost to the pleural surface. Histologically, peripheral airways are almost totally absent[4].

'Kartagener's Syndrome' comprises a triad of situs inversus, bronchiectasis and nasal sinusitis. It may be familial and is due to a generalized abnormality of ciliary function. The bronchiectasis may be localized or diffuse.

Tracheobronchopathia Osteoplastica may be an incidental finding at autopsy or the patient may present, usually over the age of 50 years, with dyspnoea, hoarseness, productive cough or haemoptysis. The lower two thirds of the trachea and often major bronchi show submucosal osseous and cartilaginous masses which occur independently of the tracheal and bronchial cartilages (Figure 1.4).

Heterotopic Tissues

Adrenal cortical tissues, striated muscle or brain tissue have been observed occasionally in the lungs of fetuses and newborn infants, particularly those with severe abnormalities of the central nervous system.

Pulmonary Cysts

Cysts may contain air or fluid and may be single or multiple. Congenital cysts are rare, whilst acquired post-infectious cysts or pneumatoceles are more common.

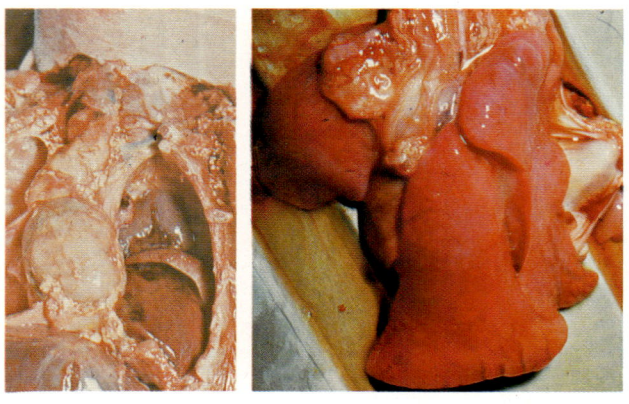

Figure 1.1 *Left:* A male infant who died shorly after birth with respratory distress. Part of the liver, spleen and bowel have entered the left thoracic cavity. The left lung, which is very small, can just be seen near the apex of the left thoracic cavity. *Right:* Another case with a congenital diaphragmatic hernia. A posterior view of the thoracic organs shows the much smaller size of the left lung compared with the right lung.

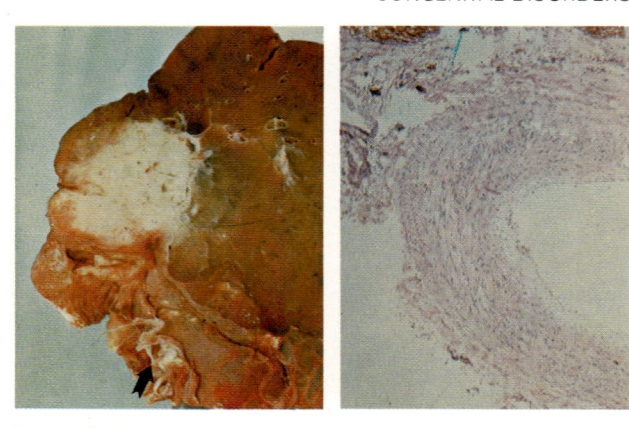

Figure 1.2 *Left:* Lower lobectomy specimen of a previously undiagnosed intralobar sequestration presenting as pulmonary suppuration. They may also present clinically as a 'neoplasm'. A large systemic vessel (arrow) is entering the diaphragmatic aspect. *Right:* This shows the 'systemic nature' of the vessel. H&E × 38.4.

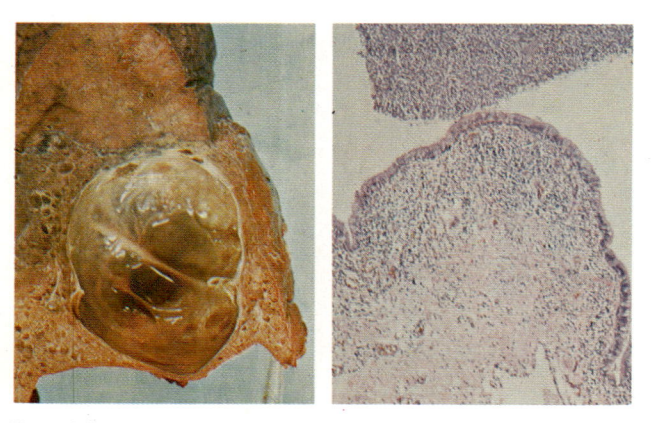

Figure 1.3 *Left:* An intralobar sequestration showing a large multilocular cyst with smaller cysts in the background. *Right:* Microscopy reveals a respiratory type lining to one of the cysts and inflammation in its wall. H&E × 38.4.

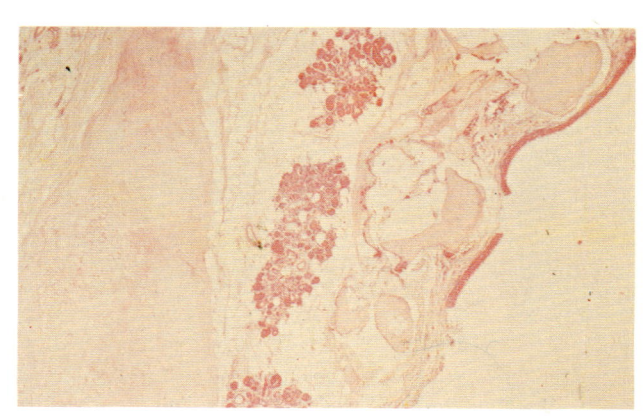

Figure 1.4 Submucosal formation of bone between the tracheal cartilage (left) and respiratory epithelium (right). H&E × 24.

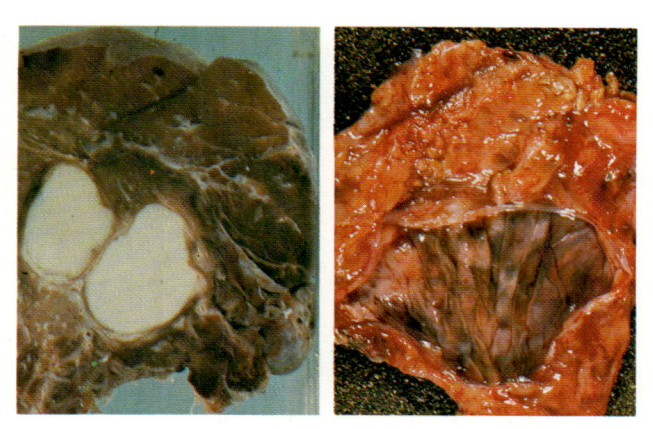

Figure 1.5 *Left:* Two bronchogenic cysts which are filled with mucin. *Right:* Another bronchogenic cyst with the contents removed to show a smooth grey wall.

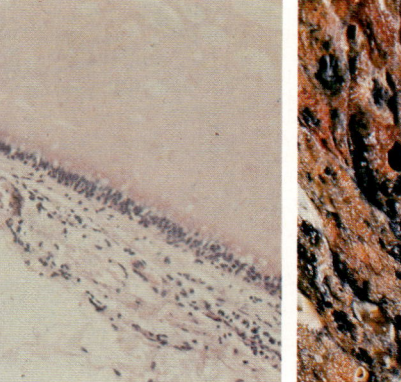

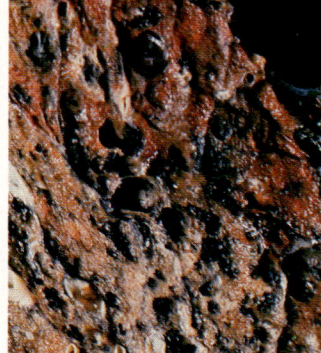

Figure 1.6 *Left:* The wall of the bronchogenic cyst is lined by respiratory type epithelium containing numerous goblet cells. H&E × 96. *Right:* A coal worker with several peripheral congenital cysts found incidentally at autopsy.

CONGENITAL DISORDERS

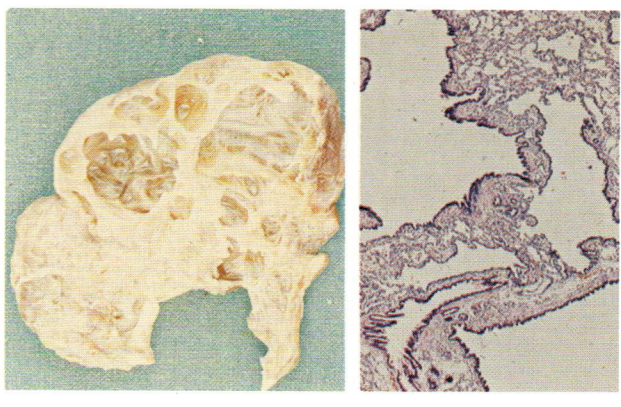

Figure 1.7 *Left:* 5-week old male infant presenting with cough, dyspnoea and cyanosis. Right thoracotomy revealed large multicystic mass in the position of the posterior segment of right upper lobe. *Right:* Microscopy reveals the appearance of congenital cystic malformation. H&E × 24.

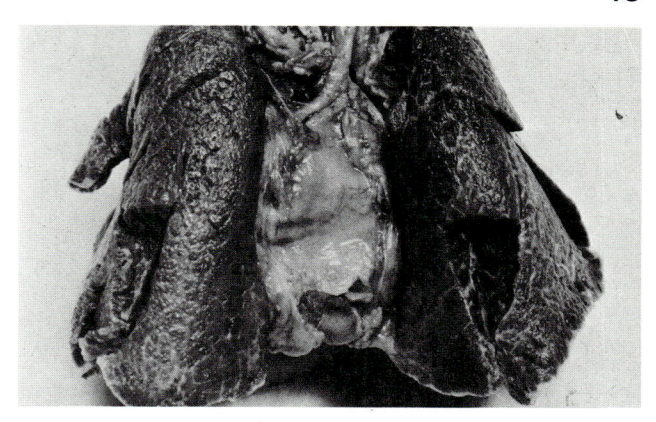

Figure 1.8 The lungs of a male infant who died a few hours after birth. There are prominent subpleural lymphatic vessels giving the lung a resemblance to liver. Some collapsed cysts can be seen subpleurally.

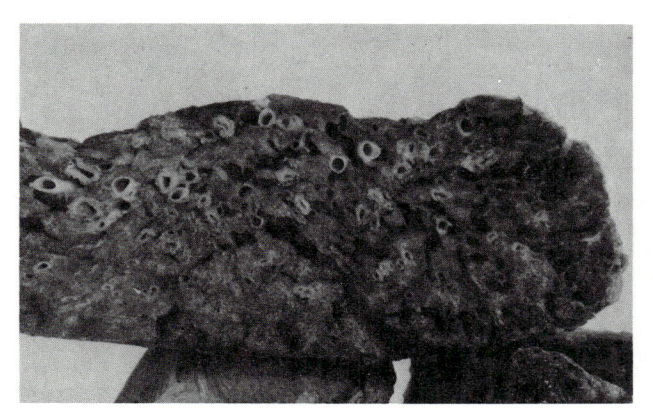

Figure 1.9 The cut surface of a case of congenital pulmonary lymphangiectasis showing numerous rounded cysts.

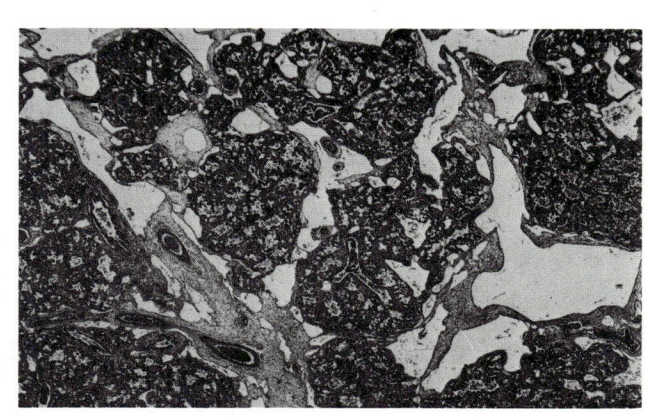

Figure 1.10 Microscopy of the previous case (Figure 1.9) revealed the cysts to be lined by non-stratified endothelium. The cyst walls are composed of a delicate network of collagen, elastic and smooth muscle. H&E × 38.4.

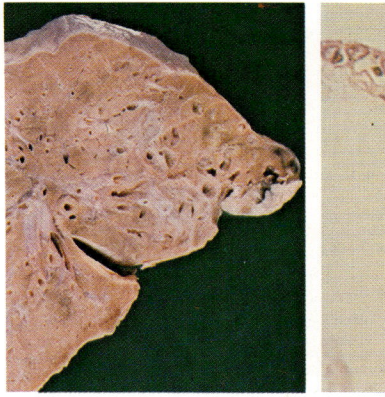

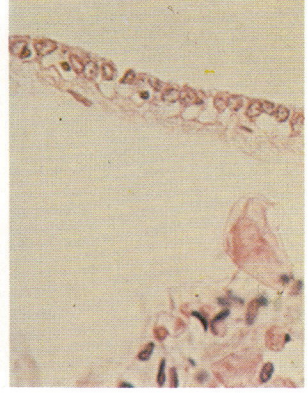

Figure 1.11 *Left:* A young male who experienced repeated respiratory infections due to cystic fibrosis. Macroscopic examination of the lung reveals bronchiectasis. *Right:* The pleural mesothelium shows characteristic clear intra-cytoplasmic and intercellular vacuoles which do not stain histochemically for mucin. H&E × 384.

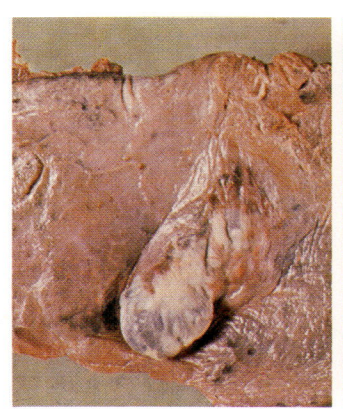

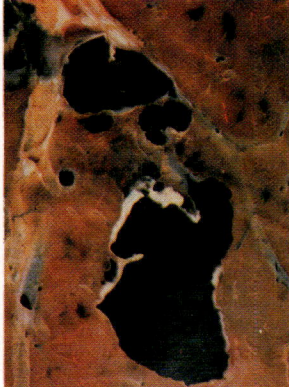

Figure 1.12 This patient presented with haemoptysis and an ill-defined radiological opacity, the diagnosis being made at thoracotomy. *Left:* A protuberant lesion on the pleural surface and the cut surface. *Right:* Reveals large complex vascular channels filled by a gelatin – Indian ink mixture.

Congenital Cysts

Spencer[4] divides these into two types:

(1) *Central (bronchogenic)* cysts are usually solitary, are lined by respiratory-type epithelium, contain mucous glands, cartilage, muscle and elastic in their wall, and have no bronchial connection (Figures 1.5 and 1.6). They may reach a size of several centimetres and are located in the mediastinum, lung hilum or in the oesophageal wall.

(2) *Peripheral* cysts are frequently multiple, may affect both lungs, a whole lung, a lobe or part of a lobe (Figure 1.6). They may be lined by ciliated or non-ciliated columnar epithelium; mucous glands, cartilage and smooth muscle are usually absent.

Infection of these cysts frequently occurs, making histological distinction from acquired cysts sometimes impossible.

Congenital Adenomatoid Malformation

This consists of an intrapulmonary tumour-like mass containing multiple or multilocular, irregular, thin-walled cysts. The cysts have a bronchiole-like epithelium without cartilage in their walls. The intervening tissue resembles very immature fetal 'alveoli'. This occurs in oedematous stillborn and premature infants[5].

An overlapping variant, termed congenital cystic malformation[5], occurs in term infants and children, and shows predominantly cystic bronchioles with interspersed mature alveoli (Figure 1.7).

Congenital Cystic Lymphangiectasis

This is a rare condition; death usually occurs within the first week of life.

Macroscopically the lung appears enlarged, nodular, hard and resembles cirrhotic liver. Close inspection reveals small smooth-walled cysts which are due to distention of lymphatic channels within the septa and pleura[6] (Figures 1.8–1.10).

In 50% of cases other congenital malformations co-exist, including asplenia, cardiac malformations, accessory pulmonary lobes and anomalies of blood supply and venous drainage to the lungs.

Enterogenous Cysts

Intrapulmonary cysts lined by gastric or intestinal mucosa have been occasionally described. They may communicate with a bronchus.

Cystic Fibrosis

This is an inherited generalized disorder causing dysfunction of the exocrine glands. In the bronchial tree there is an abnormality of epithelial mucin production resulting in an increased viscosity of the mucus. Clearance of secretions is therefore impaired, with consequent bronchopneumonia, bronchiectasis and bronchiolectasis. Ninety per cent of the patients die of respiratory disease before the age of puberty. Histologically the bronchi are filled with mucus which may be seen to be continuous with the mucus filling the gland ducts. The bronchi usually show marked inflammatory changes and often squamous metaplasia. A characteristic metaplasia of the pleural mesothelium is sometimes present[7] (Figure 1.11).

Congenital Lobar Emphysema

This is characterized by overdistension of a lobe, due to a ball-valve mechanism, usually an upper lobe. There is compression of the remainder of the ipsilateral lung, mediastinal shift and atelectasis of the contralateral lobe. A variety of anatomical lesions affecting the bronchus supplying the emphysematous lobe have been described, including absence or malformation of cartilaginous rings, flaps of bronchial mucosa, mucus plugs, and extrinsic compression of the bronchus by abnormal blood vessels or a bronchogenic cyst.

Histologically, the affected lobe shows uniform distension of bronchioles, atria and alveoli.

Wilson–Mikity Syndrome

A syndrome of unknown pathogenesis particularized by progressive respiratory distress affecting premature infants soon after birth and reaching a peak of severity 4–8 weeks after onset. Approximately 25% die within this period.

The lungs of such infants show alternating areas of extreme hyperinflation and atelectasis – best observed with a Gough-Wentworth section[8].

Anomalies of the Pulmonary Vessels

Pulmonary arteriovenous malformations may occur in isolation or in association with cutaneous and mucosal telangiectasis (Rendu-Osler-Weber disease)[2]. Within the lung they may be single or multiple. Patients usually present in adult life with polycythaemia, finger clubbing or haemoptysis. They may occur in any segment of the lung (Figure 1.12). They may calcify which sometimes leads to a false diagnosis of tuberculosis.

References

1. Levine, M. I. and Mascia, A. V. (1966). *Pulmonary Disease and Anomalies of Infancy and Childhood*. (New York: Harper & Row)
2. Weir, J. A. (1960). Congenital anomalies of the lung. *Ann. Int. Med.*, **52,** 330
3. Landing, B. H. (1979). State of the art. Congenital malformations and genetic disorders of the respiratory tract. *Am. Rev. Resp. Dis.*, **120,** 151
4. Spencer, H. (1977). *Pathology of the Lung*. 3rd Edn, Chap. 3. (Oxford: Pergamon Press)
5. Bale, P. M. (1979). Congenital cystic malformation of the lung. A form of congenital bronchiolar ('adenomatoid') malformation. *Am. J. Clin. Pathol.*, **71,** 411
6. Laurence, K. M. (1959). Congenital pulmonary lymphangiectasis. *J. Clin. Pathol.*, **12,** 62
7. Dunnill, M. S. (1954). Metaplastic changes in the visceral pleura in a case of fibrocystic disease of the pancreas. *J. Pathol. Bacteriol.*, **77,** 299
8. Askin, F. B. (1975). Lungs. In Kissane, J. M. (ed.) *Pathology in Infancy and Childhood*. 2nd Edition (St. Louis: C. V. Mosby)

Chronic Bronchitis and Emphysema

by Dr J. G. Leopold

The pathological findings in chronic bronchitis are highly variable. Features of an inflammatory bronchial disease are predominant in cases with recurrent clinical bacterial infections, but not in others. The symptoms of the disease place it under three headings: mucous catarrh (simple chronic bronchitis), infective bronchitis and bronchitis with airway obstruction and the pathology cannot be described without regard to these groupings.

Cases may show predominance of one clinical form over the others, pointing, without precision, to the pathological changes which typify each aspect of the disease. There is a close clinical relationship between mucous catarrh and the infection, and noteworthy is the frequent successful culture for *H. influenzae* in cases, during even the catarrhal phase. On the other hand, Fletcher et al.[1] have provided evidence that airway obstruction is not due to the direct progression of chronic bronchitis defined in terms of its mucoid and infective features. They believe that the relationship is complex, cigarette smoking being a shared factor in the aetiology. The morphological change in the lungs responsible for air-flow difficulty has not been established, but it remains a possibility that accompanying emphysema could be the cause. There is no direct relationship between bronchitis and emphysema and the description of these diseases is best kept separate.

Chronic Bronchitis

Mucous Hyperplasia and Chronic Bronchitis

The hypersecretion of mucus, symptomatic of the disease, is mirrored in pathology by the finding of hyperplasia of the bronchial mucous glands and the goblet cells in the lining epithelium[2] (Figure 2.1). It has also been known for a long time[3] that an equivalent hyperplasia may characterize the lungs of chronic asthmatics. Dunnill et al.[4], by accurate morphometry of various components of bronchial structure, have given added quantitative data confirming both the bronchial gland hyperplasia of chronic bronchitis and the bronchial-gland hyperplasia of asthmatics. The claim which has been made for an abrupt separation of bronchitic from non-bronchitic on this basis is no longer tenable.

Evaluation of the changes in the population of goblet cells has the inherent difficulty that the level in the bronchial tree is the all important factor in assessment. In health, goblet cells are not seen at the terminal or pre-terminal bronchiole level, whereas they may be found there in the lungs of chronic bronchitics.

The Inflammatory Aspects of Chronic Bronchitis

Many cases of non-specific, chronic inflammatory lung disease die during an attack of acute bacterial bronchial infection. Purulent bronchial contents with a complement of shed cells of the bronchial lining, bronchiolitis and bronchopneumonia of varying degree are all frequent findings. Bacteriology has clearly established the principal role of *H. influenzae* and the commensal types of pneumococci in these events [5,6]. It is also common to find other changes often taken to be indicative of persistent inflammation, but these have not been accurately correlated with the separation into catarrhal and infective cases.

The changes that fall within this category are plasma–lymphocyte cell infiltration of the bronchial submucosa, hyaline thickening of the epithelial basement membrane and squamoid metaplasia of the lining epithelium. All these findings are duplicated in the bronchi of patients with persistent, recurrent asthma and therefore are not necessarily indicative of an infective basis. Despite the frequent usage of the term infective asthma, Brumfitt and Willoughby[7] noted significant difficulty in culturing *H. influenzae* and pneumococci in bronchial aspirates from cases of asthma in contrast with cases of chronic bronchitis.

Metaplasia of surface epithelia often follows repeated cell loss in other situations, and both bronchial infection and asthma result in shedding of the columnar cell layer leaving only the basal cells, from which regeneration occurs. A noteworthy feature of the pathology of more-severe cases of chronic bronchitis is the frequent finding of peripheral tubular bronchiectasis, predominantly but not exclusively at the base of the lung (Figure 2.2).

Clinical bronchography bears out this finding. I am not aware that there has been an accurate correlation of cases showing this feature with those having infection in their clinical background. It is clear that no separation exists between such examples and the few cases in which the extreme severity of the changes, occurring in a localized area, justifies the additional diagnostic label bronchiectasis. All the features of classical bronchiectasis, barring extreme muscle and elastic destruction, are shared by the more diffuse changes, including bronchial arterial hypertrophy.

Bronchial Diverticula

Simon and Galbraith[8] reported the findings on clinical bronchography of cases of chronic bronchitis. Incomplete filling due to accumulated secretions,

CHRONIC BRONCHITIS AND EMPHYSEMA

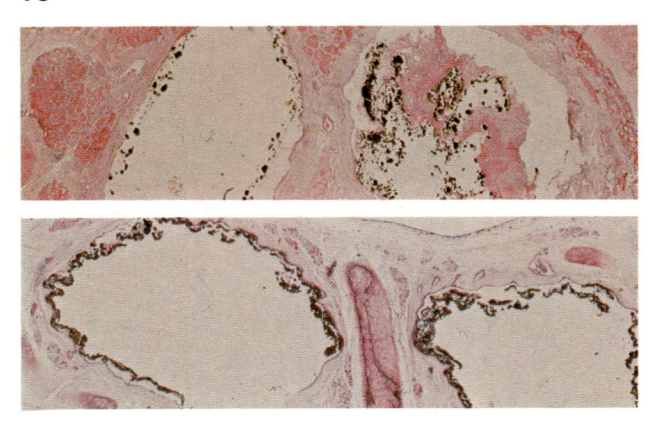

Figure 2.1 Comparative sections of the 1st divisions of inferior apical bronchus. *Bottom:* Normal lung, *Top:* Chronic (mucous) bronchitic lung. The gross increase in bulk of glandular tissue (PAS stained) is the notable feature. Black surface deposits are from post-mortem bronchography, using lead dust.

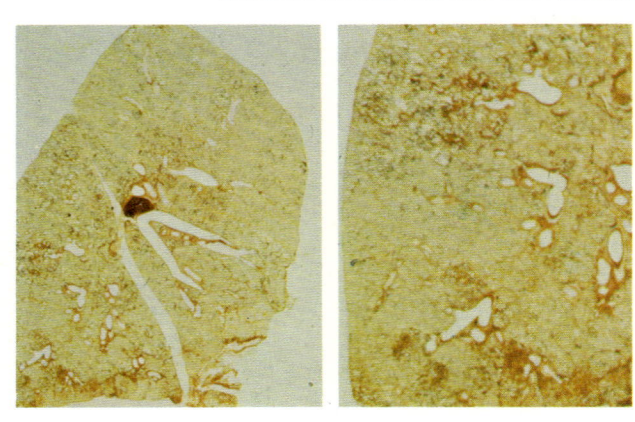

Figure 2.2 *Left:* Slight panacinar emphysema with severe, peripheral, bronchiolar, tubular dilatation, most evident at the base.

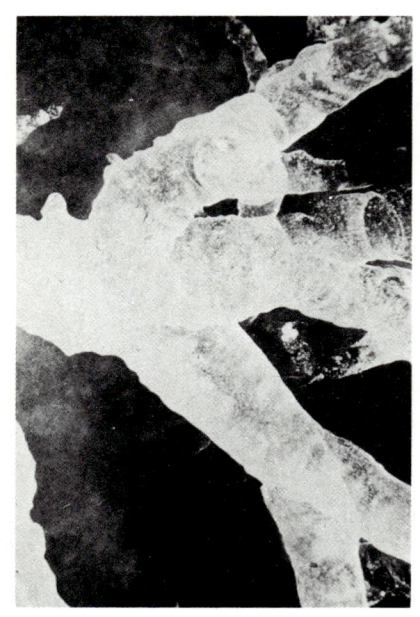

Figure 2.3 Part of post-mortem bronchogram using lead dust, showing two bronchial 'diverticulum' on the posterior apical bronchus.

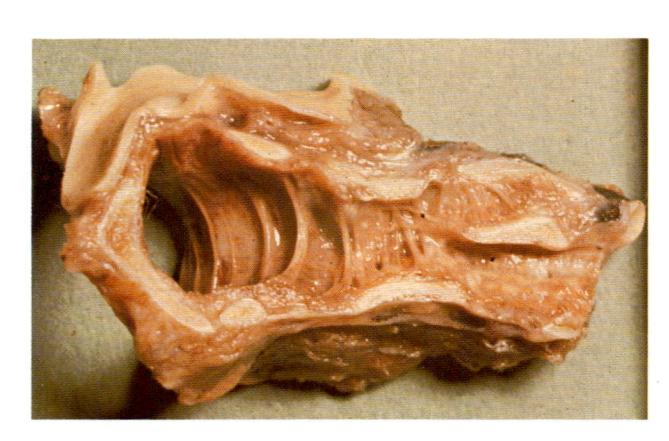

Figure 2.4 Same bronchus as in Figure 2.3 cut longitudinally showing that the indented 'silhouette' is formed by encircling folds of mucosa with deeply pocketed troughs between. The orifice of a mucous-gland duct is seen as a pin-hole aperture near centre.

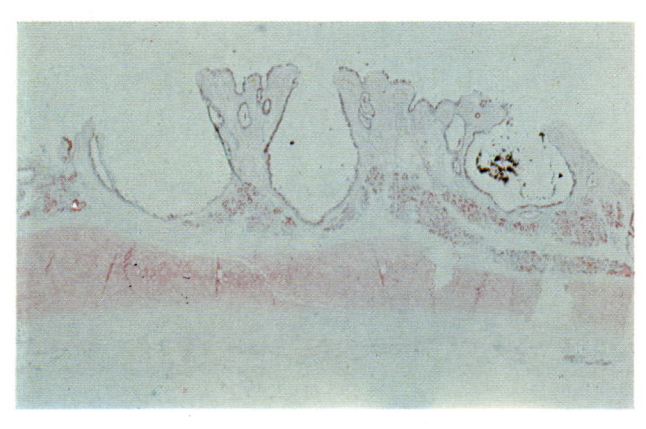

Figure 2.5 Longitudinal section of bronchus depicted in Figures 2.3 and 2.4 (PAS stain) (black material lead dust). The folds of mucosa carry hypertrophied bands of smooth muscle at their apex and also contain some mucous gland ducts.

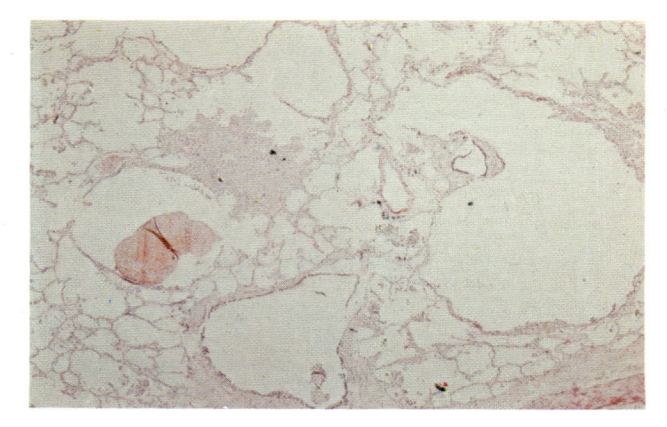

Figure 2.6 The definition of emphysema as enlargement of air-spaces distal to the terminal bronchiole is not sound, any more than is the definition of a cyst as an expansion with a defined non-respiratory wall. The majority of cysts are expanded bronchioles but, as in this case of neurofibromatosis affecting the lung, the cystic changes can spill over to involve the respiratory tissue.

CHRONIC BRONCHITIS AND EMPHYSEMA 17

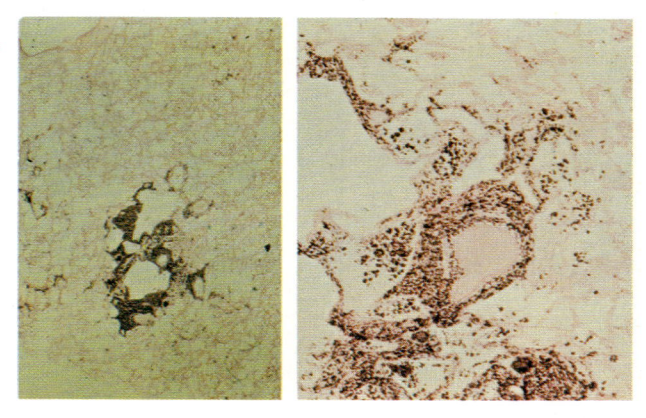

Figure 2.7 26-year-old coal miner; died of meningitis. Dust is aggregated around respiratory bronchioles. The latter show no significant dilation (focal emphysema).

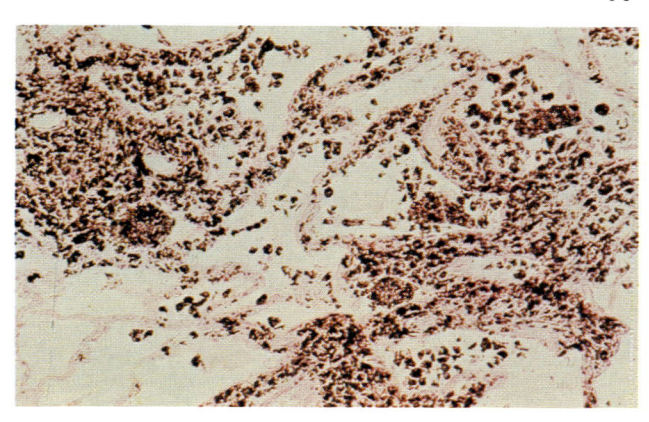

Figure 2.8 Same case as Figure 2.7. Much of the dust is within free macrophages clustered in alveoli bordering the respiratory bronchiole. Some dust lies in the interstitial tissue. Features typical of minimal and recent exposure.

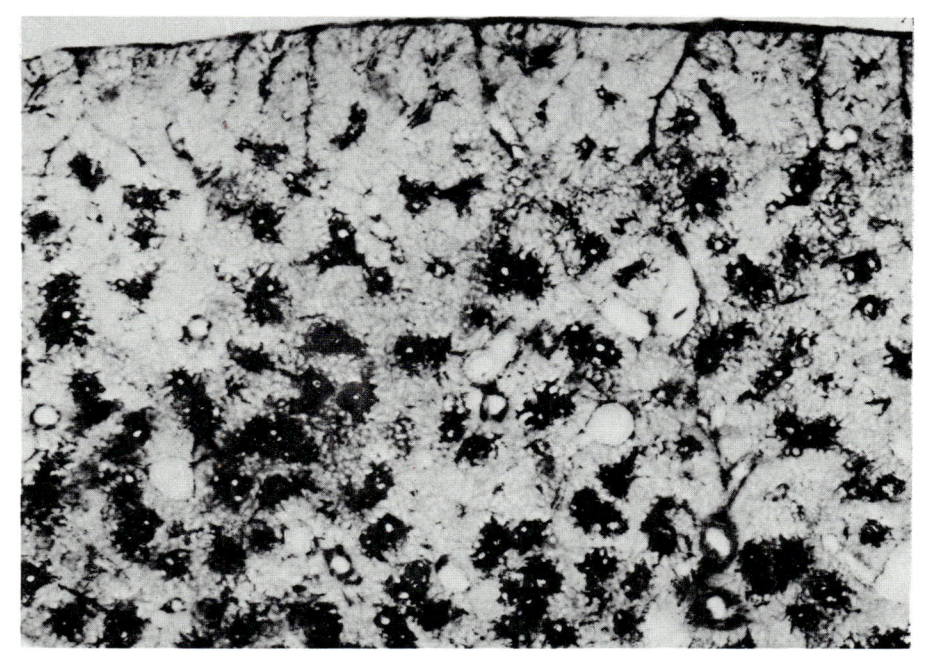

Figure 2.9 Coal-miner aged 43 years; Died of tuberculosis. Well-formed dust foci with minimal focal emphysema. Typical of the foci seen in younger age groups. B&W × 2.

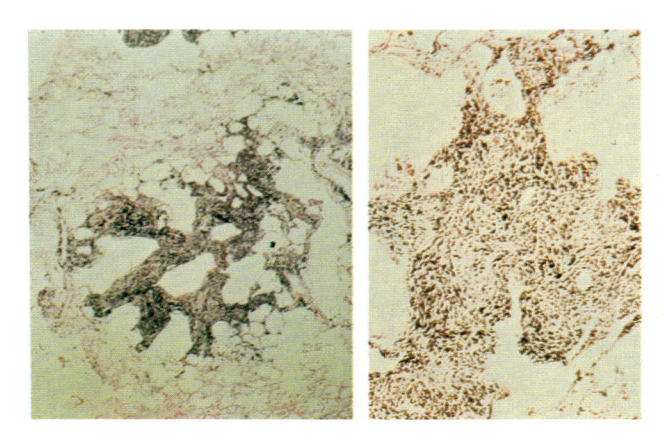

Figure 2.10 Low magnification of lung shown in Figure 2.9. Note the generally stellate form of the lesion, the broad bands of dust consolidation and only slight dilatation of the respiratory bronchioles.

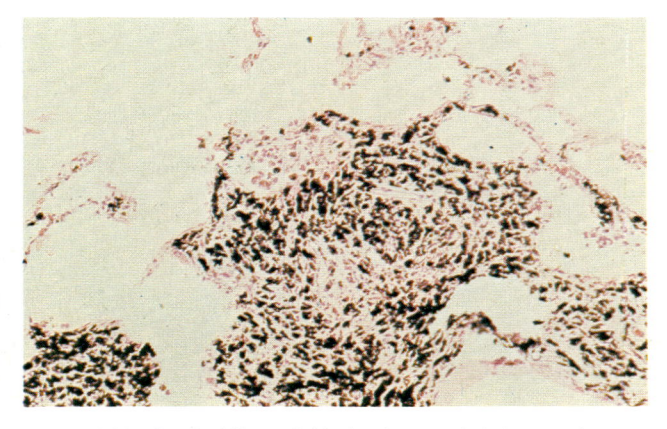

Figure 2.11 Detail of Figure 2.10 showing rounded clusters of macrophages 'free' but trapped by dust-consolidated interstitial tissue.

bronchial dilatation and 'berry'-shaped protusions from the surfaces of the major bronchi, termed diverticula, were amongst the major findings. Reid[9] regards the latter as dilatations of the orifices of the mucous gland ducts. Dilatation of these structures occurs, although personally, I doubt that the major-sized radiological diverticula develop in this way. The orifice of normal bronchial-gland duct is of the order of approximately 0.5 mm, whereas diverticula encountered personally in a postmortem bronchographical study have exceeded 1–3 mm in diameter and have not been diverticula in the pathological sense at all.

The diverticula of my experience have been a series of transverse mucosal troughs with circularly arranged bands of hypertrophied smooth muscle pulling up ridges of the mucosa between (Figures 2.3–2.5). The recognizable orifices of bronchial ducts show, in comparison, as mere pin points. Hypertrophy of the bronchial muscle in the mucosa in chronic bronchitis is an inconstant finding[4]. There is no reason to equate it with infection; the possible correlation with symptoms of obstruction has not been tested.

Atrophic Bronchitis

Since reference to it in German literature of the early part of this century, so called atrophic chronic bronchitis has had scant attention, being overshadowed by the far more frequent cases with bronchial-gland hypertrophy. There is no doubt that cases of chronic bronchial inflammatory disease with atrophic changes in the bronchial glands exist, but their relationship to the more common finding or the possibility that this disease is allied to the sicca syncrome is unsettled.

Emphysema

The pathology of emphysema is bound up with that of bronchitis, broncho-pneumonia and lung scarring. There lies an indefinable boundary where the fibrotic changes in emphysematous lungs become paramount and the character of the problem passes from the enigma of 'disappeared lung' to the readily understood expansion of spaces necessitated by foci of overt contraction. Ideally, the boundary should correspond with that set during physiological testing of lung compliance (the compliance of emphysema and fibrotic lung are opposite sides of the norm), but rarely is that possible. The truly surprising feature of non-scar related emphysema, despite the clear cut evidence of lung damage, is how little appears in the form of fibrous lung.

Modern investigative effort is concentrated at cellular and enzymic levels of study but broadly, there are two traditional pathological approaches to the study of emphysema. One approach attempts to subclassify the disease anatomically , hopefully to throw light on the mysteries of its pathogenesis and aetiology. To this end painstaking microscopic study, often in serial sections, of small, selected volumes of lung tissue is the method of precision. The second approach aims to provide quantitative anatomical data primarily for comparison with physiological tests of lung function. This requires whole lung assessments, which, in terms of ability to discriminate between type and type, is necessarily crude by comparison. Experience in microanatomical study confers a certain expertise which sometimes makes it possible to recognize emphysema in its various types without resorting to laborious micro-methods, and this expertise can be applied to whole-lung studies in which naked-eye or low power examination is the only practical method. Unfortunately, the conversion is far from precise – few persons have experience of serial section studies. Judgement upon examination at low power and one-section level is common and the literature on emphysema abounds with pathological studies which ignore the limitation that this places upon precision. Combinations of types of emphysema are a frequent finding and statements about proportions, distribution and grades cannot be made with accuracy.

An essential prerequisite for any pathological study of emphysema is to fix the lung in expansion. The method is of secondary importance, but it is more convenient to use fluid rather than vapour. It has been found that the pressure of filling is not critical unless, perhaps, the aim is to study the borderland between normality and disease.

The determination of the part of the acinar anatomy affected by emphysematous enlargement is the basis for subclassifying the disease and, despite misgivings about the methodology that has at times been adopted, initial hopes of separating types with different aetiology and pathogenesis have broadly been realized and become accepted. The history of attempts to find universally acceptable names for these types is a less happy one (see Table 2.1). In the absence of concensus, the only logical course is to use the names given when the entities were first formally described.

Focal Emphysema[10]

It has been recognized for a considerable time that coal-miners and others whose work exposes them to heavy concentrations of coal dust suffer a lung disease in which fibrosis and emphysema are combined. Descriptions of the dust foci and their surrounding zone of emphysema appear early in these accounts. The first substantial pathological account was given by Heppleston[10]; this was a milestone because it was the first study of emphysema based upon micro-anatomical analysis using serial microscopy. Heppleston found that the rounded emphysematous spaces, which in random section appear as a cluster around stellate dust scars (the foci), were traceable into elongated, roughly tubular spaces which represented expansions of orders of respiratory bronchioles.

His idea of the pathogenesis was that the sites of dust accumulation (which fringed the respiratory bronchioles) became fixed structures subject to excess tension on inspiration, but impaired in expiratory recoil. He had shown loss of both elastic and smooth muscle from their structure[11].

Duguid and Lambert[12] took a different view. Their concept of pathogenesis hinged on an observation of long-standing. Namely, the dust foci typical of men who had recently commenced in the mines and those of elderly, often retired, miners took a difference in form and in the proportion of tissue formed by the dust macule compared with tissue expanded to form emphysematous space (Figures 2.7–2.14). The results seemed paradoxical. The former component was proportionately smaller, drawn into narrow strands and tongues between the emphysematous surround, in the lesions of the older group; however, fibrosis within the dust tissue was more advanced, and the degree of dilatation of emphysematous spaces was great. Their proposition was simple: focal emphysema is an example of compensation to volume changes, which occur over a long period of time, as the widely distributed and numerous foci of dust contract with increasing fibrosis. It is different from other forms of compensatory emphysema only in that the contracting tissue is a regular, defined, anatomical component and this determines that the expanding spaces too are regular, defined parts in the anatomy of the acinus.

The implications of Duguid and Lambert's ideas on focal emphysema find universal application in the understanding of emphysema. Firstly, events of contraction and expansion occur over a long period of time. Secondly, when developed, the contracted parts become relatively less conspicuous than at earlier stages of their development, but with he development of emphysema it is impossible to evaluate what fraction of original volume they represent.

From 1952 large lung sections were collected in this department: from lungs of the general population as supplement to the earlier start of a study of coal-miners' lungs. Contrary to popular view, Cardiff is a relatively clean, unpolluted city. However, it became apparent that the lungs of many town-dwellers, females as well as males, often show a few scattered macular collections of dust, each surrounded by emphysema; counterpart of the focal lesion in miners. The few lungs received from cities more industrialized and polluted than Cardiff suggested that the problem of the focal, urban dust lesion might be more important elsewhere. We did not anticipate that this simple fact would cause such confusion as subsequently occurred when we described centrilobular emphysema.

Centrilobular Emphysema (Leopold and Gough[13])

Examining the lungs from the general population, it was possible to see that there was a type of emphysema in which dust was either absent or minimal, which shared with focal emphysema the feature of emphysematous spaces arranged in clusters (Figure 2.15). It was named centrilobular emphysema out of recognition of the position of the clusters in the lobules and because of the necessity to avoid the term 'focal' which already had a special connotation. Serial section microscopy revealed both similarity and difference from the focal dust lesion.

In focal emphysema, it had been Heppleston's experience that the major basic components of the arborizing structure of the acinus were identifiable, although distorted. However, when tracing from terminal bronchiole to the respiratory bronchioles and beyond in centrilobular emphysema, no such unambiguous path exists (Figures 2.16 and 2.17). The irregularly shaped emphysematous spaces are a zone of architectural destruction; beyond lie varying amounts of intact peripheral acinar tissue. Of the spaces themselves, only a meagre hint at loculation by membranes, in which lie the branchings of the acinar artery, remains to testify to which components have disappeared. Any dust deposits present are to be found in these grossly incomplete partitions. The balance between spaces and fibrotic tissue lies heavily in favour of the former; far more so than in the focal emphysema of even the longest surviving coal miners. It is obvious from this that while distinction between focal and centrilobular emphysema can be made on the criteria discussed, the more dust accumulated in the lung, the harder it is to draw firm conclusions.

In short, the similarity between focal emphysema and centrilobular emphysema rests upon one cardinal point; namely, in both either respiratory bronchioles themselves, or the territory where respiratory bronchioles are the major anatomical units, are the site of emphysematous changes. For the reason that centrilobular emphysematous spaces occupy a central zone of the lobular tissue, so, of course, do the spaces of focal emphysema. To bring the two under the same title[14], descriptively accurate although it is, blurs the issue, militating against the original purpose of subclassifying emphysema, namely the hope of separating what are aetiologically and pathogenetically totally different processes. McLean[15] had described emphysema central in lobules, associated with scarring, organizing peribronchiolitis and obliterating bronchiolitis. This combination, in my experience, is an occasional finding and rarely widespread in the lungs, but it serves to indicate that, if titles are to be followed solely because they have an element of descriptive accuracy, progress in the understanding of emphysema may be impaired.

A second problem, already mentioned in reference to focal urban dust emphysema, has been the frequent misidentification of the latter as the entity of centrilobular emphysema[16]; presumably centrilobular disease was regarded as essentially non-industrial and the other as uniquely industrial. There is no escaping the fact that up to diameters of approximately 6 mm the emphysematous clusters in focal emphysema have spaces unitarily separate from each other[17] and that as Duguid and Lambert's analysis has shown, there is a relationship in focal emphysema between pigmented, condensed, fibrosed lung tissue and the expanded state of the surrounding lung. The same pattern of relationship is far less obvious in centrilobular emphysema; evidence of condensed lung tissue, if it exists at all, is minimal. Because scientific measurements of pre-disease volumes is impossible it is understandable that some feel the separation of focal and centrilobular emphysema to be unjustified. Impressions are the only means for making the judgement required, but readers should try to apply their own judgement to the examples illustrating this account (Figures 2.9, 2.10, 2.12, 2.13, 2.15 and 2.16).

What cannot be ignored in discussion of the pathogenesis of centrilobular emphysema is the tissue-destructive nature of the lesions, even at their smallest size. Bronchial and bronchiolar imflammatory changes are a dominant feature[13] of lungs with centrilobular emphysema, confirming the diagnosis of bronchitis; a diagnosis conferred clinically, on

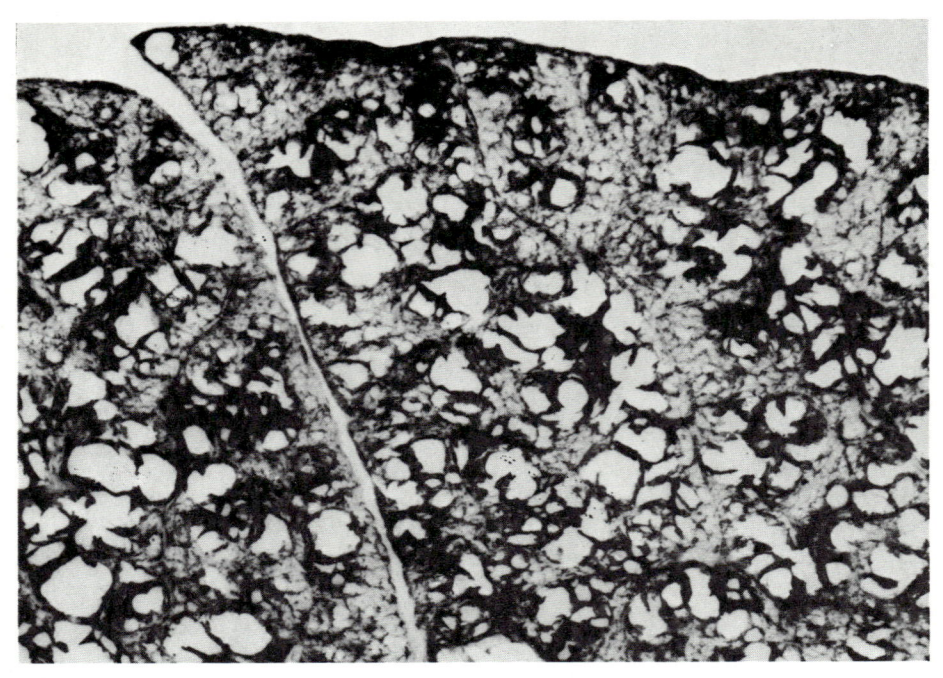

Figure 2.12 Portion of large section of lung. 78-year-old miner who had stopped working in the pits 21 years previously, after 17 years of dust exposure. B&W × 2.

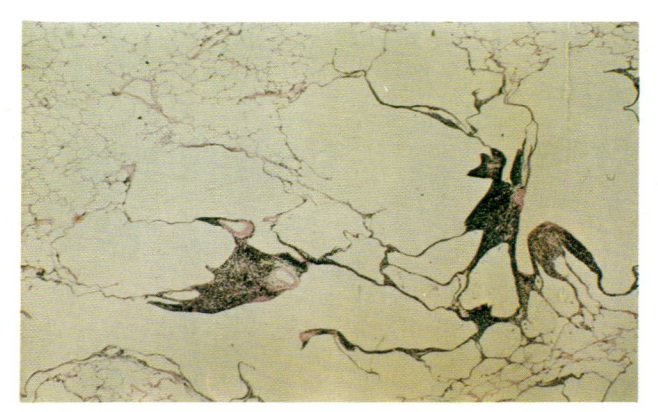

Figure 2.13 Two nearly confluent dust foci from the lung seen as Figure 2.12. Contracted dust foci with stretched, spidery limbs and extensive focal emphysema.

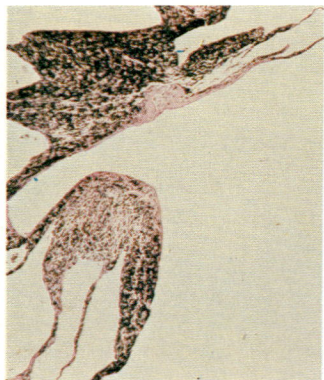

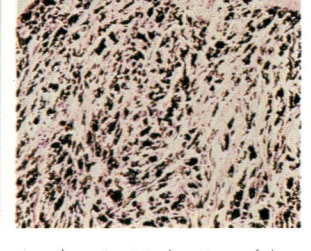

Figure 2.14 Detail of figure 2.13 showing the orientated pattern of dust particles, all contained in the interstitial tissue, with a well formed pink-stained collagenous base. Typical of the mature dust lesions. No free macrophages.

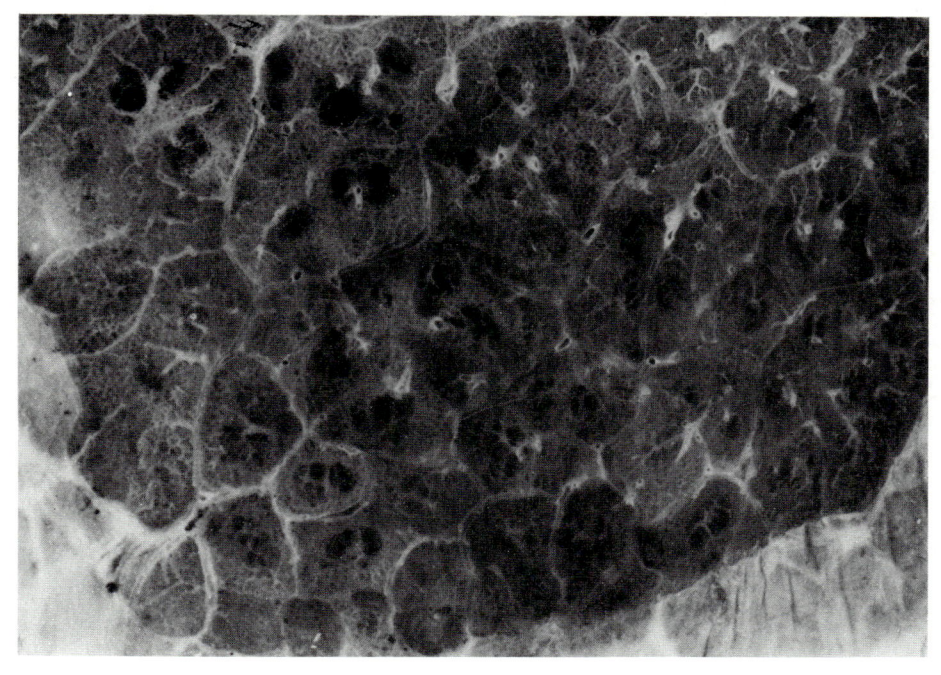

Figure 2.15 Photograph of a portion of lung surface with well-marked lobular outlines and centrilobular emphysematous spaces. There is negligible dust. Male, 52 years; company director. Heavy cigarette smoker. Dyspnoea since an attack of 'pneumonia' 8 years previously. Died cor pulmonale. B&W × 2.

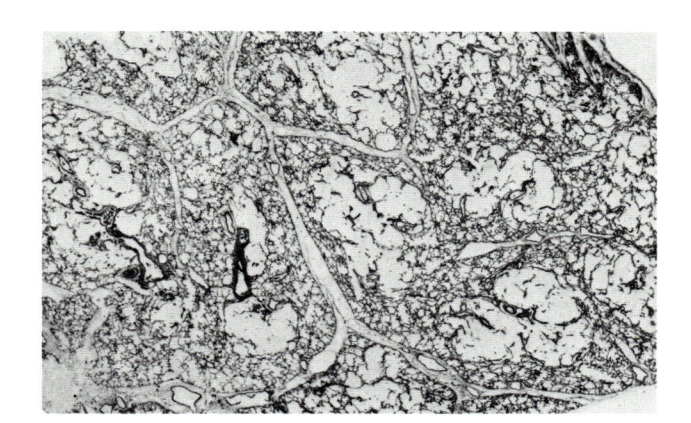

Figure 2.16 Central destructive lesions in lobules. Minimal dust and minimal evidence of scar tissue. Bronchioles are thickened by bronchiolitis. B&W × 4.

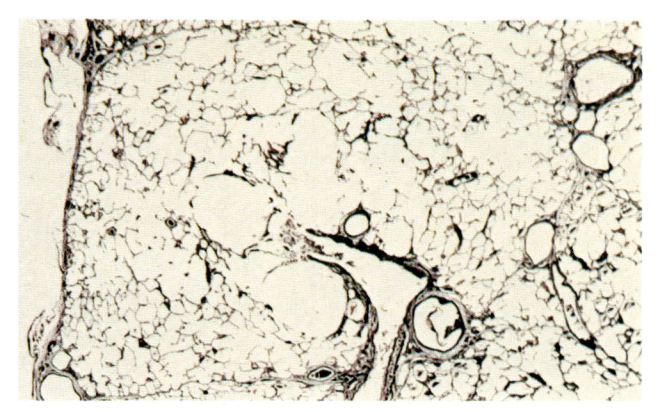

Figure 2.17 Centrilobular lesion of emphysema of small dimension. Peripheral lobular tissue is preserved but the three loculi forming the centrilobular cluster of emphysematous spaces intercommunicate. Minimal scar residue. Reticulin impregnation.

most cases of emphysema, but substantiated with far less regularity on solid pathological evidence of an inflammatory process.

The cause of tissue destruction may be, as originally postulated, infective bronchiolitis, and this is now supplemented by the knowledge that leukocytes bring increased quantity of proteolytic enzymes. Attention has also been drawn to the frequent, some say invariable, habit of cigarette smoking on the part of sufferers of emphysema, particularly of this variety. Perhaps so, if one assumes accuracy in the ability to separate focal emphysema, industrial or non-industrial, from emphysema of the centrilobular variety. Carbon from cigarette smoke is an absorptive medium and potential carrier into the lungs of more noxious constituents. The location of damage in centrilobular emphysema is consistent with that which results from contact between respired agent and the lung tissue viz. chlorine and phosgene poisoning in World War I; possibly supported by the centrilobular pattern of emphysema in chronic cadmium emphysema[18], which is the single case I have had opportunity to examine.

Panacinar Emphysema (Ciba[14])

There is no doubt that this pattern of emphysema has long been recognized and that vesicular, hypertrophic and other, now defunct titles and adjectives in prior use, related more particularly to this pattern of emphysema than to any other (Figure 2.18). It was the form of non-dust related emphysema that Heppleston took as model for comparison with focal emphysema. He described it as an enlargement seen at the terminal units of the acinus. At the Ciba Conference a concensus of view developed, which he shared, that the changes extend proximally (presumably, with increased severity of the disease), resulting in widening of spaces through all units of which the acinus is composed, hence panacinar (Figure 2.19). The general ideas on nomenclature set out at that conference passed widely into acceptance and use, but Wyatt[16] in America chose the term panlobular instead of panacinar because it was a tidier counterpart to centrilobular. In macrophotographic studies, Heard[20] showed progression of the early, non-architecturally destructive stage of panacinar emphysema through to extensive, sometimes total, lobular destruction.

On the matter of pathogenesis, nothing positive was known. Repeated hyperinflation did not seem to be an answer – life-long asthamatics were no more susceptible than the general population[3] and the stages in the development of emphysema in the opposite lung post-pneumonectomy have not been reported with precision.

Most sufferers from emphysema have clinical chronic bronchitis, although sporadically clinicians have claimed the existence of primary emphysema in which bronchitis either does not develop, or did so only as a late complication.

Recognition that inherited defects in the antiproteolytic enzyme defence of the body predispose to emphysema has opened a new avenue of research into so-called primary emphysema, which would be especially interesting if associated with emphysema of a particular pattern. Owell and Mazodier[21] reviewed the cases in the literature of α_1-antitrypsin deficiency and emphysema, and added six cases of their own. The data in the previously reported cases were rarely complete but, in their own examples, Owell and Mazodier provided complete clinical data, including history of cigarette smoking, measurement of α_1-antitrypsin activity and pathological data with large lung sections. In all their cases emphysema was severe and destructive and the pattern, assessed of necessity in the areas of lesser damage, panacinar (panlobular). Basal predominance occurred in three of the six cases. These findings were broadly consistent with data of previous cases, although showing a lesser emphasis of the much quoted basal predominance. However, the role of the anti-proteolytic enzyme deficiency is still unclear. All cases had clinical bronchitis, supported by pathological evidence. Four cases had peripheral cylindrical bronchiectasis which is most often seen only in the more severe cases of chronic bronchitis. These results, therefore, pull the curtain back a little way with some hope of solution to the aetiology and pathogenesis of panacinar emphysema. A wider view of the role of protease mechanisms in emphysema as a whole, is more speculative and is expressed in the *Lancet*[22]: 'What role do they play in bronchitis?'.

Distribution of Emphysema

Emphysema is more often a mixture of types than it is seen in pure form and, as has been indicated, accuracy in identifying and grading component types is difficult to achieve. Generalized statements based upon examples of relatively pure type are also unsound, in that exceptions can be found to any rule. It is remarkable, when one views the large lung sections cut from both right and left lungs, how similar in type, severity and distribution are the changes of emphysema in opposed lungs. Of all types, the most regular and uniform in pattern is undoubtedly panacinar emphysema. In terms of the size of the spaces, but not necessarily in their number, all types of emphysema show the most severe changes in the upper half of the lung. Segments of lung severely affected by bronchiectasis show more extensive destruction by emphysema than others and this is a common cause of reversal of the more usual upper-lung predominance.

Atrophic Lung

It is common experience that the lungs of the elderly deflate slowly, are pillowy in substance, and often referred to as showing senile emphysema. Indeed, if the lungs are fixed in expansion by any standard technique they become easily hyperexpanded, retain that state rather than recoiling, and in gross volume as well as in the size of the air spaces could be said to be emphysematous. None of this takes into account the fact that physiologically determined, normal lung volumes, if anything, decline with age (Figure 2.20).

Since emphysema is defined in terms of air-space size and not in terms of decline in tissue substance, the senile lung is atrophic but not emphysematous. The atrophy can be seen in many constituents of lung structure, elastic tissue included.

Table 2.1 Nomenclature changes in emphysema

Reference	Hypertrophic	Atrophic (senile lung)	
Heppleston[10]	Vesicular emphysema	–	Focal emphysema
Leopold and Gough[13]	Generalized	Centrilobular emphysema	Focal
Ciba Conference[19]	Panacinar	Centrilobular	Focal
Wyatt[16]	Panlobular	Centrilobular	–
Reid[14]	Panacinar	destructive ←―― Centriacinar ――→ dilation		

References

1. Fletcher, C., Pinto, R., Tinker, C. and Spiezer, F. E. (1976). *The Natural History of Chronic Bronchitis and Emphysema.* (Oxford University Press)
2. Reid, L. (1960). *Thorax,* **15,** 132
3. Leopold, J. G. (1964). *The Nature of Asthma.* Symposium, King Edward VII Hospital, Midhurst
4. Dumill, M. S., Massarella, G. R. and Anderson, J. A. (1969). *Thorax,* **24,** 176
5. Stuart Harris, C. H. (1968). *Abstr. World Med.,* **42,** 649, 737
6. May, J. R. (1972). *Chemotherapy of Chronic Bronchitis and Allied Disorders.* 2nd Ed. (London: English University Press)
7. Brumfitt, W. and Willoughby, M. L. N. (1958). *Lancet* **1,** 132
8. Simmons, G. and Galbraith, H. J. B. (1953). *Lancet* **2,** 850
9. Reid, L. (1954). *Lancet* **1,** 275
10. Heppleston, A. G. (1953). *J. Pathol. Bacteriol.,* **66,** 235
11. Heppleston, A. G. (1954). *J. Pathol. Bacteriol.,* **67,** 51
12. Duguid, J. B. and Lambert, M. W. (1964). *J. Pathol. Bacteriol.,* **88,** 389
13. Leopold, J. G. and Gough, J. (1957). *Thorax,* **12,** 219
14. Reid, L. (1967). *The Pathology of Emphysema,* p. 47 (London: Lloyd-Luke)
15. McLean, K. H. (1956). *Aust. Ann. Med.,* **5,** 73
16. Wyatt, J. P. (1959). *Am. Rev. Resp. Dis.,* **80,** 94
17. Heppleston, A. G. Personal communication
18. Lane, R. E. and Campbell, A. C. P. (1954). *Brit. J. Ind. Med.,* **11,** 118
19. Ciba Guest Symposium, 1959. *Thorax,* **14,** 286
20. Heard, B. E. (1969). *Pathology of Chronic Bronchitis and Emphysema* (London: Churchill)
21. Owell, S. R. and Mazodier, P. (1972). In Pittman, C. (ed.) *Pulmonary Emphysema and Proteolysis,* p.69 (New York: Academic Press)
22. Editorial (1980) *Lancet,* **1,** 743

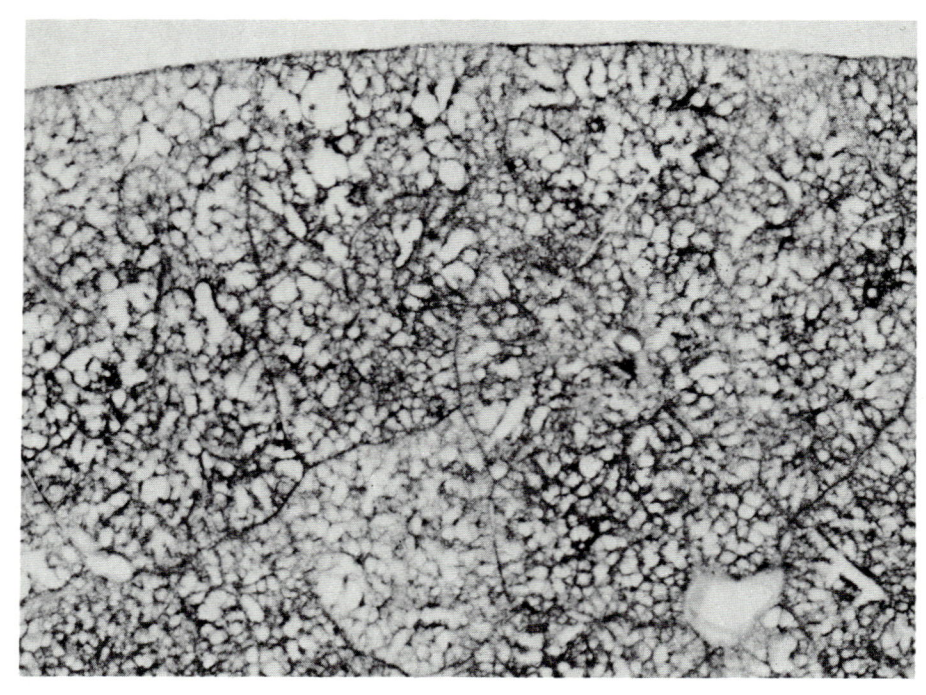

CHRONIC BRONCHITIS AND EMPHYSEMA

Figure 2.18 Portion of large lung section – mild panacinar emphysema. 68-year-old ex-busconductor. Heavy smoker, suffered from clinical chronic bronchitis, died of anoxic heart failure. B&W × 2.

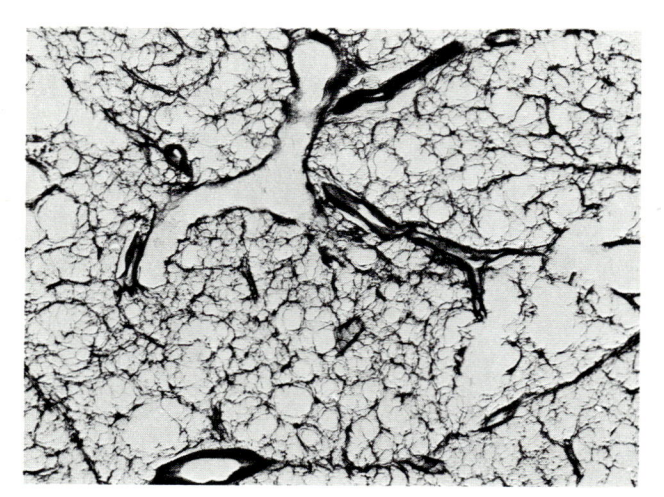

Figure 2.19 Portion of lobule with similar degree of panacinar emphysema as Figure 2.18. Dilatation exists of respiratory units near the septum; involving alveolar ducts and distal respiratory bronchioles.

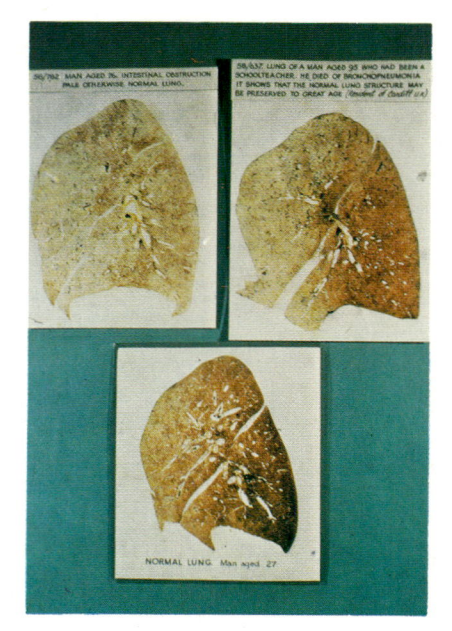

Figure 2.20 Composite of three male, normal lungs aged *(bottom)* 27 years, *(top left)* 76 years and *(top right)* 96 years. There is a progressive increase in general lung size with age and the air spaces show modest increase in size. All lungs were comparably fixed by formalin inflation – false emphysema (lung atrophy).

Bronchiectasis

Bronchiectasis means irreversible dilatation of bronchi and usually affects the middle- and small-order bronchi. There is evidence of an obstructive inflammatory process in many cases. Bronchiectasis may be unilateral or bilateral, may affect more than one of the lobes or be confined to one or more bronchopulmonary segments and is frequently focally distributed within a segment.

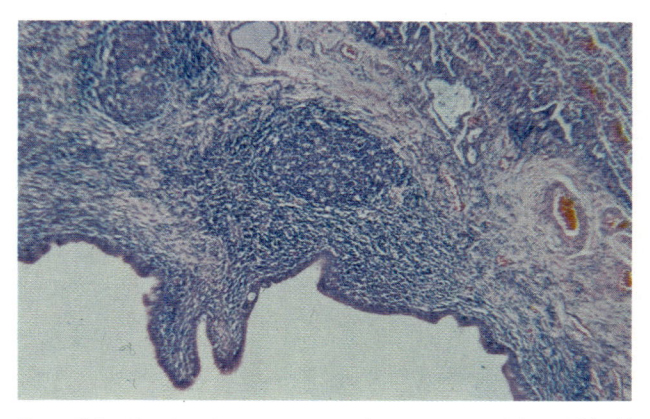

Figure 3.1 Histology from a lobectomy for bronchiectasis in a child with respiratory symptoms following measles. The dense lymphoid infiltrate with lymphoid follicles typical of follicular bronchiectasis can be seen. H & E × 24.

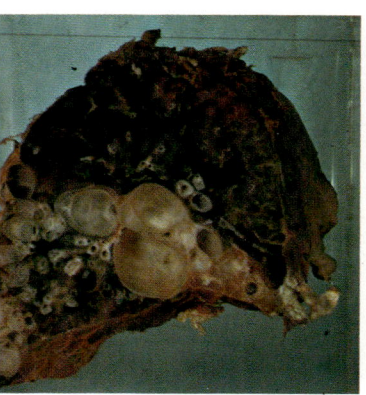

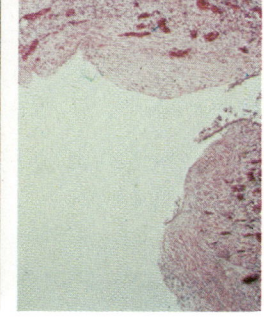

Figure 3.2 *Left:* A museum specimen of a pneumonectomy specimen for saccular bronchiectasis, affecting middle and lower lobe. *Right:* This illustrates atrophy of bronchial wall, with almost total loss of epithelium and atrial disease of purulent exudate – so called 'dry bronchiectasis'. H & E × 24.

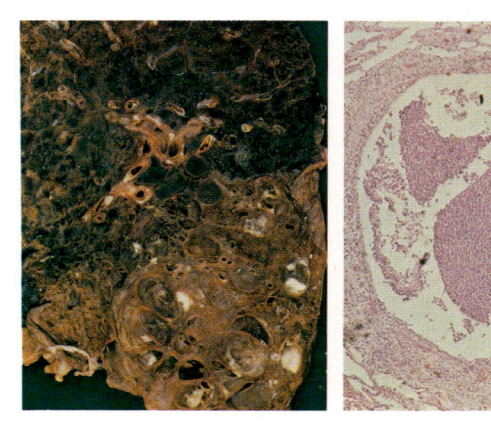

Figure 3.3 *Left:* Part saccular, part cylindrical bronchiectasis of lower lobe devoid of pigment, the bronchi containing mucopus. *Right:* Bronchus again showing atrophy but containing a purulent exudate. H & E × 24.

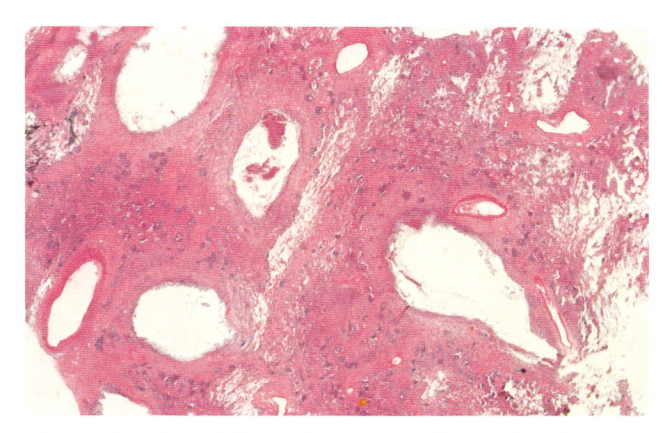

Figure 3.4 Collapsed, fibrosed lung composed largely of ectatic bronchi. There is some thickening of pulmonary arterial walls. The prominent vessels in the bronchial walls represent hypertrophied bronchial arterioles.

Whitwell[1] separates bronchiectasis into four main types:

(a) Congenital (see Chapter 1)
(b) Follicular
(c) Saccular
(d) Atelectatic.

Follicular Bronchiectasis

This has acquired its name from the presence of numerous lymphoid follicles within the affected bronchi. The disease may vary from slight involvement of a single bronchopulmonary segment of an otherwise normal lobe to diffuse involvement and concomitant severe abnormality of a whole lobe. The left lobe is the most frequently affected and there is usually conspicuous hilar lymph-node enlargement.

The smaller bronchi and bronchioles are the major site of involvement, but in severe disease the process extends more proximally. Microscopically, numerous lymphoid follicles, some with germinal centres, are present within the walls of bronchi and bronchioles and among the surrounding alveoli (Figure 3.1). There is also destruction of bronchial elastic tissue, cartilage, muscle and mucous glands. There is interstitial pneumonia in the parenchyma situated around affected bronchioles.

The advent of the condition is in early childhood and is thought to be a consequence of childhood infections, particularly whooping cough, measles or a primary bronchopneumonia.

Saccular Bronchiectasis

As its name implies, this is characterized by the formation of saccules which can be seen on macroscopic examination (Figures 3.2 and 3.3). Whitwell considers that it commences as a chronic mural inflammation of the medium-sized bronchi. Microscopically, the saccules are seen to be composed of fibrous structures having no elastic, muscle or cartilage within their walls (Figures 3.2 and 3.3), lined by cuboidal epithelium. They are thought to be dilated terminations of the first to third branchings of the segmental bronchi. Squamous metaplasia, rarely observed in the other types of bronchiectasis, is often present within the saccular lining. The presaccular bronchi often evince polyposis of the epithelium, severe inflammation in their walls, but no dilatation and little destruction of supporting tissue. The surrounding alveoli usually appear within normal limits.

This type of bronchiectasis affects an older age group than the follicular type, and appears unrelated to childhood exanthemata.

Atelectatic Bronchiectasis

Bronchiectasis associated with severe pulmonary collapse (Figure 3.4) is classified as atelectatic, since collapse if absent or minimal in the follicular or saccular types. This type shows a predilection for the right lung, particularly the middle and lower lobes.

By contrast to the other varieties of bronchiectasis in which peripheral obstruction is invariable, the bronchioles are patent even in the lobules, showing partial collapse. The bronchi, in an affected lobe, reveal similar histology in all segments (Figure 3.4), varying from mild superficial inflammation, through moderate inflammation without destruction of supporting tissues, to epithelial ulceration and destruction of supporting tissues. Bronchioles reveal similar changes, but to a lesser degree. In some cases lymphoid follicles may be present within bronchial walls, but interstitial pneumonia is absent (cf. follicular bronchiectasis). Incomplete absorption, collapse of alveoli and intraalveolar haemorrhage are usually present. Whitwell found tuberculous foci in the lung parenchyma and hilar lymph nodes of a few cases.

Whitwell postulated that the bronchiectasis was a consequence of collapse, which in turn was a result of lobar bronchial obstruction. He theorized that it might be a result of pressure by enlarged lymph nodes, due to a variety of causes, which might explain the high incidence of middle lobe involvement.

Patients between 5 and 30 years of age are mainly affected, and they may relate their symptoms to measles or whooping cough infection in childhood.

Reference

1. Whitwell, F. (1952). A study of the pathology and pathogenesis of bronchiectasis. *Thorax*, **7**, 13

Pneumonias

There are three useful ways in which pneumonias can be classified: (1) anatomical, (2) pathogenetic and (3) aetiological, each of which is helpful to the comprehension of the disease process (Plate 4.1).

Anatomical descriptions (Figures 4.1 and 4.2) are useful, in that they give a clue to the organism(s) involved, although it should be remembered that organisms beside *Streptococcus pneumoniae* can occasionally cause lobar pneumonia, for instance, and that antibiotic adminstration frequently modifies the course of the disease.

Pathogenetic consideration (Figures 4.3-4.7) may give a clue to the organisms involved and also demonstrates the importance of the host in governing the pulmonary response. Although, in a sense all organisms causing pneumonia may be considered opportunistic, it is usual to reserve this term for infections occurring in immune compromised hosts, e.g. patients receiving chemotherapy for malignant diseae and organ transplantation. The clinician is making increased use of lung biopsy in these diseases and the pathologist is often required to determine whether a pulmonary infiltrate is infective, drug induced or neoplastic. Certain pitfalls must be kept in mind. Infections are not infrequently mixed and successful treatment requires that all organisms are identified. Secondly, immune compromised hosts may not mount the typical pathological reaction to an infective agent.

Aetiological classification is the most helpful, but cannot always be determined; not all organisms produce a specific picture. The most important agents and those that pose particular problems are discussed.

Viral Pneumonias

Many viral infections give rise to similar appearances in the lungs, and diagnosis depends upon additional techniques such as antibody studies and viral cultures. Since viral infections predispose to bacterial infection, it is common for the pathological appearances to reflect a combination of bacterial and viral insults. The general features of these pneumonias will be described, taking influenza as the main example. In addition, certain features will be described which are suggestive or diagnostic of particular viruses.

Influenza

This serves as a model for many viral pneumonias. It occurs in pandemic, epidemic and sporadic forms. Most human influenza is due to infection by type A strains. Secondary bacterial infection of the lung is common in influenza and of particular importance is *Staphylococcus aureus*. We have also seen secondary infection by *Aspergillus* spp. which resulted in the death of a patient.

In acute deaths due to influenza the lungs are heavy, bulky, reddish-purple in colour and on cutting, blood-stained frothy fluid exudes from the surfaces (Figure 4.8). The alveoli are filled with fibrinous oedema, red blood cells and macrophages. Hyaline membranes may be evident in the alveoli and alveolar ducts, and the alveolar lining cells are swollen. The interstitium usually contains a mononuclear infiltrate (Figure 4.2). From the description, it will be realized that the changes are those of diffuse alveolar damage (Chapter 5, Figures 5.1-5.4).

The bronchial and bronchiolar epithelium show superficial necrosis; sometimes only the basal layer remaining[1]. There is oedema and lymphocytic infiltration of the bronchial and bronchiolar walls.

In those dying, after about five days evidence of epithelial regeneration will be seen and stratified epithelium may be seen in bronchi and bronchioles[1].

In subacute deaths, the findings will be mainly due to secondary infection such as staphylococci; greyish yellow focal areas of bronchopneumonia which may break down to form abscess cavities.

Giant-cell Pneumonia

In addition to the general changes of a viral pneumonia, giant cells may be found at all levels in the respiratory epithelium in this condition. The majority, if not all, are caused by measles virus. Intranuclear and intracytoplasmic inclusions are present in the giant cells and in the epithelium of bronchioles and alveoli (Figure 4.8).

Cytomegalovirus Pneumonia

This is an increasingly important cause of opportunistic infection in immune compromised hosts. It results in focal or diffuse interstitial pneomonitis, with the appearance of diffuse alveolar damage or there may be scattered macrophages containing the typical inclusion bodies but no accompanying inflammatory reaction. The characteristic inclusions are found within macrophages, pneumocytes and endothelial cells – the affected cells are typically enlarged and contain intranuclear inclusions with a surrounding halo (Figure 4.9). Occasional small basophilic intracytoplasmic inclusions may also be seen[2].

Wherever cytomegalovirus infection is seen, pneumocystis should be looked for and vice versa, since they frequently coexist.

PNEUMONIAS

ANATOMICAL PATHOGENETIC AETIOLOGICAL

Lobar
Segmental
Broncho
Interstitial

Obstructive
Aspiration
Embolic
Ag Ab

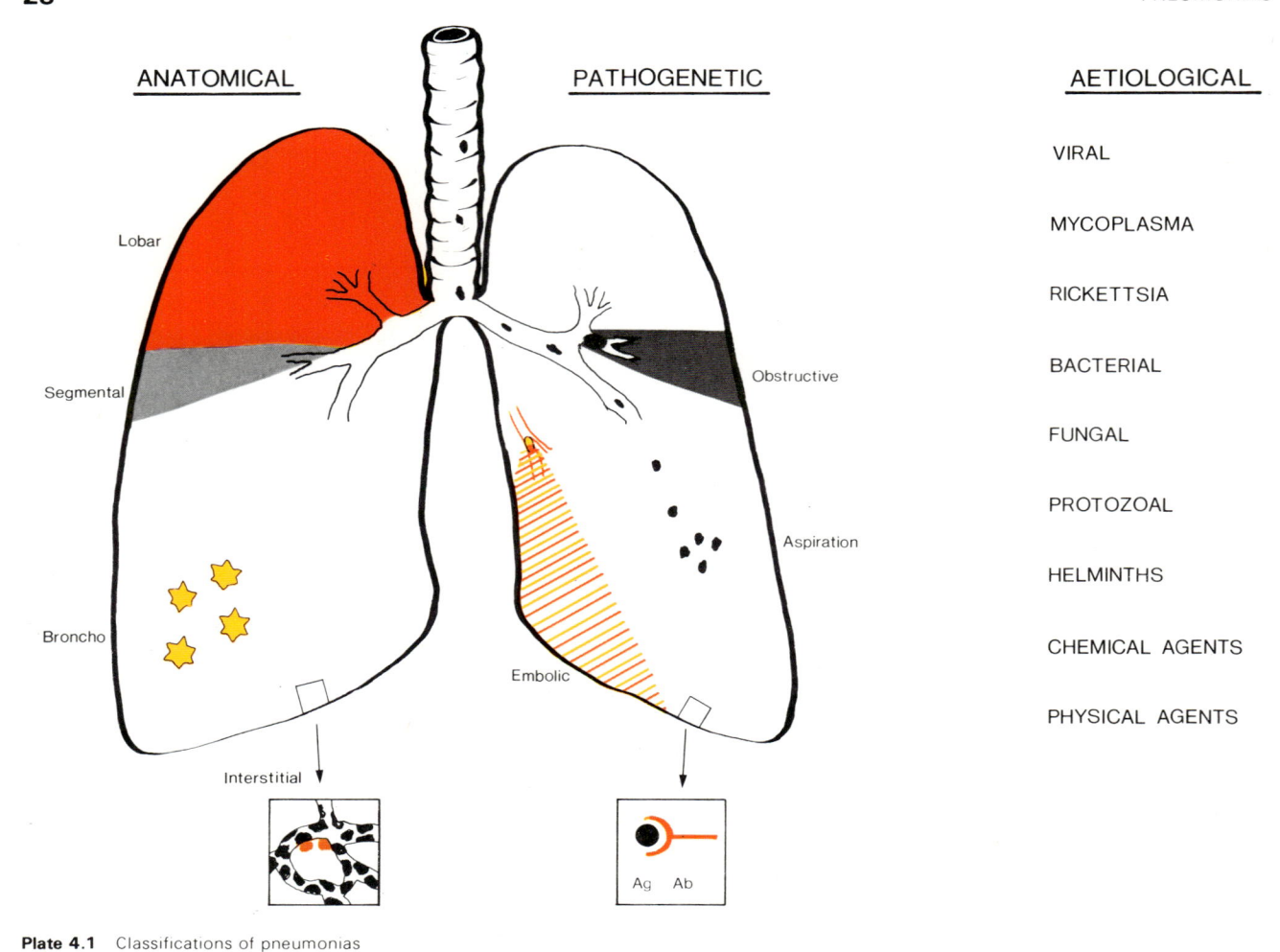

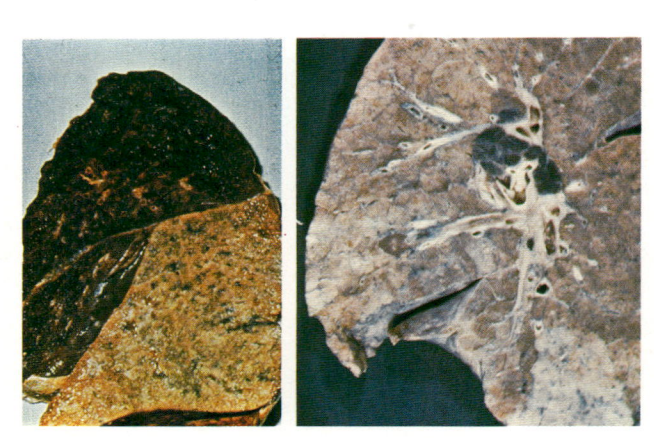

VIRAL

MYCOPLASMA

RICKETTSIA

BACTERIAL

FUNGAL

PROTOZOAL

HELMINTHS

CHEMICAL AGENTS

PHYSICAL AGENTS

Plate 4.1 Classifications of pneumonias

Figure 4.1 *Left:* Right lower lobe completely consolidated by yellow-grey pneumonic exudate. There are also some caseous necrotic lesions in the upper lobe and on Ziehl Nielsen staining there were innumerable acid-fast bacilli. *Right:* A basal segment is grey and consolidated, yielding a mixed growth of Gram negative organisms.

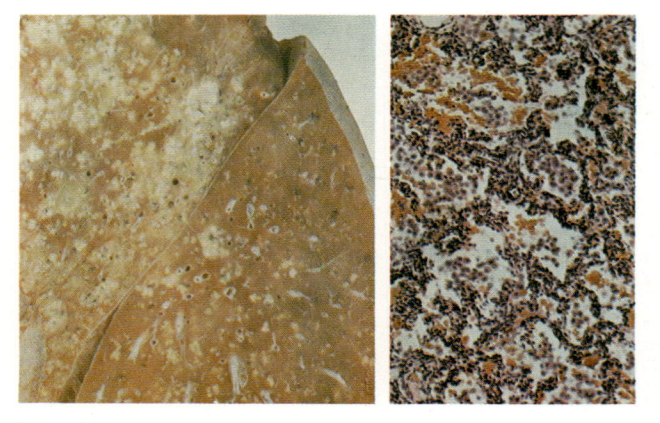

Figure 4.2 *Left:* The centre of several lobules contain grey-yellow acinar lesions, confluent in places, and more marked in upper lobe. There was a tuberculous cavity in the contralateral lung. Numerous AFB seen in this bronchopneumonia. *Right:* An interstitial lymphoid infiltrate with some exudation of larger mononuclear cells – presumed viral interstitial pneumonitis.

PNEUMONIAS

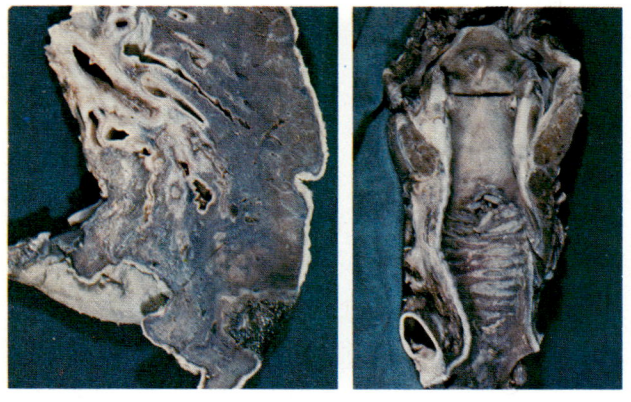

Figure 4.3 *Left:* The left lung of same patient with confluent aspiration bronchopneumonia and a septic posterior basal infarct, responsible for the fibrinopurulent exudate of an empyema. *Right:* An infected tracheostomy stoma with ulceration overlying cartilage rings.

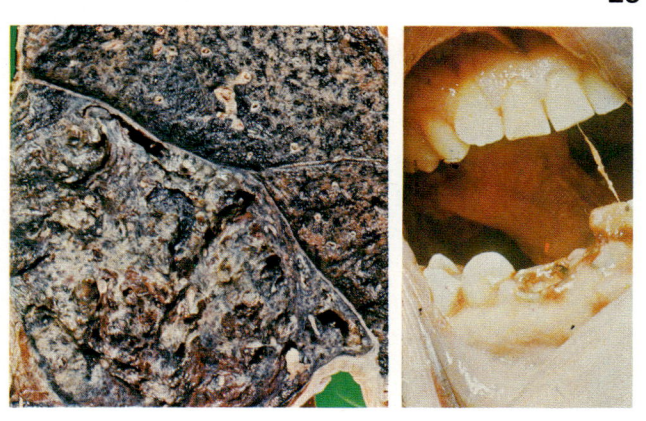

Figure 4.4 *Left:* A miner's lung with organizing, suppurative lower-lobe pneumonia, probably resulting from aspiration of infected material from gross dental caries *(right)*.

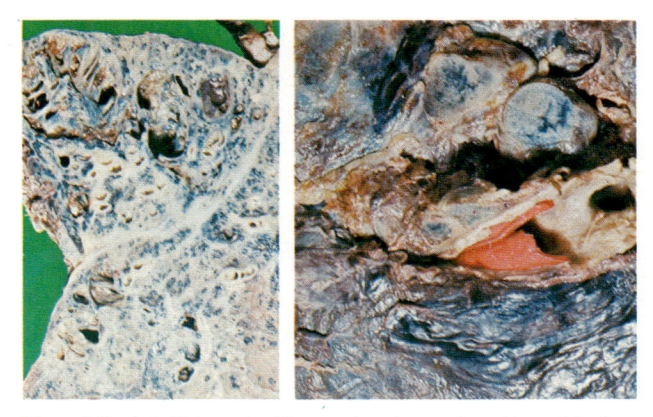

Figure 4.5 *Left:* This resulted in complete destruction of lower lobe from organizing pneumonia with extensive bronchiectasis. *Right:* Part of the cap of a ball point pen lodged in major bronchus of an epileptic.

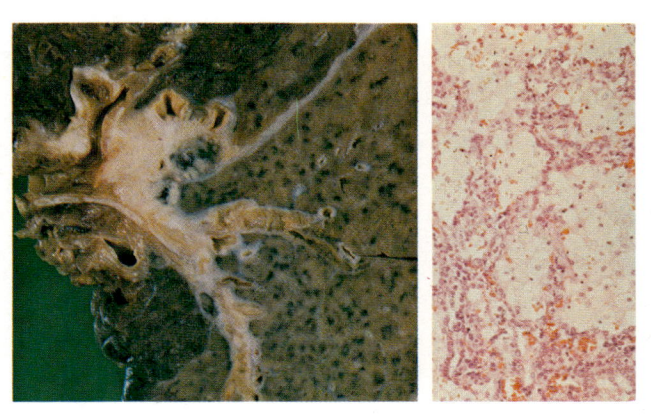

Figure 4.6 *Left:* Cut section of a pneumonic right lower lobe, resulting from obstruction of lobar bronchus by a carcinoma which can be seen extending within central bronchi. The pneumonic area reveals prominence of interlobular septa. *Right:* Obstructive pneumonitis with interstitial mononuclear infiltrate and alveoli filled with foamy macrophages. H & E × 96.

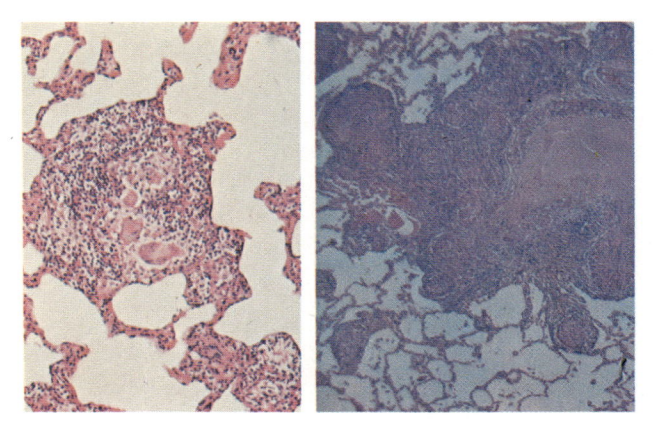

Figure 4.7 *Left:* Granulomatous interstitial pneumonitis in extrinsic allergic bronchioloalveolitis, which later resolved. H & E × 38.4. *Right:* A beryllium worker with interstitial disease – also numerous granulomata but mild interstitial pneumonitis. H & E × 96.

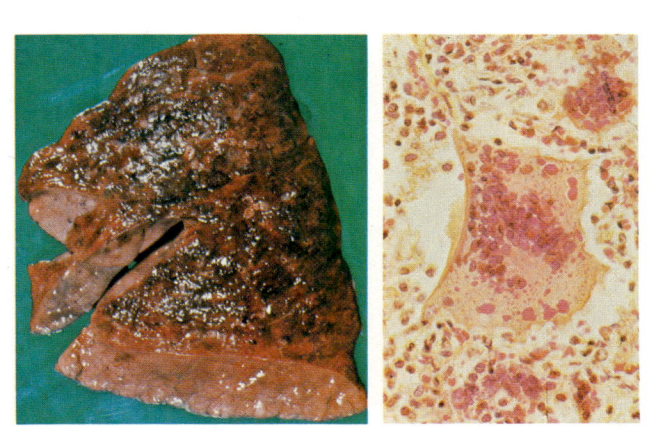

Figure 4.8 *Left:* Typical appearance of acute fatal influenza in the viraemic stage, which occurred in (1969) 'flu' epidemic. *Right:* Measles pneumonia showing a mononuclear interstitial infiltrate and giant cells within the alveoli. Intranuclear and intracytoplasmic intrusions are seen within the giant cells and alveolar lining cells. Phloxine tartrazine × 384.

Other Viral Pneumonias

In addition to the general features of viral pneumonia, adenovirus, varicella, respiratory syncytial virus and herpes simplex may evince inclusion bodies within epithelial cells[3].

Mycoplasma Pneumonia

Mycoplasmae pulmonary infections show non-specific histological features, similar to those of viral pneumonias. The features are essentially those of diffuse alveolar damage – combinations of oedema, red blood cells and hyaline membranes within alveoli and interstitial lymphocytic infiltrates (Figure 4.9). The bronchioles show chronic inflammatory changes.

Rickettsial and Bedsonial Infections

Pneumonias due to rickettsiae and bedsoniae show similar histological changes to viral pneumonias. In psittacosis intracytoplasmic inclusions, demonstrated by prolonged Giemsa staining, may be present within desquamated lining alveolar cells[3].

Bacterial Pneumonias

Pneumococcal (Streptococcus pneumoniae) *Pneumonia*

The majority of severe pneumococcal pneumonias in Britain[4] are caused by types 3, 1, 8, 14, 5 and 9, whereas in the USA the order of frquency is 1, 7, 8, 4, 3 and 12. Type 3 is particularly associated with fatality.

Lobar Pneumonia

S. pneumoniae is classically associated with causing lobar pneumonia, although this is less often seen now than it was formerly due to the advent of antibiotics. It nowadays more frequently causes bronchopneumonia.

Lobar pneumonia is also occasionally caused by staphylococcus, streptococcus, *Klebsiella* and *Legionella*. Lobar pneumonia can be divided into four stages, although it must be remembered that different stages may be seen at the same time in different areas of the same lung:

Stage 1. *Inflammatory oedema.* Seldom seen, this stage is characterized by pulmonary oedema which contains numerous pneumococci and a few polymorph neutrophils. It lasts 1–2 days.

Stage 2. *Red hepatization.* The lung appears firm, red, airless and there is a thin fibrinous pleurisy. Microscopically the alveoli contain numerous red blood cells, fibrin and scanty polymorph neutrophils. There is intense capillary congestion. This takes place between the 2nd and 4th days.

Stage 3. *Grey hepatization.* Still firm and airless, the lung now appears greyish-yellow in colour with a thick pleural fibrinous exudate. This is because there are larger number of polymorph neutrophils, fibrin and fewer red blood cells within the alveoli. Also the alveolar capillaries appear inconspicuous. This lasts from the 4th to the 8th day (Figure 4.10).

Stage 4. *Resolution.* This commences with the appearance of macrophages in the alveoli, which steadily increase in number. These ingest polymorph neutrophils and destroy them, along with their contained pneumococci. This stage lasts from 1–3 weeks.

The usual consequence of pneumococcal lobar pneumonia is complete resolution, but occasionally the fibrinous exudate becomes organized, instead of absorbed, which results in filling of the alveoli with a proliferating mass of fibroblasts and collagen. These masses communicate with similar areas in adjacent alveoli through the pores of Kohn. Other complications include lung abscess and empyema which are most likely to occur with type 3 pneumococci.

Bronchopneumonia

This is the most common anatomical type of pneumonia encountered by the pathologist (Figure 4.2). It tends to occur at the extremes of life and it is a common mode of death in a range of conditions. A wide variety of agents may cause bronchopneumonia, pneumococci, staphylococci, streptococci and *Haemophilus* being the most common.

Macroscopically, it is characterized by foci of consolidation which at first, are discrete, multiple, yellowish-grey in colour and may affect more than one lobe, and later become confluent, sometimes involving a whole lobe to mimic lobar pneumonia. If pyogenic organisms are the cause, abscesses may form.

Histologically, the inflammatory exudate, consisting mainly of polymorph neutrophils, is seen to be situated mainly around bronchioles and small bronchi with involvement of their adjacent air spaces. Gram staining may reveal the causative organism, but bacteriological cultures and typing are necessary for accurate designation of the organism.

Complete resolution is uncommon in bronchopneumonia, because of the damage of the bronchiolar walls by the inflammatory process. Small foci of fibrosis usually result, but if extensive, bronchiectasis may result.

Staphylococcal Pneumonia

Staphylococcus aureus is a very important cause of pneumonia, especially because many of its strains show considerable antibiotic resistance. The majority of cases of staphylococcal pneumonia occur on a pre-existing viral pneumonia. It has a particular propensity for causing tissue breakdown and the development of abscesses (Figure 4.9). Empyema may result.

Klebsiella Pneumonia

Pulmonary infection by *Klebsiella pneumoniae* may cause a dense lobar consolidation in which the exudate is characteristically sticky and mucinous. It shows a propensity for affecting the right upper lobe. Microscopically, the alveoli are filled with oedema fluid containing numerous encapsulated bacilli admixed with polymorph neutrophils and red blood cells. As the disease progresses, tissue destruction occurs and abscesses form. Delayed resolution with fibrosis is a common sequel to *Klebsiella* infection[5] (Figure 4.12).

Gram-Negative Organisms

Administration of broad-spectrum antibiotics and steroids, tracheostomy and neoplastic processes are particular predisposing factors in the development of Gram-negative pneumonias.

In *Pseudomonas aeruginosa* pneumonia the lungs may reveal firm haemorrhagic infarct-like areas or greenish-yellow, irregular consolidated areas which may have a haemorrhagic border (Figure 4.13). These may go on to develop abcesses. The tracheobronchial tree is usually very haemorrhagic and may show areas of necrosis.

Histologically, the lesions are necrotic, fibrinous and haemorrhagic and there is a variable amount of polymorph neutrophils and nuclear debris. The organisms characteristically invade and destroy the walls of pulmonary arteries. Appropriate stains will reveal the Gram-negative organisms within the vessel walls.

Legionella Pneumonia (Legionnaire's Disease)

Infection by a recently recognized organism, *Legionella pneumophila*, sometimes occurs in epidemics as well as sporadically. It is often linked with a particular building. Immune compromised hosts are especially prone to serious consequences of this infection, which may result in death. Rising serum titres of antibodies to this organism are useful in diagnosis.

Infection by *Legionella pneumophila* can result in bronchopneumonia, which may become confluent to affect a whole lobe, simulating lobar pneumonia[6]. The lungs are heavy and, consolidated areas, which are grey, granular and friable, may be bilateral. The lungs appear congested but not haemorrhagic. *Legionella* pneumonia should be suspected by the pathologist wherever conventional microbiological and staining procedures fail to demonstrate an organism in an apparent bacterial pneumonia. Microscopically, there are varying combinations of acute fibrinopurulent pneumonia – intra-alveolar neutrophils, macrophages and fibrin in varying proportions (Figure 4.14) – and diffuse atveolar damage. The latter is probably a secondary phenomenon. Occasionally there may be large fields of necrosis. Dietrle's silver-impregnation technique stains the organisms whch are short, pleumorphic bacilli (2–4 μm in length and less than 1 μm in width). The organisms may be seen both lying free and within macrophages and neutrophils. We have also found Levaditi's stain useful (Figure 4.14). Care must be exercised in interpreting these silver impregnation stains, since there is variable affinity for formalin pigment, haemosiderin, melanin and other bacteria as well as the *Legionella* organisms. Confirmation can be obtained by direct immunofluorescence of lung tissue using fluorescein conjugated antibody for *Legionella pneumophila*. This technique works satisfactorily on formalin-fixed mterial. This antibody does, however, cross react with a few other rare organisms which are not usually a problem in differential diagnosis.

Patients may die in the acute phase of *Legionella* pneumonia or a few weeks after the initial onset of respiratory failure. In the latter, varying degrees and combinations of intra-alveolar and intersittial fibrosis may be observed and the organisms may not be demonstrable[8].

Mycobacteria

Mycobacterial infection is discussed in Chapter 6.

Actinomycosis

Pulmonary actinomyosis may be a primary infection, or in a smaller proportion of cases results from spread of infection from below the liver or from a cervico-facial infection. The lungs classically show numerous abscess cavities interdigitated by dense fibrous tissue. Less commonly, a single large abscess results. Microscopically, the characteristic colonies of *Actinomyces israeli*, which stain intensely by haematoxylin, are evident within the centre of the abscesses (Figure 4.15).

Nocardiosis

Nocardiosis is more likely to develop in the immune compromised host and *N. asteroides* is the most common species involved. The most common organ affected is the lung, but the brain is also often involved. In the lung there are usually abscesses and occasional cavities[9]. The brain may show similar abscesses. Microscopically, the abscesses may be surrounded by histiocytes, epithelioid cells, lymphocytes and fibroblasts. The organisms are not visible on H&E staining, but on Gram or acid-fast stains appear in sections as beaded, branching filaments. Non acid-fast branching forms or occasional microscopic granules may be found[10].

Patients with alveolar proteinosis show a particular susceptibility to this infection. Rarely nocardia may colonize a pulmonary cavity to form a mycetoma[9].

Fungi

Aspergillosis

The lung may show a wide variety of responses to infection by aspergillar species (Chapter 8, Plate 8.1); the most common pathogen is *Aspergillus fumigatus*, but other species are sometimes responsible.

Pre-existing cavities due to tubercle, lung abscess, sarcoid, bronchiectasis, etc. may become colonized by aspergillus to form aspergillomas (fungus balls). The fungus produces a dense mycelium which fills the cavity, with little or no invasion of the cavity wall. In mycetomas due to *Aspergillus niger*, doubly refractile calcium oxalate crystals may be observed.

In the immune compromised host, invasive aspergillar infection occurs which results in a combination of infarction and necrotizing pneumonia[11-13] (Figure 4.17). The necrotic areas contain cellular debris, a small quantity of inflammatory cells, and fungal hyphae which may be observed even in H&E sections (Figure 4.17). The fungal hyphae are also discerned within thrombosed blood vessels. Around the periphery of the necrotic areas there is a zone of organizing pneumonia which may contain a prominent component of plasma cells and eosinophils. Multiple abscesses may also occur which contain hyphae and are surrounded by giant cells (Figure 4.18).

Rarely, invasive aspergillosis takes the form of a granulomatous reaction with abundant multinu-

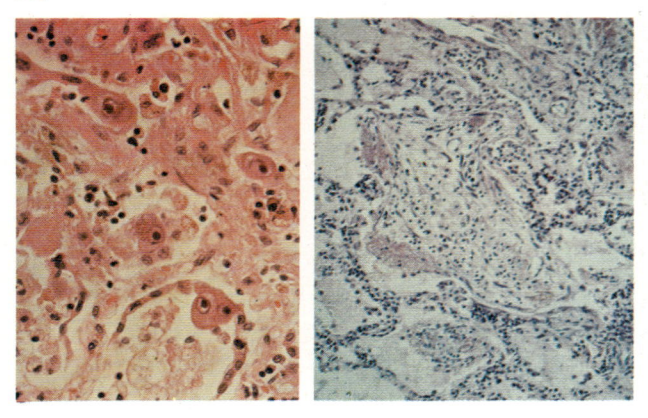

Figure 4.9 *Left:* Interstitial pneumonitis with prominent alveolar lining cells. The typical 'owls eye' intranuclear inclusions are seen in lining cells and in alveolae. H&E × 480. *Right:* A mycoplasmic pneumonia with interstitial mononuclear infiltrate and a fibrin-rich intra-alveolar exudate which is beginning to organize. Illness of three-weeks duration. H&E × 96.

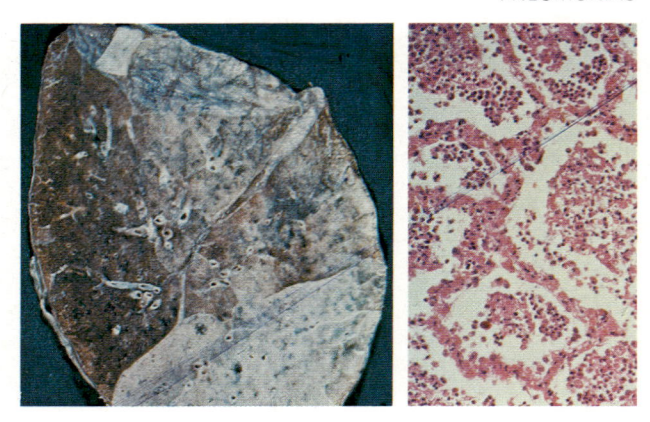

Figure 4.10 *Left:* Shows right upper lobar pneumonia in stage of grey hepatization. Encapsulated diplococci were seen. *Right:* Lobar pneumonia regarded as transitional in appearance between red and grey hepatization, with mainly polymorphonuclear exudate with 'shrinking' from alveolar walls which are still however somewhat congested. H&E × 240.

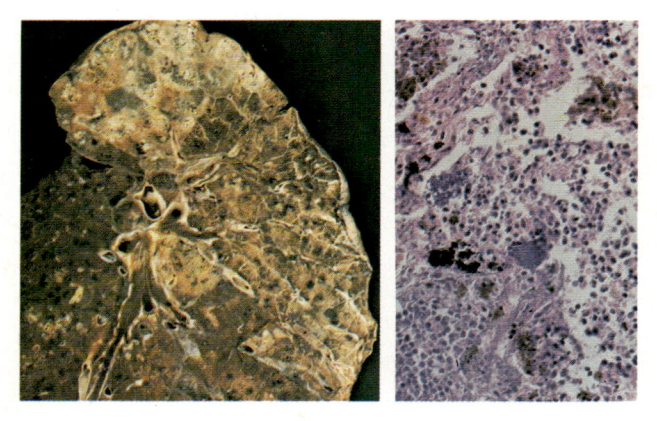

Figure 4.11 *Left:* A patchily consolidated, mainly upper lobe, pneumonia with areas of suppuration, which followed an influenza A infection. *Right:* Microscopy of an abscess showing organisms even on haematoxylin and eosin. H&E × 96.

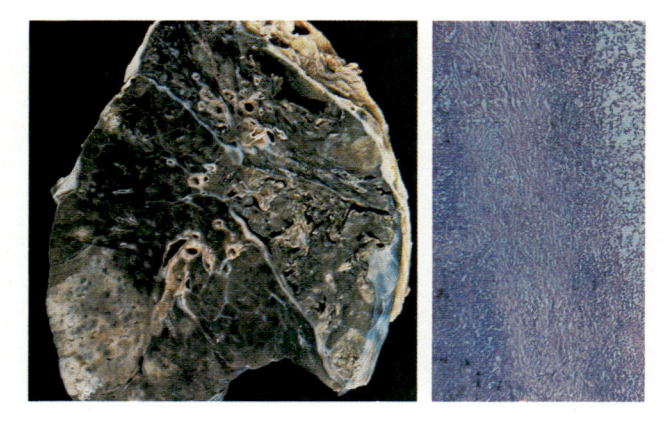

Figure 4.12 *Left:* Post-mortem right lung revealing upper lobe cavities, residual from a *Klebsiella* infection one year previously. The new infection is breaking down into abscess formation in middle lobe, but is a confluent area of consolidation in LL posteriorly. *Right:* Microscopy reveals suppuration and fibrosis. H&E × 38.4.

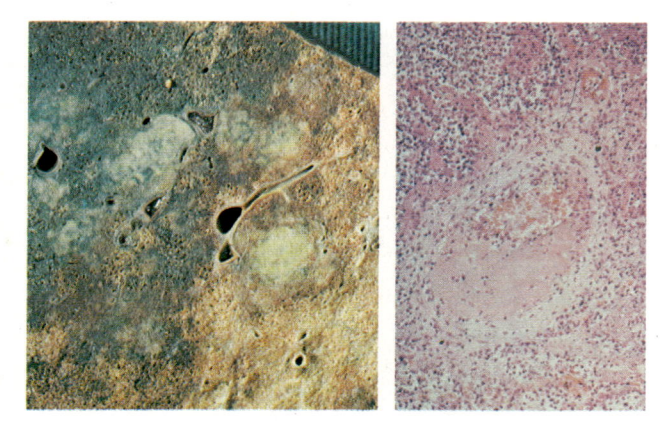

Figure 4.13 *Left:* A confluent suppurative bronchopneumonia with a characteristic green hue. A feature of *Pseudomonas* infection is the haemorrhagic infarct-like areas which are also apparent. *Right:* From an infarct-like area revealing acute inflammatory intraalveolar exudate with early thrombotic occlusion and inflammation of a pulmonary artery. H&E × 96.

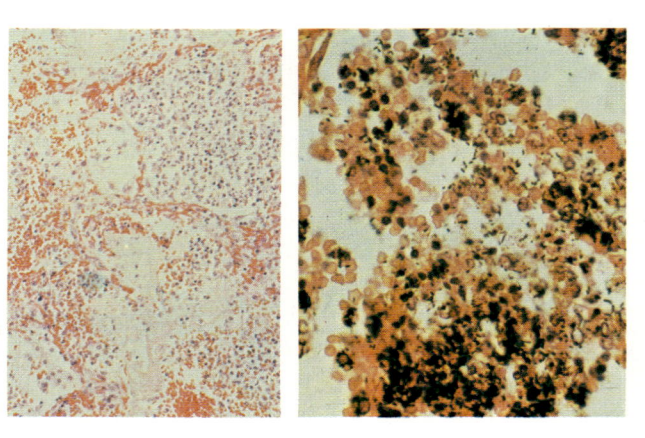

Figure 4.14 *Left:* Fatal Legionnaires disease, in spite of erythromycin therapy. This shows a collection of polymorphonuclear and mononuclear cells with alveolar congestion and haemorrhage. No organisms seen on Gram's stain. H&E × 96. *Right:* On the same tissue a modified Levaditti stain reveals numerous intra and extracellular coccobacilli. Levaditti × 384.

PNEUMONIAS

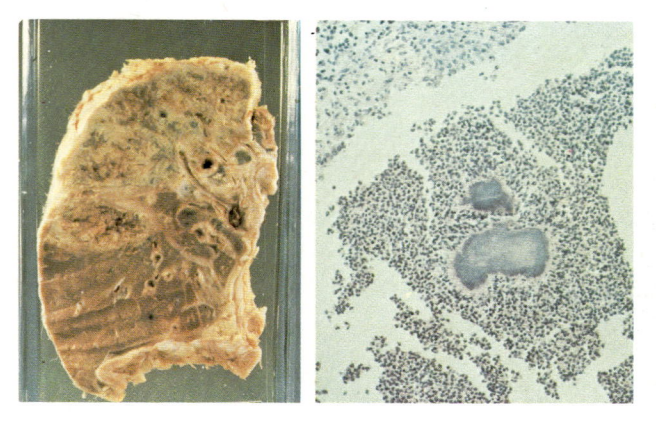

Figure 4.15 *Left:* Actinomycosis mainly affecting the upper lobe giving the appearance of ill-defined abscesses together with areas of grey organizing pneumonia – misdiagnosed as tuberculous for several months. *Right:* The characteristic 'ray fungus' in an acute inflammatory exudate. H & E × 96.

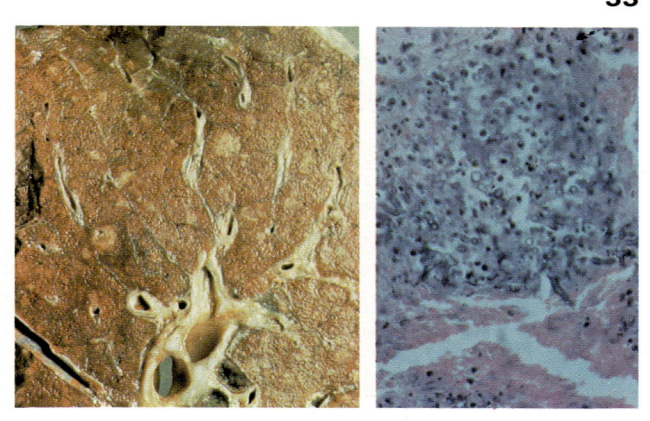

Figure 4.16 *Left:* 30-year-old patient with subacute bacterial endocarditis treated with steroids and antibiotics developing a pulmonary haemorrhagic pneumonia in which haemorrhagic lobules can be seen on the left and several grey circumscribed nodules elsewhere. *Right:* Branching septate mycelium *(A. fumigatus)* can be seen in the necrotic centre. H & E × 240

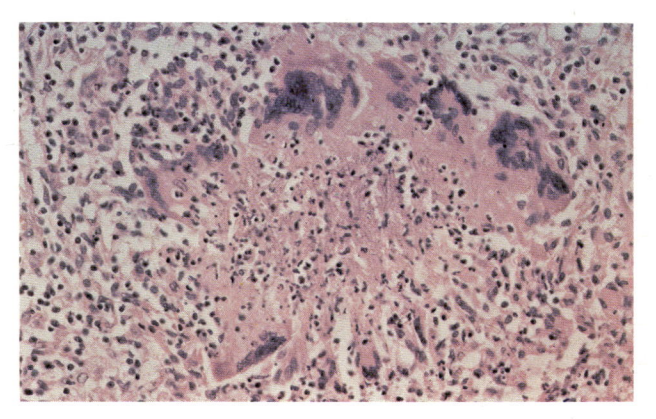

Figure 4.17 A suppurative lesion containing polymorphs and fungal hyphae surrounded by giant cells. H & E × 240

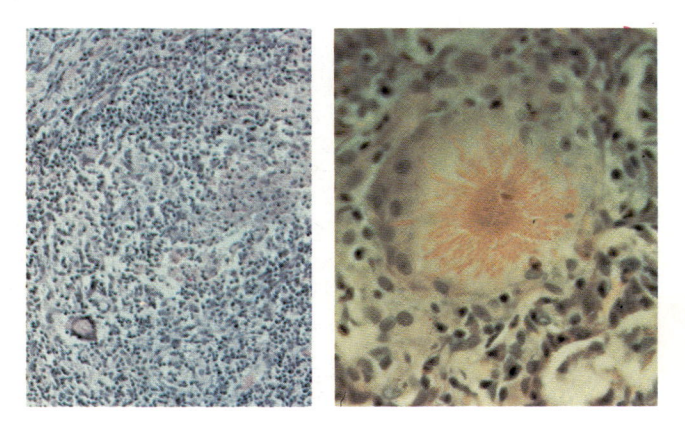

Figure 4.18 *Left:* A tuberculoid focus containing a Langhans-type giant cell in a patient with aspergillosis. H & E × 96. *Right:* An asteroid body which is due to a deposit of protein, lipids and polysaccharides – probably a manifestation of antigen–antibody reaction to the fungus. H & E × 384

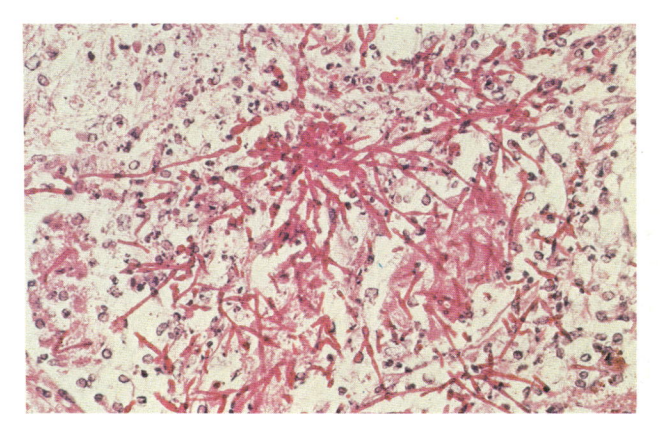

Figure 4.19 *Candida* occurring in an area of little inflammatory reaction in a patient with Legionnaire's disease. There are spores and the pseudohyphae exhibit foci of narrowing. PAS × 384

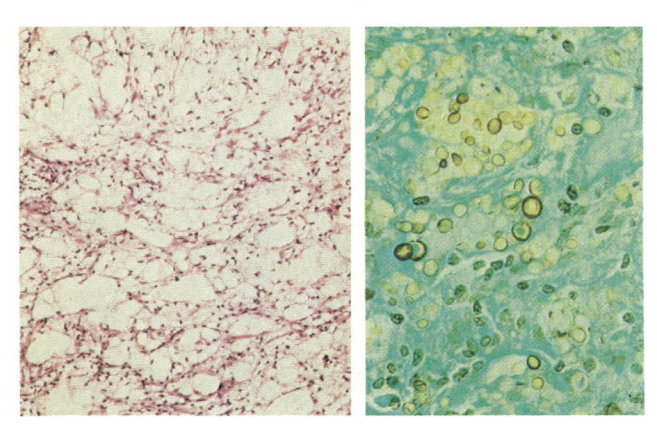

Figure 4.20 *Left:* Typical 'soap bubble' appearance of cryptococcal infection. PAS × 96. *Right:* Organisms demonstrated by Grocott's methenamine silver. × 384

cleated giant cells, many containing hyphal elements (Figure 4.19). Another rare finding is asteroid bodies (Figure 4.19).

Aspergillar hyphae are septate, less then 5 µm in thickness, and show frequent Y-shaped dichotomous branching. The blastophores of *Candida* may be simulated by aspergillar hyphae cut transversely. However, the latter have empty centres, whereas the former appear solid.

Candidiasis (Moniliasis)

The majority of pulmonary infections are caused by *Candida albicans*. Two main types of pulmonary infection occur:

(1) Monilial bronchitis – The larger bronchi are covered by a greyish-yellow membrane composed of fibrin, hyphae and spores.
(2) Invasive pneumonia – Features are similar to those of invasive aspergillosis. There may be a necrotizing pneumonia with minimal cellular reaction, microabscesses and, rarely, a granulomatous reaction[14].

Candida contain pseudohyphae, which evince focal narrowing at points and yeast forms (blastospores). When it grows on a surface (cavity or bronchus) hyphae are mainly present. Although *Candida* can be observed on H&E staining, they are more easily recognized in PAS (Figure 4.24) and Grocott's methenamine silver stains.

Phycomycosis (Mucormycosis)

Phycomycosis may be due to infection by *Rhizopus*, *Mucor* and *Absidia* species. The pulmonary changes are similar to those of aspergillosis[14]. Mycetomas and invasive phycomycosis may occur. They show striking vasoinvasive properties, so there is usually a prominent element of infarction in addition to the inflammation in the invasive type.

The hyphae are broad, varying in diameter from 5 to 25 µm, non-septate and branch at right angles. In contrast to aspergillosis which tends to show a radial arrangement, Phycomycetes show a haphazard arrangement of their hyphae. They stain with Grocott's methenamine silver method, but poorly with PAS or Gram stains.

Cryptococcosis

Cryptococcus neoformans may cause several forms of pulmonary lesions: gelatinous bronchopneumonia, miliary lesions, subpleural fibrotic nodules or a large abscess with a mucoid content and a wall devoid of fibrous tissue[3,14,15].

Microscopically, fungal bodies may be observed in the alveoli with minimal inflammatory reaction, or there may be a granulomatous reaction with some of the histiocytes and giant cells containing fungal bodies (Figure 4.21). The large chronic lesions may show considerable fibrosis.

Cryptococci are blue or pink rounded bodies in H&E sections (2-20 µm in diameter) and have weakly birefringent cell walls which stain by PAS, Alcian blue or mucicarmine. The body of the organism appears black by Grocott's methenamine silver method (Figure 4.21).

Histoplamosis

Histoplasma capsulatum is an infrequent opportunistic pathogen, but it may cause diffuse pneumonitis, miliary or cavitary lesions[14].

In diffuse pneumonitis there is organizing inflammatory infiltrate containing numerous histiocytes, in the bronchioles and alveoli.

Miliary lesions consist of epithelioid cell granulomata which may or may not show caseation.

Cavities may be single or multiple and show caseous necrosis, epithelioid granulomata and Langhans giant cells.

The major differential diagnosis is tubercle. The organisms are usually numerous and evident in H&E sections within histiocytes and giant cells as small round bodies (1-5 µm in size) surrounded by a clear halo. They are also stained by PAS (Figure 4.22) and methenamine silver. If these organisms are not demonstrated in the tissue, then this is strongly against the diagnosis of histoplasmosis.

Protozoa

Pneumocystis Pneumonia

Pneumocystis carinii has become a fairly frequent cause of opportunistic pulmonary infection [16]. It causes a very characteristic foamy intra-alveolar exudate, usually devoid of inflammatory cells (Figure 4.22). An accompanying interstitial inflammatory infiltrate composed of lymphocytes, plasma cells and histiocytes may be evident and hyperplasia of the alveolar lining cells may be seen. The crescentic or sickle-shaped cysts (4-6 µm diameter) can be demonstrated by Grocott's methenamine silver within the exudate, and occasionally within the septa. Other features sometimes include epithelioid granulatomata and calcification, the latter often surrounded by giant cells[17] (Chapter 12, Figure 12.8).

Whenever pneumocystis is identified, cytomegalovirus should also be searched for, since mixed infections frequently occur.

Helminths

Hydatid Disease

This disease is relatively common in sheep-rearing areas of the world and results from ingestion of ova of *Echinococcus granulosus* (dog tape worm). Man becomes infected by handling dogs which have become infected by eating the offal of infected sheep. The ova release embryos in the stomach and upper part of the small intestine which rapidly penetrate the bowel wall and migrate to the liver or lung where, in susceptible persons, it develops into a hydatid cyst. Children and young adults are usually affected.

The cysts may occur anywhere in the lung. They are often solitary but sometimes multiple and bilateral (Figure 4.22). The cyst consists of a single layer of cells (germinal epithelium) which is encompassed by a laminated, structureless coat (ectocyst). The latter varies in thickness according to the age of the cyst. Surrounding the ectocyst is a layer of fibrous tissue (adventitia) produced by the host (Figure 4.23). Brood capsules are produced from, and are attached to, the internal surface of the germinal layer. If the capsule bursts these may be set free to produce daughter cysts. Brood capsules are small vesicular structures within which scolices (heads of future worms) develop (Figure 4.24). The cyst contains clear fluid which frequently contain hooklets and scolices. As the cyst grows daughter cysts, which consist of a germinal layer and a poorly developed laminated layer, may originate from brood capsules or from the germinal layer and lie free within the original cyst.

Hydatid cysts may rupture into a bronchus with release of their fluid, and may result in anaphylaxis and death; rarely the collapsed cyst may be coughed up with spontaneous cure. Rupture into the pleural cavity may occur, either spontaneouly or as a result of surgery, where further cysts may arise widely throughout the pleura. Hydatid cysts may calcify if the parasite dies.

The adventitia shows only slight inflammatory reaction providing the cyst wall remains intact, but if it ruptures a severe granulomatous reaction may result (Figure 4.23). Secondary infection of a hydatid cyst may lead to formation of a lung abscess. We have also observed colonization of a hydatid cyst by *Aspergillus*.

Strongyloides

Strongyloides stercoralis may be a cause of opportunistic infection in the immune compromised host[16]. Although gastrointestinal involvement is the most prominent feature, occasionally pulmonary disease may occur without prior gastrointestinal symptoms[18]. The larvae may be seen in the sputum, bronchial washings or in lung tissue (Figure 4.25).

Lipid Pneumonias

Exogenous lipid pneumonia (including oil granuloma)

Exogenous lipid pneumonia may be a consequence of inhalation of mineral, vegetable or animal oils. The type of pulmonary reaction is similar, but the degree of damage varies with the oil responsible.

Macroscopically, part or all of a lobe may be firm and diffusely yellowish grey in colour, or there may be single or multiple focal yellowish nodules resembling neoplasms (Figure 4.27).

Histologically, lipid droplets (not seen in the endogenous type) may be found free and within the walls of arterioles and vessels, with associated distortion of vessel architecture. Numerous foamy oil-containing macrophages, lymphocytes, plasma cells and giant cells lie within the alveoli. The interstitium becomes widened by reticulin fibres and chronic inflammatory cells. Increasing fibrosis results in loss of pulmonary architecture, and enmeshed within the collagen fibres and fibroblasts are foci of histiocytes, lymphocytes and giant cells resembling tuberculoid granulomata (Figure 4.27). The arterioles containing small oil vacuoles evince increasing adventitial and medial fibrosis with fragmentation of the elastic laminae. Finally, dense fibrous tissue containing oil globules encompasses occluded arterioles and peripheral airways[19].

A pathological curiosity is the lipid pneumonia due to the inhalation of *black fat tobacco*. This tobacco is smoked in the West Indies and contains mineral oil and vasoline. A characteristic microscopic appearance occurs: there is diffuse interstitial fibrosis and vasculitis associated with lipid and amorphous black material[20] (Figure 4.27).

References

1. Hers, J. F. (1955). The histopathology of the respiratory tract in human influenza. *Verhandelkingen Von Het Nederlands Institut voor Praevertiere Geneestrunde*, **26,** 19
2. Craighead, J. E. (1975). Cytomegalovirus pulmonary disease. *Pathobiol. Annu.*, p.197
3. Spencer, H. (1977). *Pathology of the Lung*. 3rd Edn. Chap. 6. (Oxford: Pergamon Press)
4. Parker, M. T. (1980). Serotype distribution of Pneumococci. In *Pneumonia and Pneumococcus Infections*, p.11. International Congress and Symposium Series No.27. (London: R. Soc. Med.)
5. Spencer, H. (1977). *Pathology of the Lung*, 3rd Edn. Chap. 5. (Oxford: Pergamon Press)
6. Winn Jr., W. C., Glavin, F. L., Perl, O. P., Keller, J. L., Andres, T. L., Brown, T. M., Coffin, C. M., Sensecqua, J. E., Roman, L. N. and Craighead, J. E. (1978). The pathology of Legionnaire's disease. Fourteen fatal cases from the 1977 outbreak in Vermont. *Arch. Pathol. Lab. Med. Sci.*, **102,** 344
7. Blackmon, J. A., Harley, R. A., Hinklin, M. D. and Chandler, F. W. (1979). Pulmonary sequelae of Acute Legionnaire's Disease Pneumonia. *Ann. Int. Med.*, **90,** 552
8. Blackmon, J. A., Hinklin, M. D., Chandler, F. W., Special Expert Pathology Panel (1978). Legionnaire's disease; pathological and historical aspect of a 'new' disease. *Arch. Pathol. Lab. Med. Sci.*, **102,** 337
9. Murray, J. F., Finegold, S. M., Froman, S. and Will, D. W. (1961). The changing spectrum of nocardiosis. *Am. Rev. Resp. Dis.*, **83,** 315
10. Lurie, H. I. and Duma, R. J. (1970). Opportunistic infections of the lungs. *Hum. Pathol.*, **1,** 233
11. Rosen, P. P. (1976). Opportunistic fungal infections in patients with neoplastic diseases. *Pathol. Annu.*, p.255
12. Meyer, R. D., Young, L. S., Armstrong, D. and Yu, B. S. (1973). Aspergillosis complicating neoplastic diseases. *Amer. J. Med.*, **54,** 6
13. Young, R. C., Bennet, J. E., Vogel, C. L., Carbone, P. P. and De Vita, V. T. (1970). Aspergillosis, the spectrum of disease in patients. *Medicine (Baltimore)*, **49,** 147
14. Williams, D. M., Krick, J. A. and Remington, J. S. (1976). Pulmonary infection in the compromised host. Part 1. *Am. Rev. Resp. Dis.*, **114,** 359
15. Baker, R. D. and Haugen, R. K. (1955). Tissue changes in cryptococcosis. A study of 26 cases. *Am. J. Clin. Pathol.*, **25,** 25
16. Williams, D. M., Krick, J. A. and Remington, J. S. (1976). Pulmonary infection in the compromised host. Part 2. *Am. Rev. Resp. Dis.*, **114,** 593
17. Weber, W. R., Askin, F. B. and Dehrer, L. P. (1977). Lung biopsy in *Pneumocystis carinii* pneumonia. A histopathological study of typical and atypical features. *Am. J. Clin. Pathol.*, **67,** 11
18. Rassiga, A. L., Louny, J. L. and Forman, W. B. (1974). Diffuse pulmonary infection due to *Strongyloides stercoralis*. *J. Am. Med. Assoc.*, **230,** 426
19. Wagner, J. C., Adler, D. I. and Fuller, D. N. (1955). Foreign body granulomata of the lungs due to liquid paraffin. *Thorax*, **10,** 157
20. Miller, G. J., Ashcroft, M. T., Beadnell, H. M. S. G., Wagner, J. C. and Pepys, J. (1971). The lipoid pneumonia of black fat tobacco smokers in Guyana. *Q. J. Med.*, **40,** 457

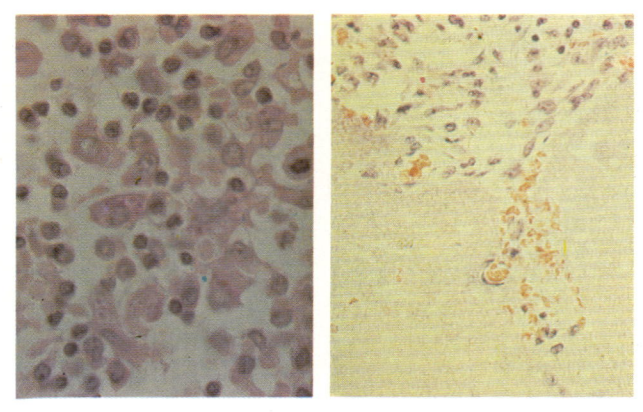

Figure 4.21 *Left:* *Histoplasma capsulatum* demonstrated within lung macrophages. PAS × 1200. *Right:* Typical foamy exudate due to *Pneumocystis carinii* infection. H&E × 240

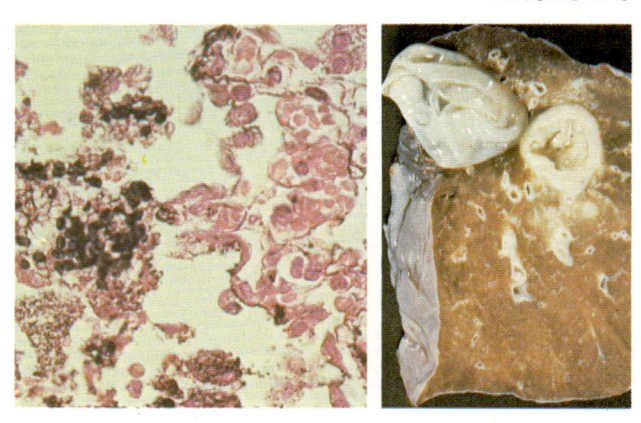

Figure 4.22 *Left:* An interstitial chronic inflammatory infiltrate is present and the pneumocystic organisms can be seen within the intraalveolar exudate. Grocott's methenamine silver × 384. *Right:* Lobectomy from a child presenting with haemoptysis, a round peripheral lesion and hilar lymphadenopathy. The consolidatd hyaline membrane (ectocyst) has been lain on the surface of the specimen. Much of the edge of the lesion consists of host inflammatory response (pericyst or adventitia)

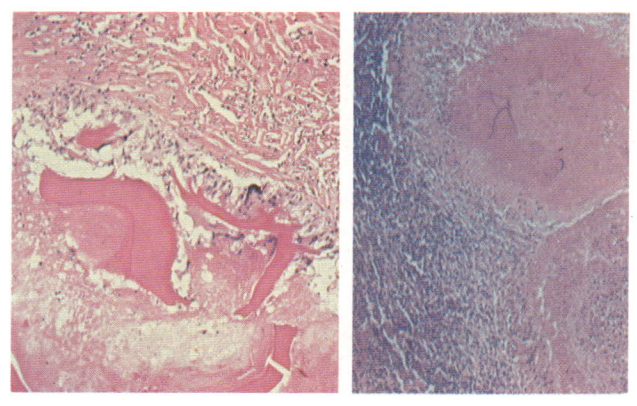

Figure 4.23 *Left:* Hyaline germinal membrane (ectocyst) surrounded by fibrous capsule (pericyst). H&E × 38.4. *Right:* The hydatid cyst is surrounded by a granulomatous reaction. H&E × 38.4

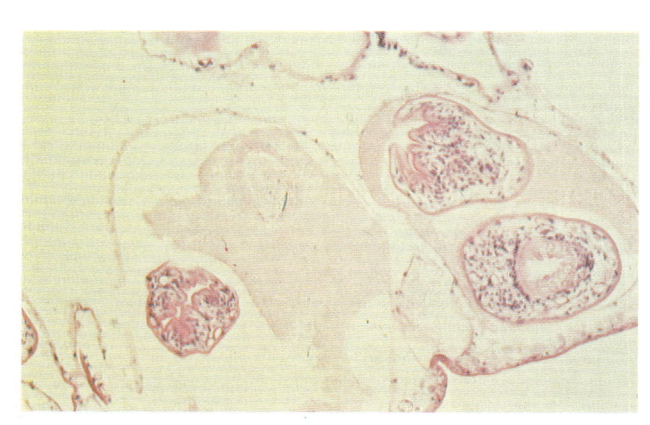

Figure 4.24 The inner germinal layer with a brood capsule and several scolices. In the pink amorphous material in the centre several scimitar shaped individual hooklets can be discerned. H&E × 384

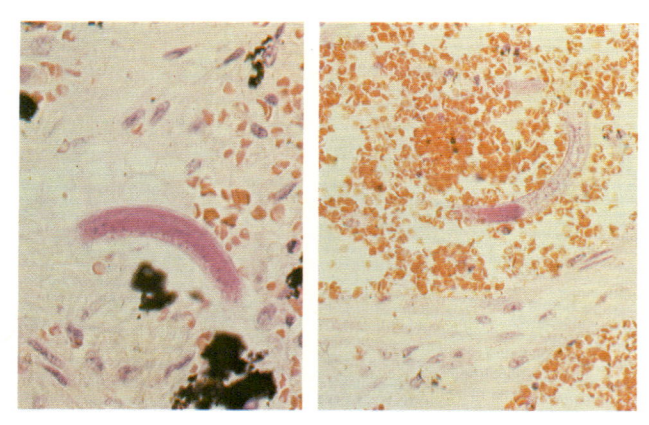

Figure 4.25 This patient has no history to suggest any immunosuppression, but disseminated strongyloidosis was found at autopsy. The larvae were present in the alveoli *(left)* bronchial mucous glands and within pulmonary vessels *(right)*. *Left:* H&E × 384. *Right:* H&E × 240

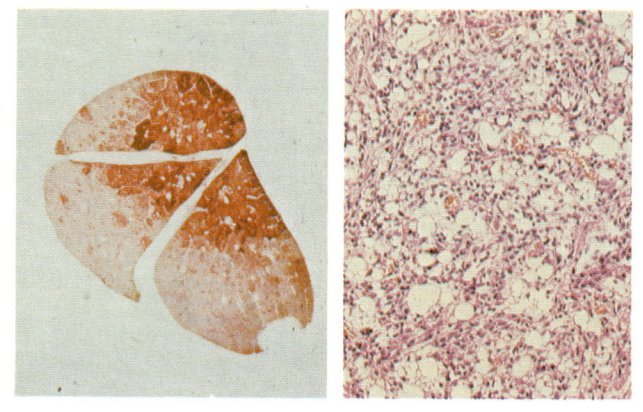

Figure 4.26 *Left:* A Gough Wentworth section of a lung from an infant who had inhaled cod liver oil stained for lipid by Oil red O. *Right:* Lipid vacuoles are seen in association with a variety of inflammatory cells and fibrous tissue. H&E × 38.4

PNEUMONIAS

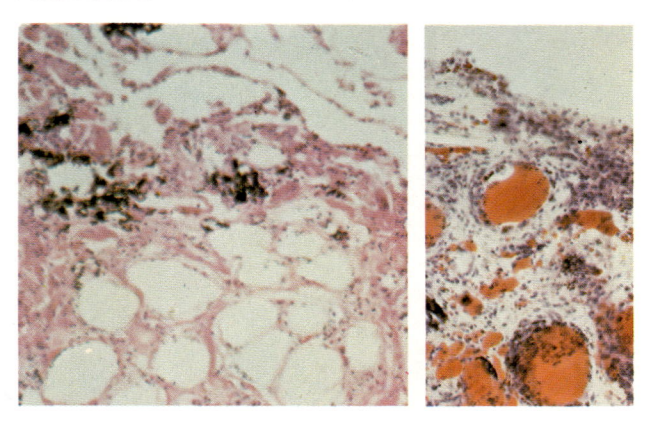

Figure 4.27 *Left:* Biopsy from a 'black fat tobacco' smoker showing fibrosis, 'cystic spaces' and black amorphous material. H & E × 96. *Right:* Oil red O stain shows the spaces to be composed of lipid. Oil red O × 96

Interstitial Pneumonias 5

Diffuse Alveolar Damage (DAD)

We shall describe the pattern of pulmonary response, known as DAD, which occurs to a variety of injurious agents (Table 5.1), and is probably the mechanism by which a significant proportion of cases of chronic interstitial fibrosis develop. Adult

Table 5.1 Some causes of diffuse alveolar damage

Oxygen

'Shock', trauma, 'perfusion lung' etc.

Sepsis

Viruses

Chemicals e.g. beryllium, cadmium and paraquat

Drugs e.g. busulphan, cyclophosphamide and bleomycin

Radiotherapy

Collagen diseases

respiratory distress syndrome, respiratory insufficiency syndrome, shock lung and traumatic wet lung are terms given to specific examples[1].

Clinically there is usually severe and life-threatening acute respiratory distress as evinced by dyspnoea and cyanosis (pronounced hypoxaemia). Radiographically bilateral diffuse infiltrates resembling pulmonary oedema are seen initially followed by the development of linear to coarse nodular opacities. Increasing hypoxia and lung stiffness is often treated by ever-increasing oxygen concentrations and ventilation pressures, in some contributing to alveolar damage. The condition is frequently fatal in the acute stage; sometimes complete resolution occurs; occasionally interstitial fibrosis or obliterative bronchiolitis is a sequel.

DAD is characterized by varying degrees of injury to alveolar lining cells, endothelial cells and probably bronchiolar cells. The temporal sequence of the pathological changes is based upon clinical and experimental studies[1-4]. The earliest microscopical changes, occurring within three days of exposure to the inciting agent, are capillary congestion, focal atelectasis and focal intra-alveolar oedema. Fibrin thrombi may be present at this time within capillaries and small arteries. Hyaline membrane formation, which occurs as a layer of protein-rich exudate at the air–wall interface of respiratory bronchioles and alveolar ducts, may be present focally as early as 22 hours after injury and may persist for up to 2 weeks (Figure 5.1 and 5.2) After 3 days interstitial oedema becomes prominent in both interalveolar and large interlobular septa. Intra-alveolar accumulation of proteinous material occurs with variable amounts of cells including both macrophages, type II pneumocytes and red blood cells. Within a few days of injury a striking interstitial mononuclear infiltrate usually accumulates consisting of lymphocytes, plasma cells and atypical cells variably interpreted as megakaryocytes, endothelial or lymphoid cells (Figure 5.3). Alveolar lining cell hyperplasia usually becomes conspicuous after one week, although focal proliferations of these cells may be seen as early as 3 days (Figure 5.4). These lining cells become enlarged, line up sometimes in syncytial sheets along either the lumina or septal sides of the hyaline membranes, and may be very atypical with bizarre, polypoid nuclei, which contain prominent nucleoli, which may be confused with malignant cells or falsely interpreted as indicating a viral aetiology. Sometimes there may be marked squamous metaplasia.

After 8 days extensive interstitial fibrosis becomes apparent, although small foci of interstitial fibrosis may be identified after as little as three days. Proliferation of smooth muscle fibres may occur and the interstitial cellular infiltrate becomes progressively less. At 2 weeks the changes may appear surprisingly chronic. Vascular changes which include muscular proliferation of arterial walls and subintimal fibrosis of veins and arteries usually occur in areas of scarring. Sometimes there is abundant loose fibrous tissue within alveolar spaces. It is possible that this organization of alveolar exudate occurs when the epithelial cells are damaged but not destroyed and the pulmonary architecture remains intact, whereas formation of interstitial fibrosis and cyst formation follows epithelial necrosis, basement membrane and alveolar collapse[5].

Using a variety of injurious agents to produce DAD ultrastructural studies have shown first oedema of the interstitium and type I pneumocytes followed later by their death[2-4]. Then type II pneumocytes undergo mitosis, maximally between 2 and 4 days after injury, first becoming plump, and then flattened to resemble type I cells, the osmiophilic bodies and surface microvilli being lost in the process. If accurate this finding supports the view that the type II cells act as the 'reserve' cells of the alveolar lining.

At no stage can inference be drawn as to the injurious agent. One feature, however, can be suggestive of aetiology, namely, the presence of foam cell-plaques in the intima of arterial walls. Seen in radiation pneumonitis, their finding is regarded as specific but Bennett et al.[6] found them in only 5% of irradiated lungs.

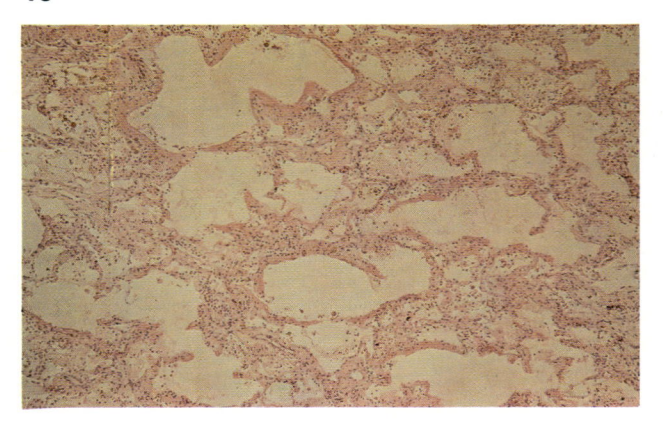

Figure 5.1 Post-mortem appearances of a patient with a rapidly progressive respiratory illness believed viral and dying before assisted respiration instituted. The non-specific picture of DAD with focal intra-alveolar oedema, minimal 'hyaline membrane' (centre and bottom), and a mild interstitial mononuclear infiltrate. H&E × 38.4.

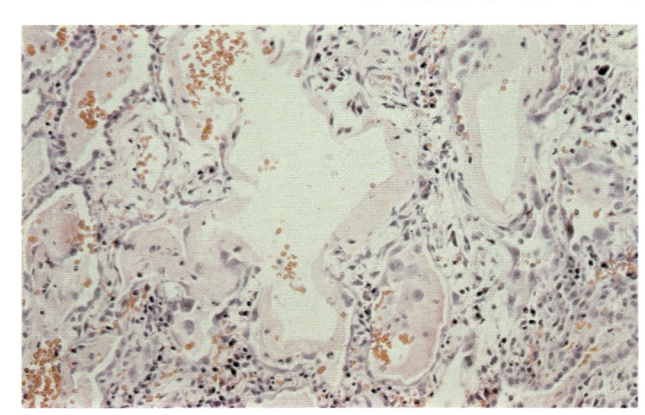

Figure 5.2 This was a patient with SLE who rapidly deteriorated; a lung biopsy to eliminate opportunistic infection revealed DAD. The prominent features are well developed 'hyaline membranes' and marked cuboidal cell metaplasia. H&E × 240.

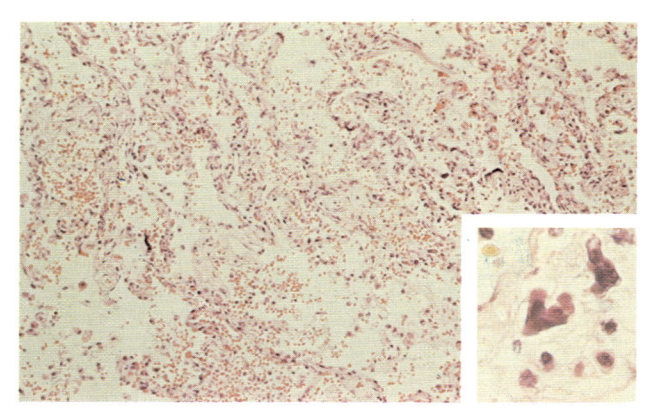

Figure 5.3 Another example of diffuse alveolar damage illustrating some large hyperchromatic cells (enlarged in inset). H&E × 96.

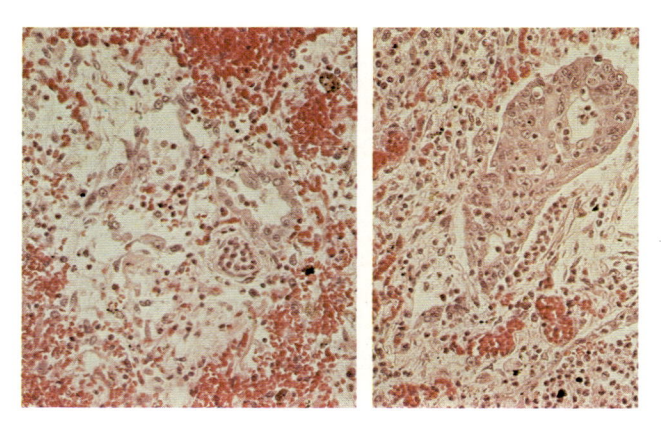

Figure 5.4 An example of paraquat ingestion leading to DAD emphasizing a prominent haemorrhagic component (left) and development of metaplastic epithelium and early fibrosis of interalveolar septum (right). H&E × 300.

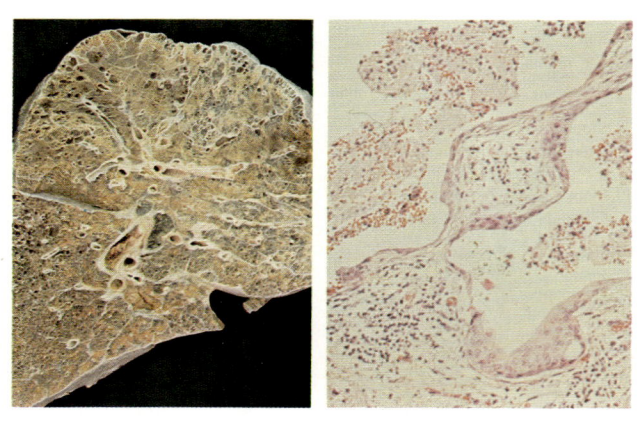

Figure 5.5 Left: Photograph of a ICIP lung after barium sulphate impregnation which emphazises the fine nature of the fibrosis in a lower lobe but with fine honeycombing also involving upper lobe. Right: This shows the interstitial fibrosis with squamous metaplasia lining the walls of terminal airways. There is a mild lymphocytic infiltrate. H&E × 384.

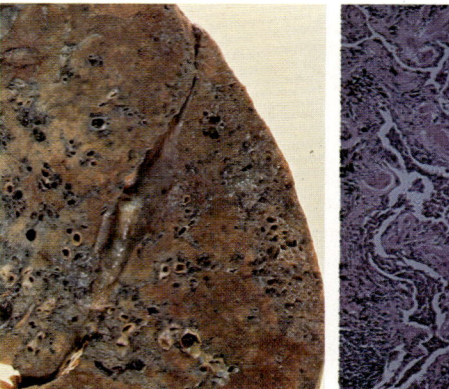

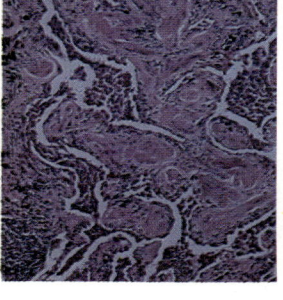

Figure 5.6 Left: Cut surface of lung. Whilst there is honeycombing posteriorly in lower lobe there are areas of more ill-defined induration. Right: Taken from an indurated area showing marked muscle hyperplasia and desquamation of pigment laden cells only some of which were Perl positive. H&E × 96.

INTERSTITIAL PNEUMONIAS

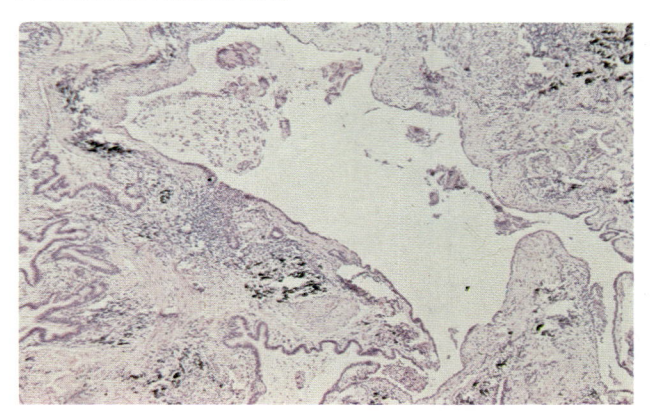

Figure 5.7 A honeycombed area from a case of ICIP demonstrating that the enlarged spaces consist of dilated respiratory bronchioles with fibrosis in their walls. H&E × 78.

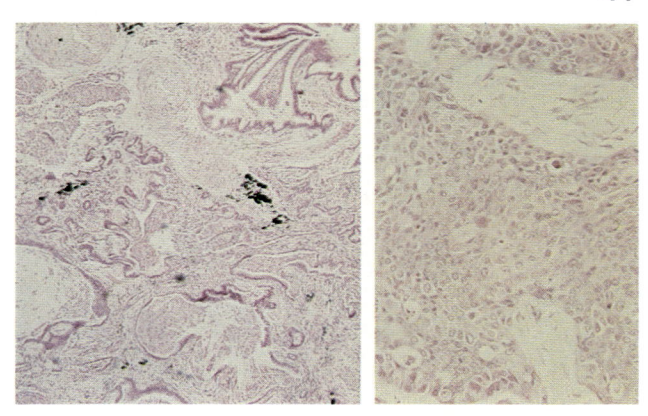

Figure 5.8 *Left:* A patient with ICIP showing marked metaplasia of bronchiolar and alveolar epithelium. H&E × 78. *Right:* Biopsy of another patient with ICIP showing an area of diffuse severe dysplastic/in-situ carcinomatous change. The patient developed an overt squamous carcinoma 18 months later. H&E × 192.

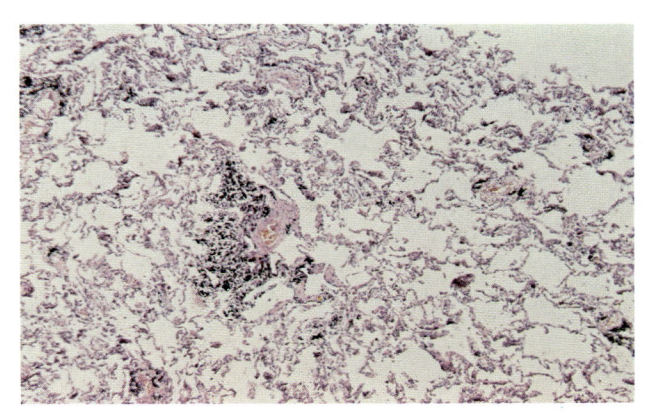

Figure 5.9 Lung biopsy fom a 33-year-old coal miner showing the unmodified central dust focus and fine mural fibrosis H&E × 78.

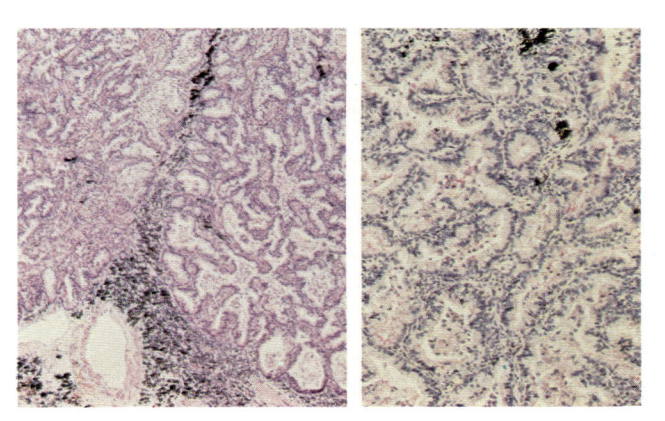

Figure 5.10 The same patient as in Figure 5.9 developed a peripheral localized tumour which was diagnosed as bronchioalveolar carcinoma. *(Left)* H&E × 78. *(Right)* PAS diasase × 192.

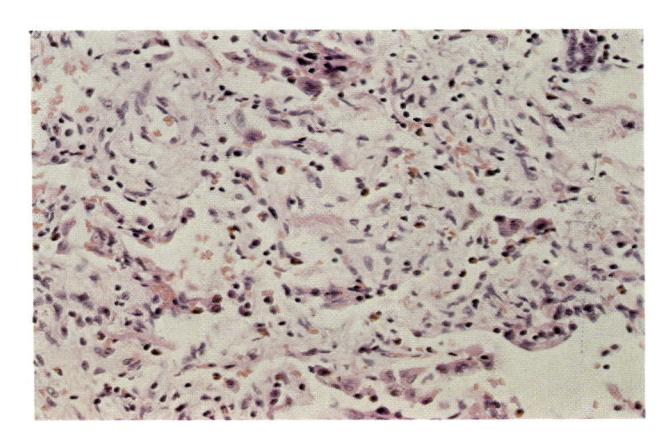

Figure 5.11 A case of ICIP showing scattered eosinophils within the interstitium, raising the problem of the number of eosinophils permitted before contemplating the alternative diagnosis of histiocytosis X and eosinophilic pneumonia. H&E × 480.

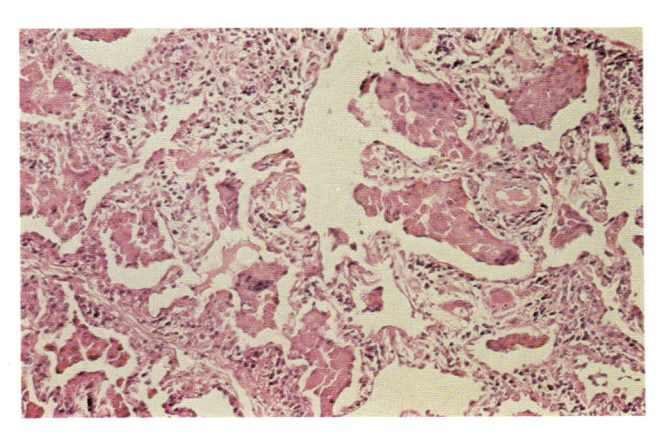

Figure 5.12 Open lung biopsy of a clinically ICIP revealing interstitial fibrosis with lymphoid infiltration and a marked desquamative component.

Interstitial Pneumonias

The interstitium which is the supporting tissue of the lung, includes the tissue lying between the alveolar lining cells and endothelial cells and the tissue in contact with the bronchiolar walls and interlobular septa. It comprises collagen, reticulin and elastic fibrils and a variety of mesenchymal cells. The term interstitial pneumonia implies that the inflammatory process exclusively involves the interstitium but in fact there is nearly always concomitant alveolar involvement, and on occasion this may be the dominant feature, e.g. in desquamative interstitial pneumonia.

The terminology used to define the spectrum of insterstitial disease is confusing. Attention was first drawn to a group of patients who developed interstitial disease, some of whom died within a few months of onset and others running a more protracted course ending in interstitial fibrosis, by Hamman and Rich in 1935[7] and 1944[8]. For some time this idiopathic condition was referred to eponymously as chronic Hamman–Rich syndrome, objected to by many on the basis that most of these patients were not of the protracted type. Recognition that the end stage fibrosis of alveolar walls was the consequence of a diffuse interstitial inflammatory process resulted in the use by Scadding and Hinson[9] in Britain of the term cryptogenic fibrosing alveolitis and by Liebow[10,11] in the USA of the concept of interstitial pneumonia of usual type (UIP). Though clinicians in Britain have adopted cryptogenic fibrogenic alveolitis (CFA) and have extended the use of the term fibrosing alveolitis to such an extent that it frequently implies no more than the broad group of interstitial diseases, as pathologists in Britain have been loath to depart from the use of the term 'interstitial' we prefer the term idiopathic chronic interstitial pneumonia which will clearly allow a varying degree of fibrosis. Table 5.2 shows the variety of terms that have been used for the condition. Whilst UIP is regarded as a rather clumsy term for this entity there are merits in utilizing some of the other entities Liebow[11] has separated off (Table 5.3).

Table 5.2 Other terms given to idiopathic chronic interstitial fibrosis

Usual interstitial pneumonia
Fibrosing alveolitis
Hamman–Rich syndrome*
Cryptogenic fibrosing alveolitis
Muscular cirrhosis of the lung
Interstitial pulmonary fibrosis
Diffuse pulmonary fibrosis
Classic interstitial pneumonitis–fibrosis
Chronic interstitial pneumonia
Adult respiratory distress syndrome

*Hamman–Rich syndrome is usually applied to the rapidly progressing and fatal form of the disease, death occuring within three months of the onset.

Table 5.3 Liebow's classification of interstitial pneumonias

Usual Interstitial pneumonia (UIP) – The most common type of interstitial pneumonia which has been referred to by others as (cryptogenic) fibrosing alveolitis.

Broncholitis Obliterans and Diffuse Alveolar Damage (BIP) – This combines the features of UIP and bronchiolitis obliterans. In our opinion, it serves no useful purpose to include under the heading of interstitial pneumonia, bronchiolitis obliterans.

Desquamative Interstitial Pneumonia (DIP) – Characterized by packing of alveoli with mononuclear cells (macrophages and type III pneumocytes) with a minimal interstitial component.

Lymphoid Interstitial Pneumonia (LIP) – Characterized by a diffuse lymphoid infiltrate of the interstitium with focal collections of mature lymphoid cells with germinal centres. It is discussed fully in Chapter 20.

Giant Cell Interstitial Pneumonia (GIP) – A very rare variant with interstitial pneumonitis and large bizarre giant cells in the alveoli.

It is accepted in general that some of these represent types of reaction to injurious agents but there is argument as to whether they are distinct entities or aspects of a spectrum of changes.

Idiopathic Chronic Interstitial Pneumonia (ICIP) – Cryptogenic Fibrosing Alveolitis (CFA)

As the title implies no aetiological agent can be identified but it is probable that any agent producing diffuse alveolar damage may lead to chronic interstitial fibrosis. However, this may not be the only pathway and other mechanisms may be involved. The 'collagen group' of disorders – rheumatoid disease, systemic lupus erythematosus, dermatomyositis and scleroderma – result in pulmonary changes indistinguishable from those described in this entity. They are best designated by the appropriate term, e.g. rheumatoid disease, with interstitial involvement.

On gross examination the lungs are usually reduced in size and show numerous fine or coarse fibrotic bands. Sometimes the lungs just feel indurated with no obvious macroscopic interstitial fibrosis but microscopy reveals a surprising degree of interstitial fibrosis. Honeycombing with rounded cystic spaces, varying in diameter from a few millimetres to a centimetre or more, may or may not be present. The changes are usually bilateral and maximal in the lower and outer zones of the lung. This contrasts with the chronic stages of extrinsic allergic alveolitis and sarcoidosis which show changes predominating in the upper lobes. The disease is always more advanced pathologically than the radiology would suggest (Figure 5.5 and 5.6).

Microscopically, there is loss of alveoli with alteration of pulmonary architecture due to fibrosis. The cystic structures between fibrotic areas form from non-respiratory and respiratory brochioles[12]. These labyrinthine structures may be lined by cuboidal, columnar (which may be mucus secreting), or squamous epithelium (Figure 5.7). Atypia of lining epithelium is not unusual and marked atypia may remain unchanged over many years, though the development of frank carcinoma is a well recognized event (Figures 5.8-5.10). The interalveolar septa and more proximal interstitium is widened, collagenous and infiltrated by lymphocytes, plasma cells and occasional eosinophils. When eosinophils are more than occasional (Figure 5.11), the problem arises of whether another diagnosis should be entertained (see Chapter 9). Lymphoid follicles with germinal centres, often present in Liebow's DIP, are infrequent (Figures 5.12 and 5.13). If occasional microscopic fields of alveolar sacs packed with pale pink mononuclears are seen, this should be reported as a DIP component rather than the separate entity described below (Figures 5.14 and 5.15). Occasional Perl positive intracellular granules are often seen in intraalveolar mononuclears; when prolific the possibility of idiopathic pulmonary haemosiderosis (IPH) must be entertained (Chapter 13). In addition features of bronchiolitis obliterans may be present; referred to by some as BIP (Figure 5.15).

It is surprising how infrequently intra-alveolar or interstitial polymorph neutrophils are seen, considering their frequency in bronchial lavage material; high polymorph and eosinophil counts are regarded as indicating poor steroid response[13]. Occasional small intra-alveolar giant cells forming poorly defined granulomata may be evident but well formed tuberculoid granulomata are absent (cf. sarcoidosis) (Figures 5.16-5.18). Other changes sometimes seen are small foci of calcification and ossification.

When, on careful search, an occasional asbestos body is seen (Figure 5.18), a diagnosis of asbestosis is not justified, as occasional asbestos bodies will be seen in lungs of urban males with asbestos counts of 25-170000 in the absence of fibrosis (see Chapter 15).

Smooth muscle hypertrophy and hyperplasia is frequently marked and is related to the bronchiolar structures which become expanded to form the honeycomb cysts.

The muscular pulmonary arteries show intimal fibrosis and muscular hypertrophy in areas of fibrosis.

In addition to these changes, foci of fibrosis may be present, in relationship to which irregular emphysema may develop.

Whenever this pathological picture is encountered a detailed occupational history is obligatory, since the inhalation and deposition of mineral dusts and fumes can be the cause (Figures 5.19 and 5.20). Indeed, additional methods for identifying these substances, such as electron microscopy, electron and X-ray diffraction, and X-ray fluorescence and infrared spectroscopy should be used, if available, for investigation of patients with interstitial fibrosis if the cause is unknown[14].

Role of Bronchoalveolar Lavage

Examination of fluid obtained by bronchoalveolar lavage may yield useful information in patients with ICIP, both from the diagnostic and therapeutic standpoints. The results obtained are believed to reflect the inflammatory and immunological events taking place in the lower respiratory tract since bronchoalveolar lavage recovers cells and proteins present on the epithelial surface of the lower respiratory tract[15]. The fluid recovered by bronchoalveolar lavage can be examined for cellular content by light or electron microscopy, analysed biochemically and a variety of immunological tests performed. In normal non-smoking subjects diffential counts obtained by light microscopy reveal the majority of the cells to be macrophages (70% ± 7.0) with a smaller percentage of lymphocytes (15.2% ± 2,6)[16]; polymorph neutrophils comprise less than 3% of the count and eosinophils are absent[17]. Consistent results are obtained when fluid is examined from multiple pulmonary sites at the same time in the same individual[15]. In healthy individuals who smoke, however, total cell yield is increased four or five times that of the normal, with higher percentages of macrophages (95%) and consequent reduction in the proportion of lymphocytes[16]; the percentage of polymorph neutrophils may be increased particularly in the older smokers. Also seen in smokers are pigment inclusions within the macrophages. Studies in patients with ICIP have demonstrated some individuals with increased percentages of polymorph neutrophils and eosinophils and reduced percentages of lymphocytes in pretreatment lavage. Further, those with increased percentages of polymorph neutrophils and/or eosinophils and reduced percentages of lymphocytes are unlikely to respond clinically to steroids whilst those with lymphocyte percentages above 11% often show a clinical response to steroids[13,17].

Bronchoalveolar lavage may also be helpful in differential diagnosis. High proportions of lymphocytes in the lavage fluid usually indicate sarcoidosis or extrinsic allergic bronchioloalveolitis[16].

Desquamative Interstitial Pneumonia (DIP)

Liebow et al.[18] introduced this term for a disease, of unknown aetiology, characterized by a striking, uniform accumulation of large eosinophilic mononuclear cells within alveolar spaces. Since then a few cases with similar pathological appearances have been described in association with asbestos exposure[19], nitrofurantoin administration[17,20] and tungsten carbide exposure [18]. A localized similar pathological reaction has been described by Bedrossian et al.[21] around specific pulmonary lesions, such as rheumatoid nodule, eosinophilic granuloma and chondromatous hamartoma.

In his original description Liebow stated the main difference between DIP and UIP (ICIP) to be that in DIP there was little interstitial fibrosis, an absence of hyaline membranes and necrosis, uniformity of changes from field to field, and slight interstitial reaction but occasional interstitial lymphoid follicles with germinal centres.

The intra-alveolar cells in DIP are large 9-12μm), rounded or polygonal, deeply eosinophilic and may contain cytoplasmic vacuoles (Figure 5.21). There may be intracytoplasmic, yellow-brown granules but minimal anthracotic pigment. The granules are PAS-positive but negative with iron stains[18]. The nuclei tend to be rounded or ovoid and usually have prominent nucleoli. Ultrastructurally, these intra-alveolar cells have been shown to be mixtures of varying proportions of macrophages and type II pneumocytes[19]. Intra-alveolar giant cells, with similar cytological characteristics to the intra-alveolar cells, are occasionally present. If the giant cells are very numerous, large and bizarre, then there may be reason for segregation within a separate group, designated by Liebow GIP[11] (Figure 5.22). In DIP

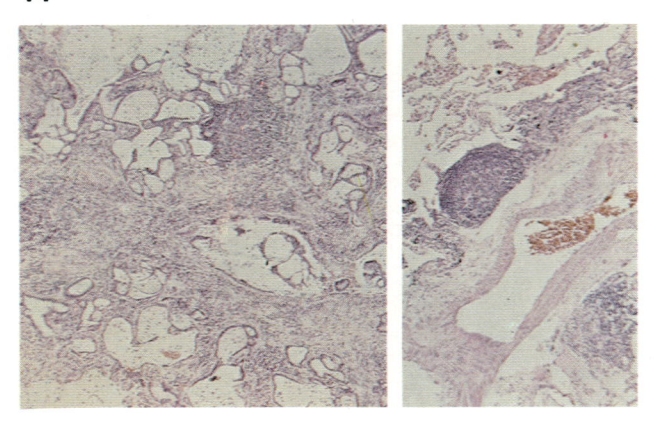

Figure 5.13 *Left:* From a honeycombed area showing marked bronchiolectasis and interstitial fibrosis with diffuse and focal collections of lymphocytes. H & E × 78. *Right:* From a relatively normal area of the same case with lymphoid follicles and minimal intra-alveolar desquamation, illustrating the difficulties of interpreting minute transbronchial biopsies. H & E × 78.

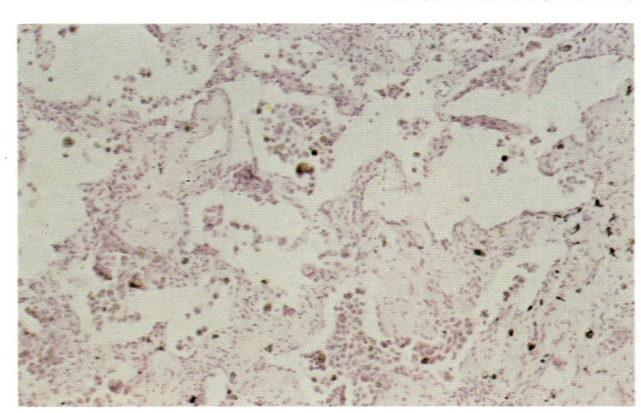

Figure 5.14 Mixed mural and desquamative features in a patient regarded as ICIP. A vague history of viral pneumonia was elicited at the onset of the symptoms 3 years previously; this represents one of the pathways in the development of ICIP. Much of the brown particulate material was PERL positive and was accepted within the spectrum of ICIP. H & E × 78.

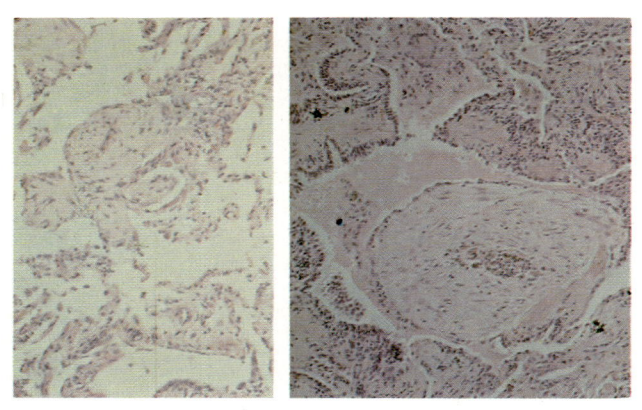

Figure 5.15 *Left:* A transbronchial biopsy from a patient with dyspnoea of a few months duration and finger clubbing. It shows 'interstitial pneumonitis' and organisation of intra-alveolar exudates. H & E × 120. *Right:* Another patient with similar history showing the appearances of bronchiolitis obliterans. H & E × 120.

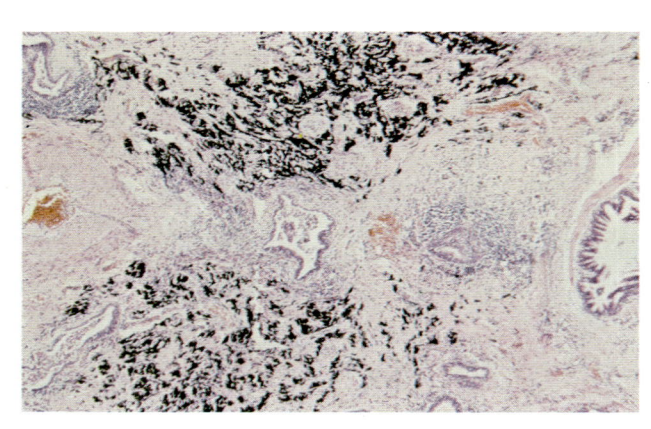

Figure 5.16 A coal miner diagnosed as ICIP with lower lobe fibrosis and 'clubbing' of many years duration. The coal dust can be seen interstitially. This case also illustrates the problem encountered when occasionally scattered poorly formed granulomata are seen. At later post-mortem there was no evidence of granulomata in hilar nodes or other organs. A hypertrophied pulmonary artery can also be seen. H & E × 78.

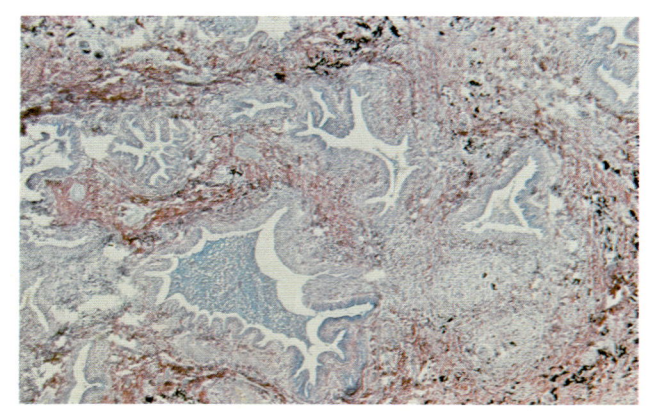

Figure 5.17 The same patient as in Figure 5.16 was also a smoker. Goblet cell metaplasia is seen in terminal airways. Alcian blue × 78.

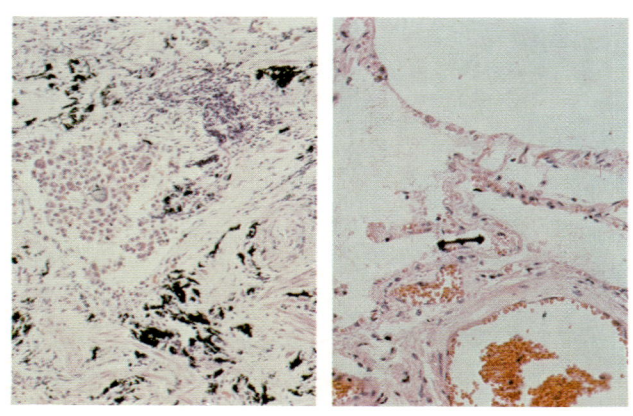

Figure 5.18 *Left:* Another example of ICIP in a coal miner illustrating fibrosis, smooth muscle hyperplasia and desquamated cells including a giant cell containing inorganic material. The presence of poorly formed granulomata and some inorganic material does not invalidate the diagnosis of ICIP. H & E × 78. *Right:* A similar problem occurs when an otherwise typical example of the disease occurs in the minimally exposed asbestos patient. The count in this patient was 56 000/g and was not considered an example of asbestosis. H & E × 78.

INTERSTITIAL PNEUMONIAS

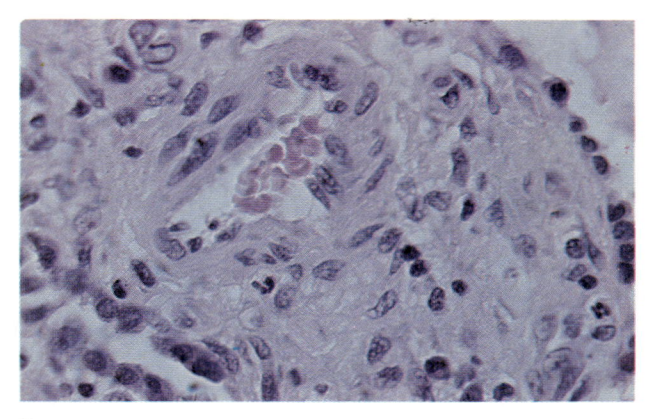

Figure 5.19 Biopsy of lung of a 22-year-old female shoe factory worker presenting with 'interstitial disease'. The biopsy reveals early interstitial fibrosis, cuboidal cell metaplasia each side of the septum and a light mononuclear infiltrate. H&E × 300.

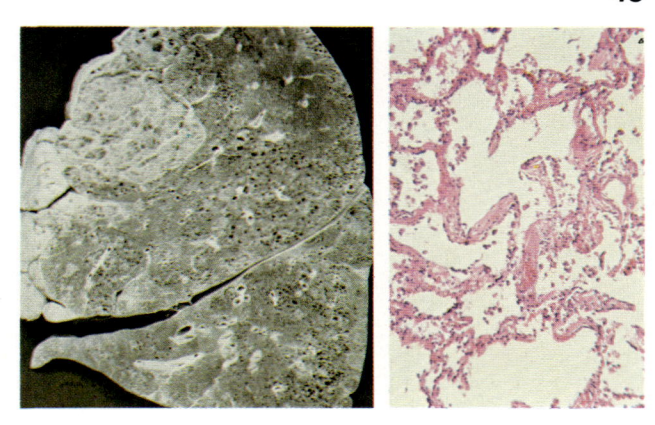

Figure 5.20 The same patient 20 years later who had progressed to interstitial fibrosis but died suddenly of coronary artery disease. *Left:* Barium sulphate impregnation showing fine uniform interstitial fibrosis. *Right:* Established mural fibrosis easily labelled ICIP. H&E × 96.

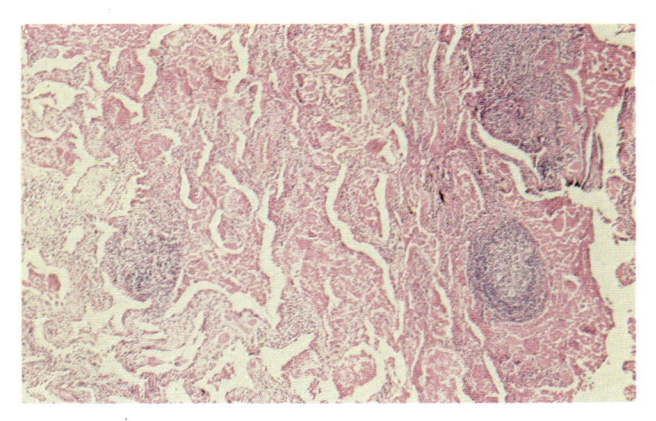

Figure 5.21 Open lung biopsy of a patient who had progressive dyspnoea, diffuse crepitations and clubbing of fingers, revealing a combination of marked desquamation of pink mononuclear cells, 'interstitial pneumonitis' with lymphoid foci and a follicle. In spite of the overt interstitial component and lymphoid collections this is regarded as DIP. H&E × 38.4.

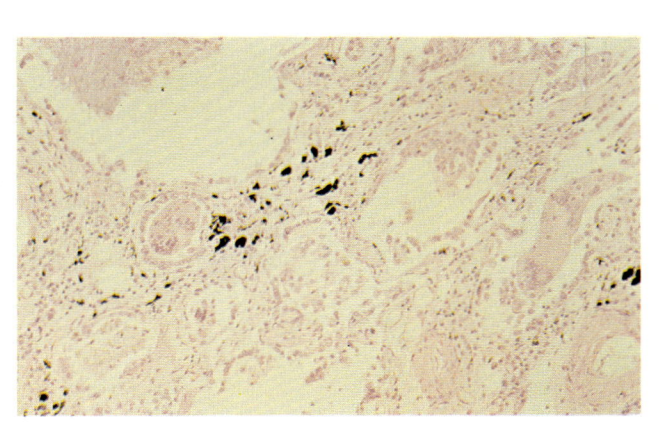

Figure 5.22 This shows interstitial fibrosis with a light lymphoid infiltrate, thickening of arterial walls and numerous multinucleated intra-alveolar giant cells meriting the designation GIP. H&E × 96.

small numbers of eosinophils, lymphocytes and neutrophils may be admixed with the intra-alveolar mononuclear cells.

Alveolar lining cells become cuboidal and prominent; mitoses may be identified both within them and the free alveolar mononuclear cells. Similar large mononuclear cells are also present in bronchioles.

In most cases, lymphoid follicles with germinal centres occur within the interstitium. Whereas in Liebow's original description[18] interstitial infiltration by plasma cells, lymphocytes, eosinophils and neutrophils was stated to be mild, later observers have commented that the interstitial infiltrate may be marked, blurring the distinction between these conditions. Similarly, different observers have continued to use this description, even when there is much interstitial fibrosis. Certainly in this event, particularly when the desquamative change is patchy, it is best to report ICIP with desquamative component and reserve DIP for those with minimal or non-interstitial component.

However, sometimes focal lymphoid collections are very prominent, to a degree where confusion with lymphoproliferative disease of the lung becomes possible. The latter lack a marked desquamative component.

Prominent groups of intra-alveolar mononuclear cells are, of course, a feature of eosinophilic pneumonia but confusion should not occur because of the presence of a large number of intra-alveolar eosinophils, eosinophilic abscesses and Touton type giant cells.

Malakoplakia of the lung, a condition unknown to us, apparently has similar appearances to DIP but the macrophages contain the pathognomonic, basophilic Michaelis–Gutmann bodies.

Obstructive pneumonitis may also lead to diagnostic confusion but the macrophages within the alveoli are strikingly foamy with fat.

References

1. Katzenstein, Anna-Louise A., Bloor, C. M. and Liebow, A. A. (1976). Diffuse alveolar damage – the role of oxygen, shock and related factors. *Am. J. Pathol.*, **85,** 210
2. Evans, M. J., Cabral, L. J., Stephen, R. J. and Freeman, G. (1973). Renewal of alveolar epithelium in the rat following exposure to NO_2. *Am. J. Pathol.*, **70,** 175
3. Adamson, I. Y. R. and Bowden, D. H. (1974). The Type 2 cell as a progenitor of alveolar epithelial regeneration: A cytodynamic study in mice after exposure to oxygen. *Lab. Invest.*, **30,** 35
4. Strauss, Ruth H., Palmer, K. C. and Hayes, J. A. (1976). Acute lung injury induced by cadmium aerosol. *Am. J. Pathol.*, **84,** 561
5. Thurlbeck, W. M. and Thurlbeck, S. M. (1976). Pulmonary effects of paraquat poisoning. *Chest,* **69,** suppl. 276
6. Bennett, D. E., Million, R. R. and Ackerman, L. V. (1969). Bilateral radiation pneumonitis, a complication of the radiotherapy of bronchogenic carcinoma. *Cancer,* **23,** 1001
7. Hamman, L. and Rich, A. R. (1935). Fulminating diffuse interstitial fibrosis of the lungs. *Trans. Am. Clin. Climatol. Assoc.,* **51,** 154
8. Hamman, L. and Rich, A. R. (1944). Acute diffuse interstitial fibrosis of the lungs. *Bull. Johns Hopkins Hosp.,* **74,** 177
9. Scadding, J. G. and Hinson, K. F. W. (1967). Diffuse fibrosing alveolitis (diffuse interstitial fibrosis of the lungs). *Thorax,* **22,** 291
10. Liebow, A. A. (1968). Interstitial pneumonias. In Liebow, A. A. and Smith D. E. (eds.) *The Lung* (International Academy of Pathology Monograph), pp.336-351 (Baltimore: Wilkins and Wilkins)
11. Liebow, A. A. (1975). Definition and classification of interstitial pneumonias in human pathology. *Prog. Resp. Res.,* **8,** 1
12. Heppleston, A. G. (1956). The pathology of honeycomb lung. *Thorax,* **11,** 77
13. Turner-Warwick, M., Haslam, P. C., Lukoszek, A., Townsend, P., Allan, F., DuBois, R. M., Turton, C. W. G. and Collins, J. V. (1981). Cells, enzymes and interstitial lung disease. The Philip Ellman Lecture. *J. R. Coll. Phys. Lon.,* **15,** 5
14. Rüttner, J. R., Spycher, M. A. and Sticher, H. (1973). The detection of etiologic agents in interstitial pulmonary fibrosis. *Hum. Pathol.,* **4,** 497
15. Hunninghake, G. W., Gadek, J. E., Kawanami, O., Ferrans, V. J. and Crystal, R. G. (1979). Inflammatory and immune processes in the human lung in health and disease: Evaluation by bronchoalveolar lavage. *Am. J. Pathol.,* **97,** 149
16. Gee, J. L. B. and Fick, R. B. Jr. (1980). Editorial–Bronchoalveolar lavage. *Thorax,* **35,** 1
17. Haslam, P. L., Turton, C. W. G., Heard, B., Lukoszek, A., Collins, J. V., Salsburg, A. J. and Turner-Warwick, M. (1980). Broncho-alveolar lavage in pulmonary fibrosis. *Thorax,* **35,** 9
18. Liebow, A. A., Steer, A. and Billingsley, J. G. (1965). Desquamative interstitial pneumonia. *Am. J. Med.,* **39,** 369
19. Corrin, B. and Price, A. B. (1972). Electron microscopic studies in desquamative interstitial pneumonia associated with asbestos. *Thorax,* **27,** 324
20. Bone, R. C., Wolfe, J. and Sobonya, R. E. (1976). Desquamative interstitial pneumonia following long term nitrofurantoin administration. *Am. J. Med.,* **60,** 297
21. Bedrossian, C. W. M., Kuh, C., Luman, M. A., Corklin, R. H., Byrd, R. B. and Kaplan, P. D. (1977). Desquamative interstitial pneumonia-like reaction accompanying pulmonary lesions. *Chest,* **72,** 166

Tuberculosis

Pulmonary Tuberculosis and Non-tuberculous Mycobacterial Pulmonary Disease

Pulmonary tuberculosis results from infection by *Mycobacterium tuberculosis*. *M. bovis* is very seldom recovered from pulmonary tuberculous lesions or from patients' sputum.

The terminology of non-tuberculous mycobacterial disease is somewhat confused, as 'opportunist mycobacterial infection' has been used but objected to because many patients seem immunologically uncompromised. Atypical mycobacterial infection is a term frequently used by clinicians. The various potential pathogens include *M. kansasii, M. xenopei* and a group consisting of *M. avium, M. intracellular* and *M. scrofulaceum,* collectively known as MAIS. All these mycobacteria account for about 3% of disease presenting clinically as tuberculosis in Britain. They may affect patients with previously damaged lungs. The tissue response is indistinguishable from that resulting from *M. tuberculosis* infection, though the authors noted that plasma cells were more plentiful when a small series was compared with resected *M. tuberculosis* lesions (Figure 6.1). The lesions may affect lung and lymph nodes, but it is unusual for the disease to disseminate widely. The histologist should always endeavour to submit tissue for bacteriological investigation prior to fixation, as *M. tuberculosis* and the atypical group may be resistant to some of the drugs available. This group will be discussed no further.

The Histological Appearances in Tuberculosis as an Index of the 'Host–parasite' Relationship

The initial response to *M. tuberculosis* is a mild acute inflammation rarely seen in practice, but histopathologists should be aware that occasionally a mainly neutrophilic inflammatory exudate may be shown to be mycobacterial when ZN stains reveal large numbers of bacilli (Figure 6.2). This is sometimes reflected in the differential count in cerebrospinal fluid, pleural and ascitic fluid when neutrophils predominate, as opposed to the more common lymphocyte predominant exudate.

The hallmark of tuberculosis is a caseo-necrotic lesion bounded by epithelioid cells and Langhans giant cells. Such a lesion, where the bacillary population is contained and the lesion does not extend, is characterized by fibroblastic proliferation outside the cellular capsule, with varying amounts of collagen and variable numbers of lymphocytes (Figures 6.3 and 6.4). As the quiescent lesion matures and the bacterial population within the caseum declines, calcium salts are progressively deposited within both the core and the capsule (Figure 6.5). Occasionally, small caseous lesions hyalinize, being difficult to distinguish from similar change occurring in sarcoid lesions (figure 6.5, right). Calcification has been shown to appear within the first year, but usually indicates greater chronicity. Sweany[1] was able to age quiescent lesions on the basis of these histological capsular changes to within ±25%.

That these histological appearances reflect the viable bacillary population within the caseum is suggested by the acceleration of the change from a cellular to a collagenous capsule after effective antituberculous therapy[2]. Modern effective bactericidal treatment, which includes isoniazid and rifampicin, sterilizes the lesions within approximately 6 months, but presumed effete organisms may still be seen on appropriate staining. This accounts for the occasional direct positive sputum microscopy but negative culture seen in treated cavitary pulmonary tuberculosis. The histological appearances of tuberculosis in the immunologically deficient, exemplified by steroid-treated rheumatoid disease and those patients treated for any reason by steroids and cytotoxic drugs, is modified in that ill-demarcated areas of necrosis may occur without any recognizable cellular response. Acid-fast bacilli abound in such lesions.

Primary Tuberculosis

Primary tuberculosis and its complications is usually a disease of childhood, but is increasingly encountered in the geriatric age group, presumably in those who have lost both cellularly induced and actively immune hypersensitivity. The commonest manifestation is the usually subpleural parenchymal component of the primary complex (Ghon focus), which is often encountered when well collagen is encapsulated and calcified. One manifestation of primary tuberculosis is the enlargement of such lesions to produce the circumscribed round focus, sometimes with a small eccentric cavity; so-called 'tuberculoma'. The cut surface of such lesions may reveal laminations and small areas of mottling, indicating the episodic mode of previous progression[3] (Figure 6.6). There may be satellite foci and the character of its limiting capsule indicates its state of activity; the more collagenous, the longer the period of quiescence. Occasionally the lymph nodes progressively enlarge (Figure 6.6), but seldom produce bilateral hilar lymphadenopathy to mimic sarcoid.

Complications of Primary Tuberculosis

Most tuberculosis effusions result from bacilli and tuberculo protein, from parenchymal or lymph-node components, entering the pleura in the primary stage. The pleural changes are diffuse, but not

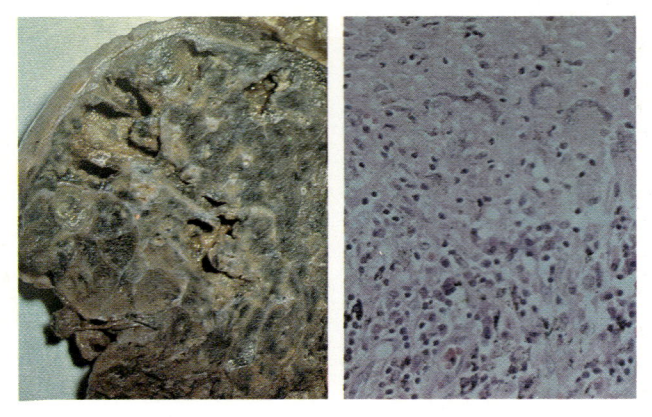

Figure 6.1 *Left:* Resection specimen of *M. kansasii* infection revealing cavities, and a few small moderately encapsulated caseous areas with sparse coal dust foci. *Right:* A caseating granuloma bounded by epithelioid cells, Langhans giant cells and a prominent external plasma cell infiltrate. H&E × 192.

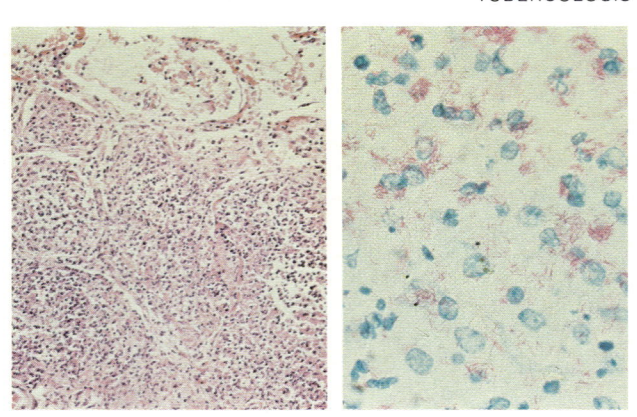

Figure 6.2 *Left:* An ill-defined bronchopneumonic lesion in which there are numerous neutrophils without any epithelioid or giant cells or caseation. H&E × 192. *Right:* Ziehl–Nielsen stain from the same lesion, revealing numerous acid-fast bacilli. × 672.

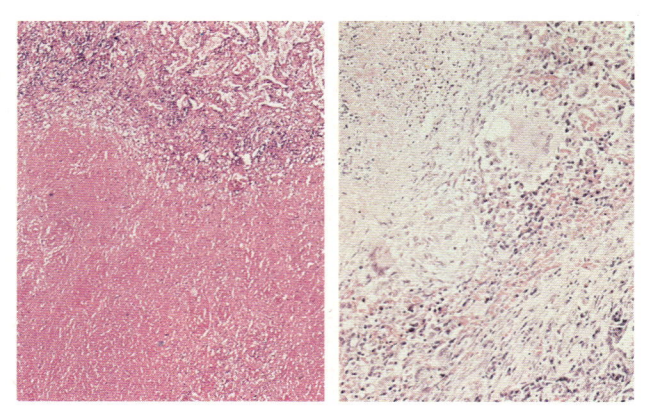

Figure 6.3 *Left:* Edge of caseous lesion, untreated, of 2–3 months duration; the caseation is bounded by a narrow epithelioid zone with only an occasional giant cell. H&E × 96. *Right:* Edge of caseous lesion, untreated, of 8 months duration, revealing caseation bounded by an epithelioid giant-cell cellular zone, external to which, fibroblasts, collagen and lymphocytes can also be seen. H&E × 192.

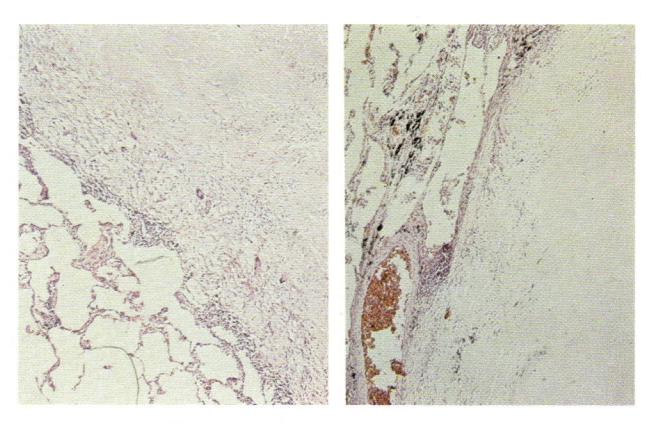

Figure 6.4 *Left:* The appearance of the capsule after several years quiescence or after chemotherapy, showing a collagenous and lymphocytic outer zone and a narrow epithelioid giant-cell zone without satellite foci. H&E × 96. *Right:* Caseous lesion, untreated, 8 years after primary infection. The caseation is entirely collagen limited. H&E × 96.

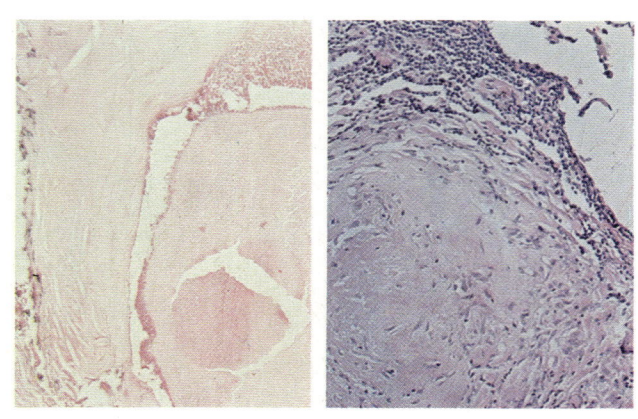

Figure 6.5 *Left:* Caseation with some calcification in core and capsule. The collagenous capsule is entirely acellular. The scalloped edge suggests an erosive process. H&E × 96. *Right:* A small lesion after prolonged treatment, showing hyalinization. An occasional giant cell with collagenous and lymphocytic capsule can be seen. H&E × 96.

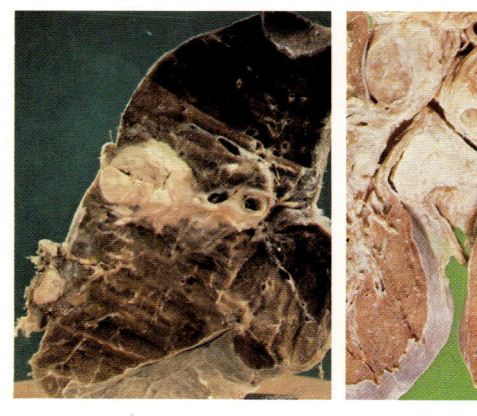

Figure 6.6 *Left:* Two subpleural parenchymal components of a primary complex; in the larger, episodic extension can be seen to have occurred, partly by concentric extension and partly by incorporation of satellite foci. *Right:* Lungs and mediastinum revealing extensive right paratracheal and subcarinal caseous lymphadenopathy.

TUBERCULOSIS

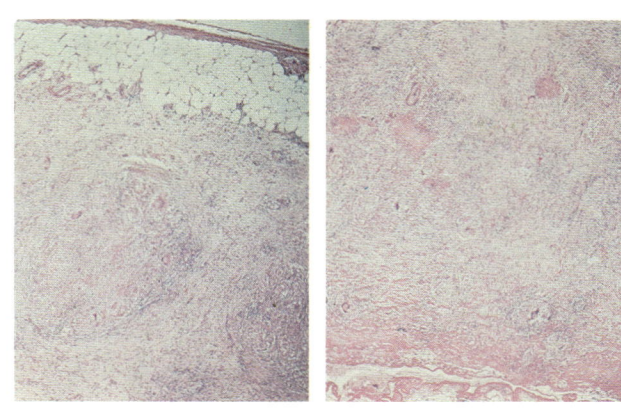

Figure 6.7 *Left:* Parietal pleural fat with a diagnostic area in the centre. H&E × 38.4. *Right:* a continuation of the transpleural appearances showing diagnostic features centrally and the non-specific fibrinous changes (inner and mid aspect). H&E × 60.

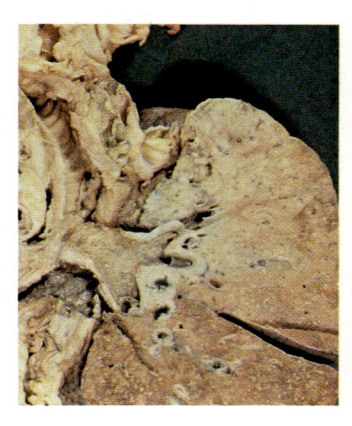

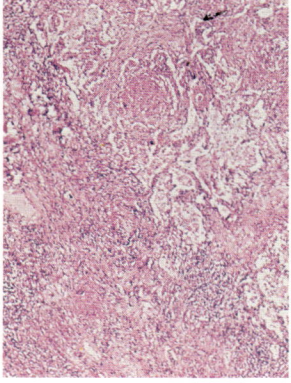

Figure 6.8 *Left:* An adult presented with a sinus over supraclavicular caseous lymphadenopathy. The lungs show the consolidated 'segmental' lesion in left upper lobe, erosion of trachea and left upper-lobe bronchus and unusual miliary dissemination, recognizable in left lower lobe. *Right:* Histology from the left upper lobe reveals thickened interlobular septa, intra-alveolar mononuclear exudation and non-caseating tubercle. H&E × 96.

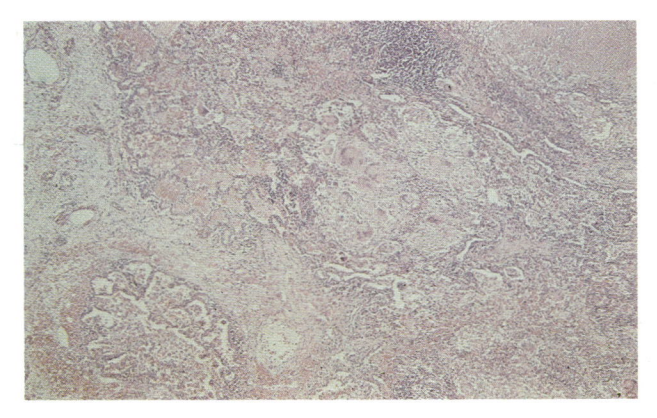

Figure 6.9 Typical appearances of a consolidated area from a segmental lesion, illustrating the inflammatory thickening of interlobular septa (left), the protein rich inflammatory oedema, caseation (top right), non-caseating tubercles (centre), some metaplastic change of alveolar epithelium and a focal collection of lymphocytes. H&E × 96.

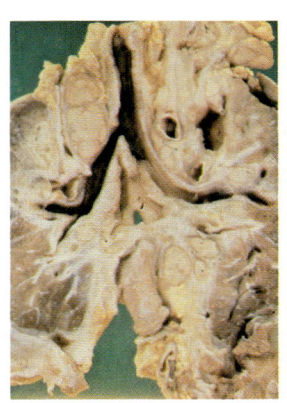

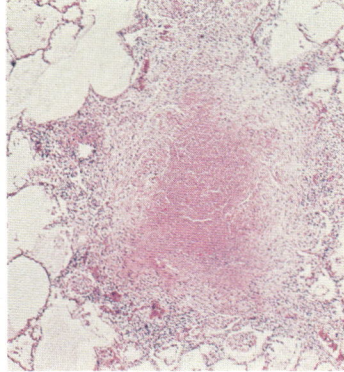

Figure 6.10 *Left:* Extensive mediastinal caseous lymphadenopathy; the subcarinal nodes have evacuated posteriorly by perforating the oesophagus (centre) and lower main bronchi. There is cavitation of the parenchymal primary focus in left upper lobe, with fatal massive haemoptysis. *Right:* Acute caseating miliary tubercle with no recognizable epithelioid or giant cells. H&E × 96.

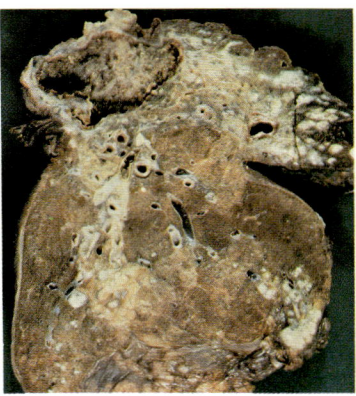

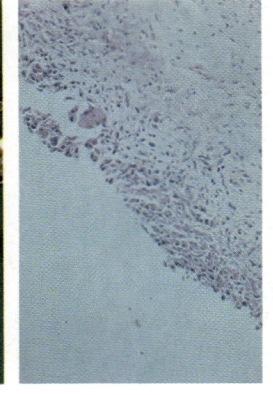

Figure 6.11 *Left:* Post-primary cavitary tuberculosis with a mainly necrotic, lined cavity wall and scattered, poorly encapsulated, caseous foci in both lobes. Hilar nodes are not involved. There is a smaller anterior cavity. *Right:* Cavity wall, part collagen lined, but with a cellular epithelioid and giant-cell zone still discernible. H&E × 96.

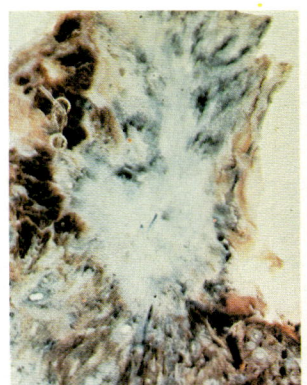

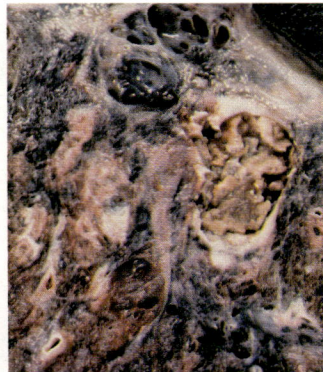

Figure 6.12 *Left:* Site of previous cavity, now a stellate scar, external to which a few small encapsulated caseous foci can be seen. *Right:* An industrial brick-layer who developed classical silicosis, complicated by cavitary tuberculosis, effectively treated, but later haemoptysis announced mycetoma formation. The largest smooth walled cavities contain brownish fungus and there are two grey silicotic nodules to the left of the mycetoma.

uniformly diagnostic to the histopathologist on examination of pleural biopsy material. Some zones contain epithelioid cell granulomata, often with necrosis, whilst others contain non-specific granulation tissue only. The inner fibrinous pleurisy is usually devoid of any specific features. (Figure 6.7).

Bronchial Involvement

The bronchus may be partially obstructed, leading to an over-inflated lobe – *obstructive lobar emphysema*, which is a non-destructive emphysema and reversible on relief of the obstruction. Foreign bodies in childhood are now the most likely cause of this entity.

The 'Segmental Lesion' (Epituberculosis)

When bronchial perforation leads to aspiration of caseous material into the distal lung, some obstruction and consolidation of lung, lobe or segment results. When first described, this lesion was termed epituberculosis; a more appropriate term is the 'segmental lesion'. It is usually, but not invariably, a lesion of childhood tuberculosis, often found radiologically in fairly well 'contacts'. The lung is grey with variable irregular areas of yellowish caseation, the interlobular septa are prominent. Histologically the lesion has some of the features of an obstructive pneumonia with protein-rich intra-alveolar inflammatory oedema, numerous epithelioid and Langhans giant cell tubercules and varying amounts of caseation (Figures 6.7 and 6.8). As the lesion is, in part, a hypersensitivity reaction (being capable of production in BCG sensitized rabbits by local introduction of killed bacilli or PPD) tubercle bacilli are difficult to identify in the lesions. The fate of such lesions is shown in Table 6.1.

Table 6.1 Fate of segmental lesions

1. Complete resolution (rare)
2. Partial resolution, leading to patchy fibrosis with irregular emphysema
3. Collapse and fibrosis
   (a) With bronchiectasis
   (b) With calcification of caseous foci
   (c) With or without some proximal bronchostenosis

The bronchial erosion usually heals uneventfuly, but a late sequel of lymph-node involvement is cicatricial bronchostenosis.

Progressive Primary Tuberculosis

Occasionally, presumably after a large infecting dose and or low natural immunity, the disease spreads extensively locally and untreated may lead to death from pulmonary progression, often bronchopneumonia and mediastinal lymph-node complications (Figure 6.10)

Haematogenous Spread

Minor spreads to other organs results in the later development (after varying intervals from primary infection) of bone and joint, and genito-urinary tuberculosis.

Miliary Tuberculosis

In miliary tuberculosis of lung the lesions are more numerous in the upper lobe, fairly uniform in size, varying from minute lesions of less than a millimetre to several millimetres in diameter. They are roughly circular in section (Figure 6.8), as opposed to the acinar bronchopneumonic lesions which are commoner in the lower lobes. Histologically, there is usually central necrosis limited by epithelioid cells; Langhans giant cells are sometimes plentiful, but may be sparse or absent. Old lesions may have fibroblasts and lymphocytes at the periphery. Occasionally, in the immuno-deficient, the lesion may be composed almost entirely of necrotic tissue with only an occasional cell of the histiocytic type; in such cases acid-fast bacilli are plentiful (Figure 6.10).

The main features of primary tuberculosis are diagrammatically illustrated in Plate 6.1.

Post-primary Tuberculosis

This variety of pulmonary tuberculosis has sometimes been termed 'adult'; this has been criticized as age is not a true arbiter. Another term used was 're-infective', either exogenous or endogenous; the latter fell into disuse when other authorities used the term to denote a second primary type infection after complete healing, with loss of hypersensitivity, usually in the geriatric age group.

The disease is characterized by usually occurring in young or older adults, a tendency to cavitate, and for hilar nodes to be spared caseous disease. Cavities more commonly occur in the apico-posterior segments of upper lobes and the apical segments of the lower lobes (Figure 6.11). The disease is frequently bilateral; either affecting both apices or with a bronchopneumonic spread to the contralateral lower lobe. Histologically, the caseous lesions and the cavity walls reveal a spectrum of changes ranging from the characteristic epithelioid and Langhans giant cell zones to fibroblastic and collagenous appearances already described (Figure 6.11). Post-primary tuberculosis in an immunologically compromised individual may also be characterized by irregular areas of necrosis and an absence of characteristic epithelioid and giant-cell cellular response, as already illustrated.

The natural history of cavitary post-primary tuberculosis prior to the chemotherapy era was episodic progression by bronchopneumonic spread, with a 5-year mortality of around 80%. Today the lesions are dramatically influenced by effective drugs, leading to cavity closure in more than 90% of patients. One possible end result is the development of a 'stellate scar' (Figure 6.12); another is the disappearance of the cavitary lesion. Open healing occurs in a small percentage, when the cavity is smooth walled and histologically may be collagen lined or occasionally may be lined by respiratory epithelium with or without areas of squamous metaplasia – 'epithelialized' cavities. Approximately a fifth of these open-healed cavities become colonized by *Aspergillus*, usually either *A. fumigatus* or *A. niger* (Figure 6.12). Over 90% of such patients possess precipitins to an extract of the fungus in their serum.

The features of post-primary tuberculosis are summarized in Plate 6.1 on page 52.

Tuberculosis with Inorganic Dust Pneumoconiosis

When round tuberculous caseous foci occur in the presence of lesser degrees of simple coal-workers' pneumoconiosis, the lesions may contain laminations representing the site of a dust-laden histiocytic capsule. These lesions must be distinguished from Caplan nodules (rheumatoid pneumoconiosis), where similar laminations occur (Chaper 13). In the absence of either the limiting capsular changes of tuberculosis or the rheumatoid process, they are indistinguishable.

In those coal workers more heavily exposed, the super-imposition of mycobacterial infection leads to areas of dust fibrosis with areas of caseation. One probable explanation for some cases of progressive massive fibrosis (PMF) is that they are caused by mycobacterial infection; certainly in miners who develop tuberculosis, areas indistinguishable from PMF may be encountered.

The incidence of tuberculosis is much higher in silicotics than in coal workers, though some coal workers ('hard headers' and other coal-face workers) may have lesions in part silicotic, in part anthracotic, sometimes called anthraco-silicosis. When tuberculosis complicates either industrial disease, the terms anthraco-tuberculosis and silico-tuberculosis are used (Figure 6.12). For compensation purposes, the effect of tuberculosis is deemed additive.

References

1. Sweany, H. C. (1941). Age morphology of primary tubercles. (Springfield, III.: Thomas)
2. Cotter, D. J., Foreman, H. M. and Seal, R. M. E. (1958). The pathology and bacteriology of resected tuberculous lung lesions after chemotherapy. *Thorax*, **13,** 150
3. Seal, R. M. E. (1971). The pathology of tuberculosis. *Br. J. Hosp. Med.* **5,** 783

(Plate 6.1 will be found overleaf)

52

TUBERCULOSIS

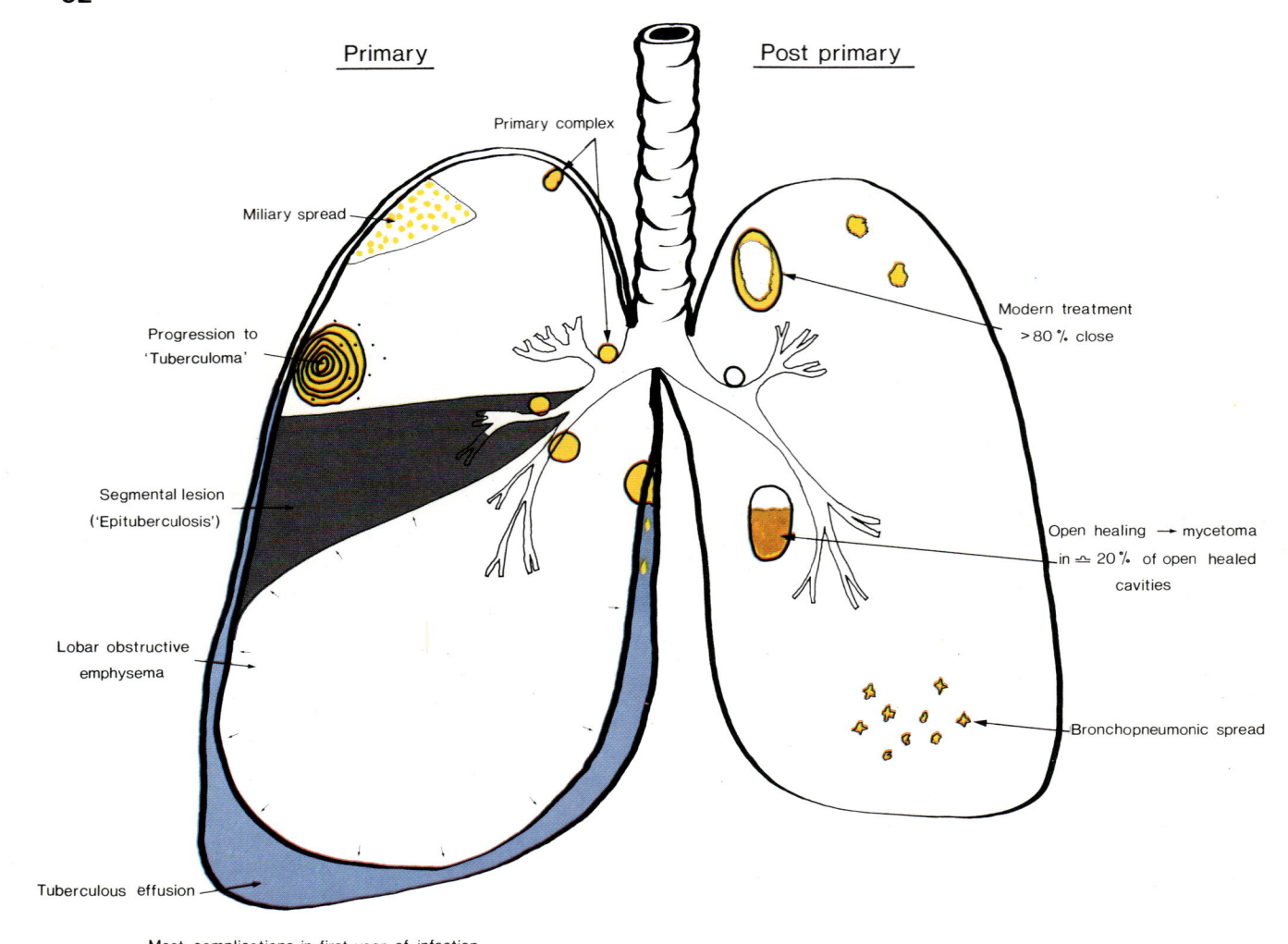

Primary | **Post primary**

- Primary complex
- Miliary spread
- Progression to 'Tuberculoma'
- Segmental lesion ('Epituberculosis')
- Lobar obstructive emphysema
- Tuberculous effusion
- Modern treatment >80% close
- Open healing → mycetoma in ≃ 20% of open healed cavities
- Bronchopneumonic spread

Most complications in first year of infection

Plate 6.1 Main features of primary tuberculosis

Non-Tuberculous Granulomatous Conditions

7

Sarcoidosis is a multisystem granulomatous disease of unknown aetiology and pathogenesis, and its hallmark is the non-caseating epithelioid cell granuloma. Whether it is a single disease or the manifestation of several different disorders is debatable.

The highest incidence is in the third and fourth decades, but no age is immune, and it has been stated to vary between 0.21 and 0.45 per 10 000 population in Great Britain[1].

The Kveim reaction is positive in about 80% of acute cases (about 38% in the chronic stage). The tuberculin and other types of delayed-hypersensitivity reaction are depressed, whereas humoral immunity is usually enhanced.

The lung is affected in over 80% of sarcoidosis patients. Macroscopically[2], the granulomata appear within the lungs as 2–3 mm diameter grey–white ill-defined lesions simulating miliary tuberculosis, as 1–2 cm diameter or larger conglomerate nodules. They are most conspicuous in relation to bronchi, septa, blood vessels and pleura. Approximately 7% of cases become chronic, in which case, bilateral diffuse fibrosis, most pronounced in the upper lobes, occurs and there is often related cystic change ('honeycomb lung') (Figures 7.1 and 7.2). Cavities occasionally develop and these may be colonized by *Aspergillus* to form 'aspergillomas'.

Microscopically[2,3], the sarcoid granuloma is composed of a focal, compact collection of pale-staining eosinophilic epithelioid cells, admixed with giant cells, of both Langhans and foreign-body type, and a peripheral rim of lymphocytes. The granuloma is usually well delineated from the background tissue. They are usually situated around bronchi, around vessels, in the subpleural tissue and in the submucosa of large bronchi (Figures 7.3–7.5). Necrosis is usually absent or minimal and shows fine

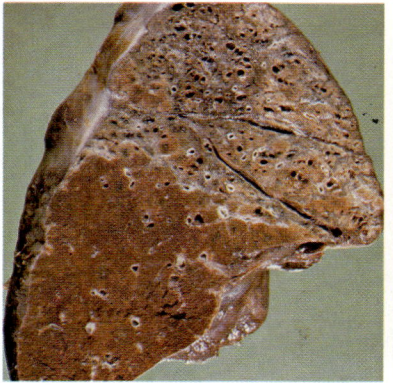

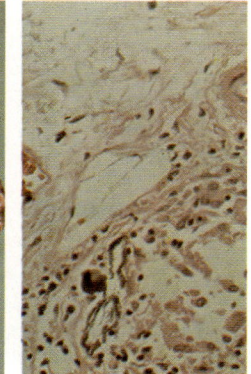

Figure 7.1 *Left:* Right lung revealing interstitial fibrosis with honeycomb change, which is sparing the lower lobe. *Right:* In the fibrotic area there was an ill-defined granuloma with Schaumann bodies and numerous lymphocytes. Patient had presented with hilar lymphadenopathy many years previously. H&E × 144.

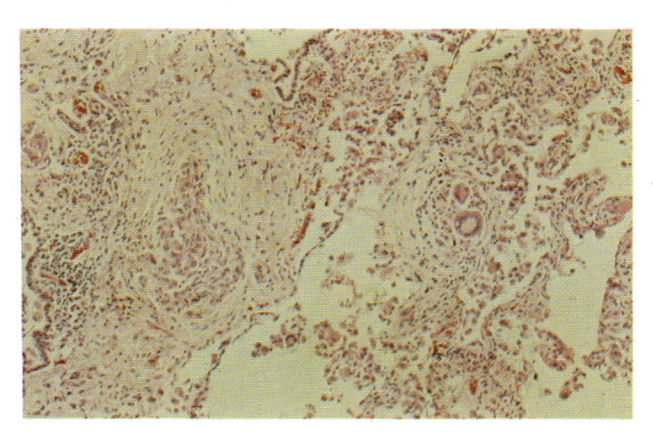

Figure 7.2 The same case as Figure 7.1, showing interstitial fibrosis with ill-defined hyalinizing granuloma. H&E × 96.

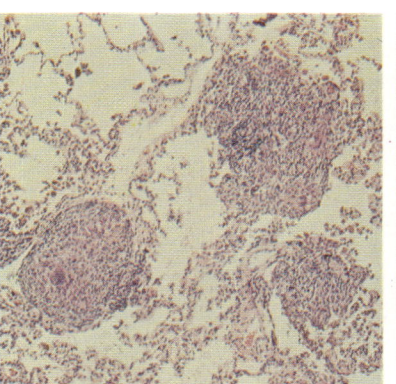

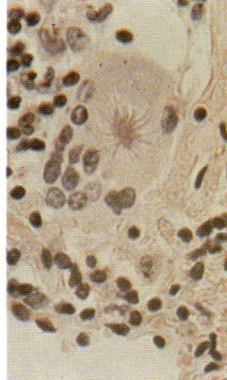

Figure 7.3 *Left:* Multiple granulomata with a minimal interstitial infiltrate. Kveim positive. Multisystem disease. H&E × 38.4. *Right:* An asteroid body within a giant cell. H&E × 38.4.

reticulin fibres which are absent in tuberculosis. On electron microscopy, both epithelioid and giant cells show intracytoplasmic mucoprotein vesicles[4] which may be the source of the raised serum angiotensin converting enzyme, of value in diagnosis[5]. Interstitial pneumonitis is usually mild in sarcoidosis (cf. extrinsic allergic bronchiolo-alveolitis). Schaumann, asteroid or Hamazaki-Wesenberg bodies may be present (Figures 7.1 and 7.3).

Schaumann (conchoidal) bodies are large (up to 100 μm diameter), concentrically laminated, birefringent, basophilic structures which contain calcium and iron. They are seen most frequently in giant cells but may become extracellular (Figure 7.1). They probably develop on a nidus of colourless, spiculated crystals which may be observed in epithelioid cells. Schaumann bodies are not specific to sarcoidosis; Jones Williams[2] found them in 88% of sarcoidosis cases, 62% of chronic berylliosis cases, 10% of Crohn's disease cases and 6% of tubercle cases. We have also observed them in occasional cases of extrinsic allergic bronchio-alveolitis and in chronic passive venous congestion due to a variety of causes. Schaumann bodies may persist long after the granulomata have healed and are therefore useful markers of previous granulomata.

Asteroid bodies are intracytoplasmic and star-shaped, having a central core with radiating curved spines[6]. They may be seen in epithelioid cells, but more frequently in giant cells (Figure 7.3). They are even less specific for sarcoidosis since they have been found in a wide variety of conditions, including tuberculosis, leprosy and histoplasmosis. They were found in 9% of open lung biopsies from sarcoidosis patients by Rosen et al.[3].

Sarcoid granulomata may disappear completely or as a consequence of fibrosis may become hyalinized (Figures 7.2 and 7.6). In contradistinction to tubercle, they rarely calcify.

Role of Biopsy

Roethe et al.[7] have found that in transbronchoscopic biopsy of the lung for suspected sarcoidosis, the diagnostic yield is close to 100% if ten biopsies are obtained. However, they suggest that five biopsies will be adequate if the most severely affected lobe radiologically is biopsied. If granulomata are obtained on biopsy, then special stains for mycobacteria and fungi should be performed to aid in the exclusion of the agents. Bronchial biopsy often yields non-caseating granuloma in sarcoid and in the usual obstructive bronchial sarcoid granulomata, where associated non-specific inflammatory change is seen.

To establish the multisystem nature of the disease, Kveim test, liver biopsy and skin scar biopsy are often employed (Figures 7.6 and 7.7). In recent years, open lung biopsy has been largely replaced by needle or drill biopsy and, more recently, transbronchial biopsy is the favoured approach.

Extrinsic Allergic Bronchiolo-Alveolitis

We prefer the term extrinsic allergic bronchiolo-alveolitis (EABA), since it is more accurate than the commonly utilized 'extrinsic allergic alveolitis' or 'hypersensitivity pneumonitis', for a group of respiratory disorders caused by inhalation of fine particulate antigenic protein-rich material, of animal or vegetable origin. Table 7.1 lists some of the antigens responsible for this group of disorders.

Table 7.1 Organic dust diseases (hypersensitivity pneumonitis = extrinsic allergic bronchiolo-alveolitis)

Disease	Process/exposure	Active agent
Maltworker's lung	Whisky production	A. clavatus
TDI	Rubber/foam production	TDI*
Fishmeal handler's lung	Fishmeal production	Piscine protein
Poultry worker's lung	Chicken/turkey breeding	Chicken/turkey protein
Woodworker's lung	Furniture production	Wood dust
Farmer's lung	Handling mouldy hay	M. faeni
Bagassosis	Handling mouldy bagasse	T. sacchari
Maple-bark stripper's lung	Stripping maple bark	C. corticale
Mushroom handler's lung	Handling mushroom compost	M. faeni
Wheat weevil allergy	Handling contaminated flour	S. granarius
Bird handler's lung	Pigeon/budgies	Avian proteins
Pituitary snuff inhaler's lung	Snuff	Hog/bovine proteins
Dog house disease	Mould on dog blanket	A. versicolor
Humidifier fever†	Contaminated humidifier water	Amoebae

*TDI = toluene diisocyanate. †Closely related entity.

The pathology is similar in each of the conditions and reveals characteristics of more than one type of response. It would appear that, in addition to a simple Arthus (type III) hypersensitivity reaction, delayed (type IV) hypersensitivity and non specific inflammatory responses may play a part[8]. It has been proposed by Edwards et al.[9] that inhalation of mouldy hay dust activates the alternative complement pathway, producing local pulmonary lesions including granulomas, thus explaining the occasional patient who develops the disease on first exposure and those acute patients in whom antibodies cannot be demonstrated.

The clinicopathological features of EABA can be conveniently divided into acute and chronic stages. Classically, symptoms in the acute stage commence a few hours after exposure to the inhaled antigen, and consist of both respiratory and constitutional (influenza-like) symptoms; wheezing is not a feature. They reach a peak after 6-12 h. Resolution within months is the usual sequel. In about 60% of patients in the acute stage, which is still reversible, the onset is much more gradual and insidious, and the episode and its relationship to the prolonged lesser exposure are less easily defined. Severe attacks or repeated low-grade exposures over weeks, months or years may progress to the chronic stage which may cause respiratory failure cor pulmonale and death. Very prolonged lesser degrees of exposure, as in budgerigar fancier's lung, may result in the patient presenting for the first time in the irreversible fibrotic chronic stage.

Acute stage

Non-caseating sarcoid-like granulomata appear within approximately 3 weeks of exposure and slowly resolve over the next few months[10]. They are most frequent in the centre of the lobule (Figure 7.8). Foreign-body giant cells containing doubly refractile material may be evident. We have observed Schaumann bodies in a small proportion of cases. Granulomata apparently resolve within months, as they are seldom seen at the latter end of an acute episode.

'Interstitial pneumonitis' consisting of an infiltrate of lymphocytes, plasma cells and histiocytes, is usually marked [10,11] (Figures 7.8–7.10). Doubly refractile material may be present within the interstitium.

'Bronchiolitis' is usually conspicuous (Figure 7.9), with inflammation and oedema of the bronchiolar walls and a luminal exudate of fluid and polymorphonucleaars. 'Bronchiolitis obliterans' may occur[10,11]. There is usually swelling of endothelial cells and muscle fibres of pulmonary arteries and arterioles and occasionally intramural inflammatory cells (Figure 7.9).

In severe cases inflammatory oedema may be marked[11]. Table 7.2 shows the major features which distinguish acute EABA from sarcoidosis.

Table 7.2 A comparison of sarcoidosis with acute extrinsic allergic bronchiolo-alveolitis

	Sarcoidosis	*Extrinsic allergic bronchiolo-alveolitis*
Exposure to antigen	Not identified	Always
Clinical state	Often well	Respiratory and constitutional symptoms
Radiographic changes:		
Parenchymal	Often extensive	Often slight
Bilateral hilar lymphadenopathy	Present	Absent
Pathological features:		
Granulomata	Persistent	Evanescent
'Interstitial pneumonitis'	Mild	Prominent
Bronchiolitis	Minimal	Moderate
Schaumann bodies	Frequent	Occasional

Chronic stage (Figures 7.11–7.15)

Macroscopically, there is usually diffuse fine interstitial fibrosis with larger focal areas of fibrosis with intercommunicating bands. Cysts varying from a few millimetres to several centimetres in diameter may later represent an end-stage honeycomb lung. These changes are more marked in the upper lobes of the lung[10], and this aids in distinguishing it from idiopathic chronic interstitial fibrosis and asbestosis, which are most marked in the lower lobes (Figures 7.12 and 7.13).

Microscopically, the focal fibrotic areas are located around bronchi (Figures 7.12 and 7.13). Granulomata are not present, unless there has been recent exposure. Organization of granulomata in the acute stage does not appear to contribute to the fibrosis. Variable degrees of interstitial lymphocytic infiltration are present (Figures 7.11–7.15). Focal collections of lymphocytes and plasma cells may be situated around bronchioles and small vessels. Intracellular doubly refractile material is a consistent finding (Figure 7.15). Hypertensive changes may be seen in the pulmonary arteries, similar to those found in other types of interstitial fibrosis[11] (Figure 7.14).

Emphysema

We have encountered nine non-smoking patients who have had documented episodes of 'farmer's lung' who developed progressive dyspnoea associated with radiological evidence of emphysema rather than fibrosis and an obstructive respiratory function profile. At autopsy, emphysema was apparent (Figure 7.15) and evidence of interstitial disease easily overlooked.

Differential diagnosis of pulmonary granulomata

Similar granulomata are found in a variety of conditions in addition to sarcoidosis. Therefore, careful correlation of the pathological with the clinical and radiological features is essential to make an accurate diagnosis of sarcoidosis. Tubercle, extrinsic allergic bronchiolo-alveolitis, berylliosis, talc, hard-metal disease, fungi, vasculitides and neoplasms are some of the disorders which may show granulomata in the lung.

The presence of caseation and acid-fast bacilli distinguishes tubercle from sarcoidosis.

Table 7.2 shows the major features of differentiating acute EABA from sarcoidosis. In the chronic phase of EABA granulomata are absent unless there has been recent exposure, whereas they tend to persist in sarcoidosis.

Chronic berylliosis produces almost identical features to sarcoidosis; however, there is a greater degree of 'interstitial pneumonitis' in the former. History of exposure is obviously important.

Industrial exposures such as talc and tungsten carbide (hard metal) may result in granulomata. The

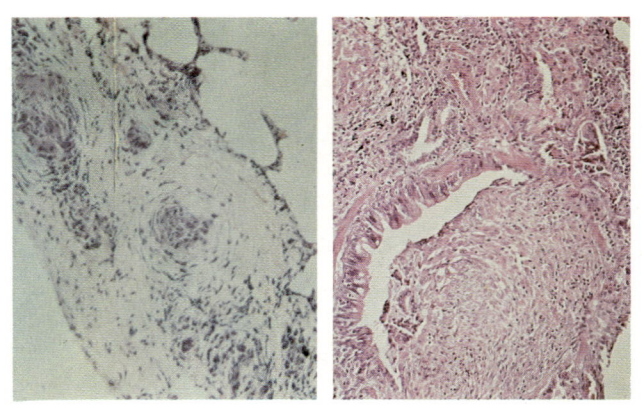

Figure 7.4 *Left:* Pleural involvement by granulomata. H & E × 38.4. *Right:* Bronchiolar involvement by granulomata. H & E × 96.

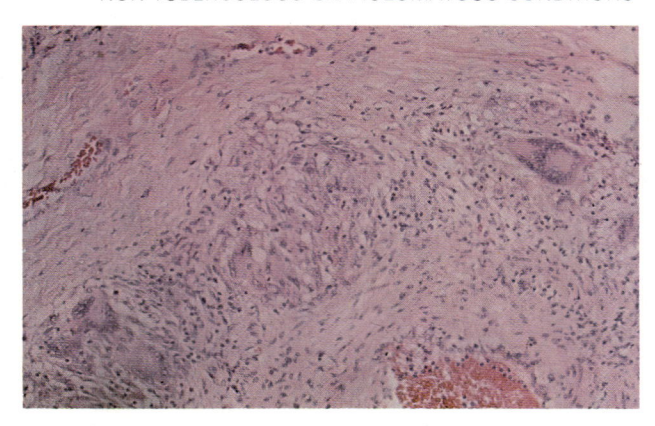

Figure 7.5 An unusual case of interstitial granulomatous disease in a Kveim-positive rubber worker. No talc was demonstrated. Microscopy illustrated the perivascular distribution. H & E × 96.

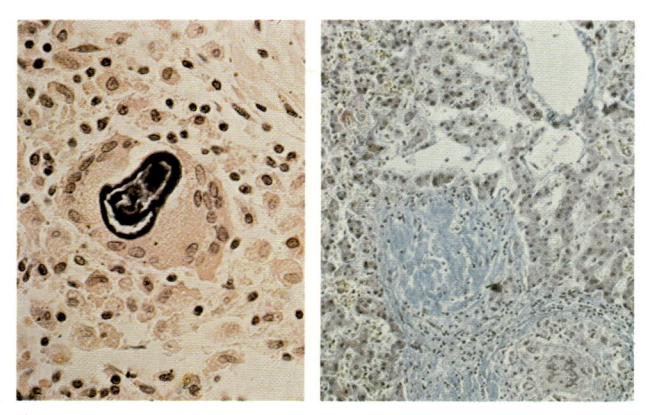

Figure 7.6 *Left:* Chronic sarcoid with fibrosis and a giant cell containing a Schaumann body. H & E × 240. *Right:* The liver from the same patient showing an already hyalinized and a hyalinizing granuloma. Trichrome × 38.4.

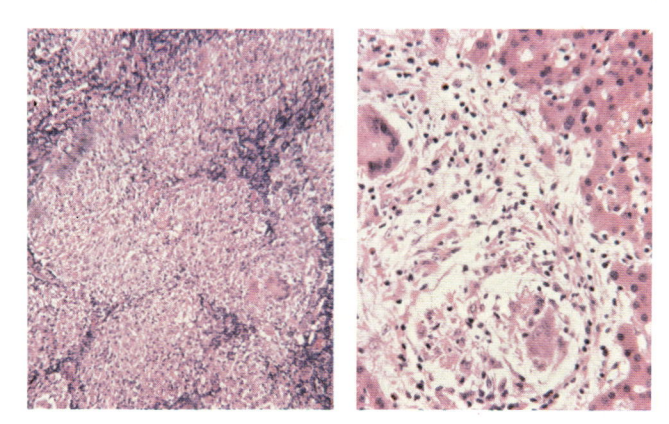

Figure 7.7 *Left:* Hilar node almost replaced by discrete non-caseating granuloma. H & E × 38.4. *Right:* Similar granulomata in the liver. H & E × 240.

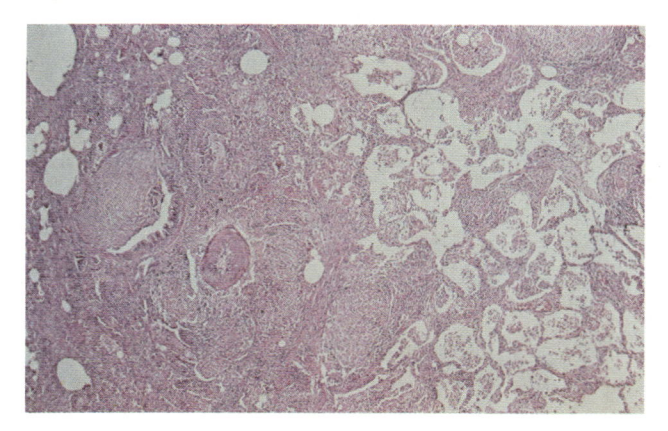

Figure 7.8 Biopsy early in second acute attack of farmer's lung, revealing interstitial pneumonitis (alveolitis) but maximal inflammatory damage in the centre of the lobule where a respiratory bronchile is involved. There is also inflammatory involvement of a nearby vessel, and granulomata are present. H & E × 38.4.

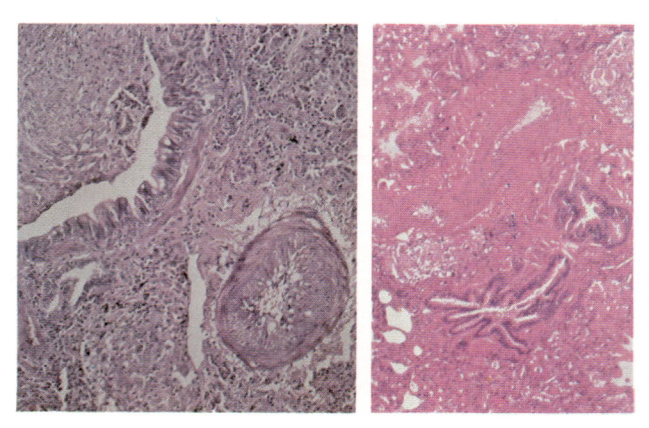

Figure 7.9 *Left:* More detailed view of a central area from Figure 7.8 revealing detail of the arteriole and bronchiole involvement. The patient progressed to the chronic stage. H & E × 96. *Right:* Similar biopsy appearance in a 22-year-old farmer who made a complete recovery and changed occupation. H & E × 38.4.

NON-TUBERCULOUS GRANULOMATOUS CONDITIONS

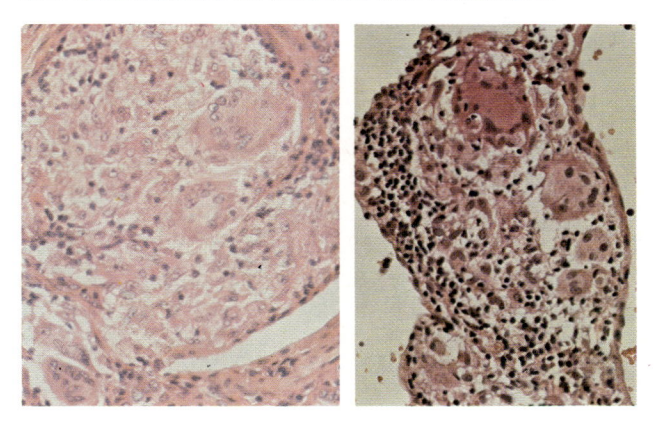

Figure 7.10 *Left:* A well-structured granuloma from the previous case. H&E × 240. *Right:* A lesser ill-defined granuloma from a third patient who progressed to the chronic stage. H&E × 240.

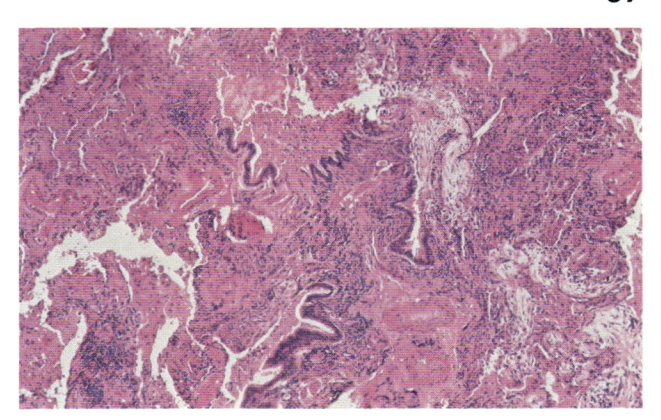

Figure 7.11 Biopsy taken several months after the onset of a severe acute attack. Lymphoid infiltrate persists, granulomata are absent, commencing fibrosis can be observed. This patient progressed to the chronic stage. H&E × 38.4.

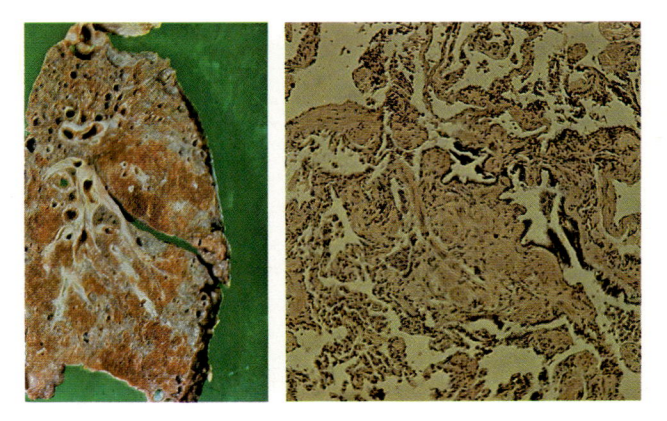

Figure 7.12 *Left:* Chronic stage farmer's lung, showing more extensive 'honeycombing' in the upper lobe. *Right:* Interstitial fibrosis with accentuation around respiratory bronchioles, suggesting an extrinsic cause. Biopsy, chronic farmer's lung. H&E × 96.

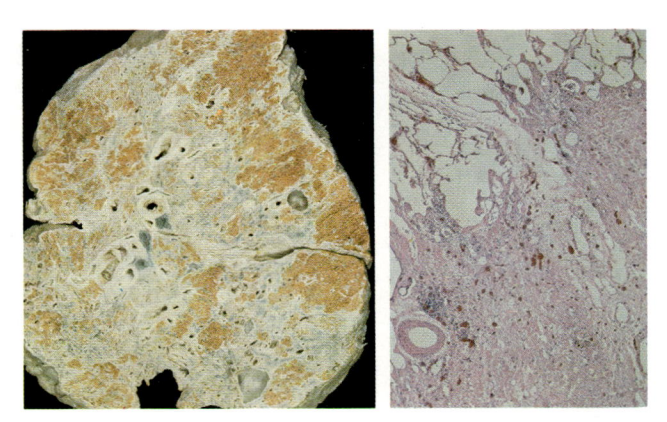

Figure 7.13 *Left:* Chronic stage farmer's lung with extensive honeycombing in upper lobes and irregular islands of focal fibrosis in the lower lobe. *Right:* The edge of a focal fibrotic lesion H&E × 38.4.

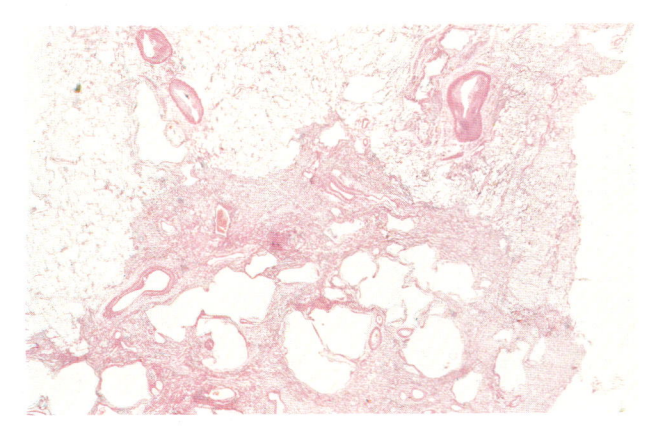

Figure 7.14 Chronic bird-fancier's lung showing extensive fibrosis with related honeycombing (left) and 'hypertensive' changes in pulmonary arteries.

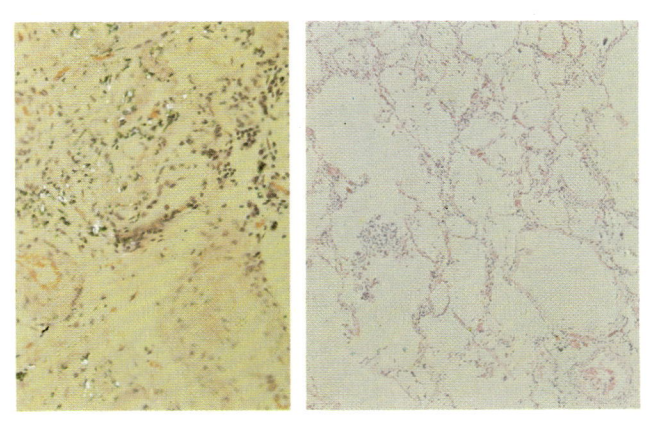

Figure 7.15 *Left:* This shows mainly intracellular birefringent material, from the same case as Figure 7.14. H&E × 240. *Right:* This patient had had typical episodes of farmer's lung but developed radiological changes of emphysema. Microscopy reveals an appearance easily interpreted as emphysema with minimal fibrosis. H&E × 24.

former shows birefringent plate-like crystals. History of exposure and EDXA analysis are important in separating the conditions.

Fungi, such as histoplasma, usually produce more necrosis in the centre of a granuloma, and are sclerosing mediastinitis and retroperitoneal fibrosis has been reported[13].

It must be admitted that occasionally, even with the most careful clinicopathological correlation, cases do not fit neatly into sarcoidosis or any of the other entities. We have experienced this problem with particular regard to EABA, granulomatous vasculitis, fungal infections and inorganic dust exposure[14] (Figure 7.5).

References

1. British Thoracic and Tuberculosis Association (1969). Geographical variations in the incidence of sarcoidosis in Great Britain: a comparative study of four areas. *Tubercle*, **50,** 211
2. Jones Williams, W. (1967). The pathology of sarcoidosis. *Hosp. Med.* **2,** 21
3. Rosen, Y., Vultetin, J. C., Pertschuke, L. P. and Silverstein, E. (1979). Sarcoidosis. From the pathologist's vantage point. Pathology Annual, Part 1, p.405
4. James, E. M. V. and Jones Williams, W. (1974). Fine structure and histochemistry of epithelioid cells in sarcoidosis. *Thorax*, **29,** 115
5. Silverstein, E., Friedland, J. and Pertschuke, L. P. (1980). Sarcoid pathogenesis. Mechanism of angiotensin converting enzyme elevation: epithelioid cell localisation and induction in macrophages and monocytes in culture. In Jones Williams, W. and Davies, B. H. (eds.) *Eighth International Conference on Sarcoidosis and other Granulomatous Diseases* p.246.(Cardiff: Alpha Omega)
6. Cain, H. and Kraus, B. (1980). The ultrastructure and morphogenesis of asteroid bodies in sarcoidosis and other granulomatous diseases. In Jones Williams, W. and Davies, B. H. (eds.) *Eighth International Conference on Sarcoidosis and other Granulomatous Diseases* p.38. (Cardiff: Alpha Omega)
7. Roethe, R. A., Fuller, P. B., Byrd, R. B. and Hafermann, D. R. (1980). Transbronchoscopic lung biopsy in sarcoidosis. *Chest*, **77,** 400
8. Seal, R. M. E., Edwards, J. H. and Hayes, M. (1975). The response of the lung to inhaled antigens. *Prog. Resp. Res.*, **8,** 125
9. Edwards, J. H., Wagner, J. C. and Seal, R. M. E. (1976). Pulmonary responses to particulate material capable of activating the alternative pathway of complement. *Clin. Allergy*, **6,** 155
10. Seal, R. M. E., Hapke, E. J., Thomas, G. O., Meek, J. C. and Hayes, M. (1968). The pathology of the acute and chronic stages of farmer's lung. *Thorax*, **23,** 469
11. Seal, R. M. E. (1975). Pathology of extrinsic allergic bronchiolo-alveolitis. *Prog. Resp. Res.*, **8,** 66
12. Laurberg, P. (1975). Sarcoid reactions in pulmonary neoplasms. *Scand. J. Resp. Dis.*, **56,** 20
13. Engleman, P., Liebow, A. A., Gmelich, J. and Friedman, P. J. (1977). Pulmonary hyalinizing granuloma. *Am. Rev. Resp. Dis.*, **115,** 997
14. Gibbs, A. R., Seal, R. M. E., Jones Williams, W. and Jannigan, D. T. (1980). The borderland of sarcoidosis. In Jones Williams, W. and Davies, B. H. (eds.) *Eighth International Conference on Sarcoidosis and other Granulomatous Diseases* p.687. (Cardiff: Alpha Omega)

Asthma and Related Conditions (Mucoid Impaction, Eosinophilic Pneumonia and Bronchocentric Granulomatosis)

The conditions described in this chapter exhibit degrees of commonality and interrelationship which make it difficult, in come cases, to decide where one ends and another begins. They can co-exist in various permutations and combinations and each can be produced by a number of agents and mechanisms, only some of which have been identified. *Aspergillus* may affect the lung in a variety of ways (Plate 8.1) and it is important in the pathogenesis of several of the disorders described in this chapter.

Bronchial Asthma

Asthma is a functional disorder characterized by generalized intermittent and reversible airways obstruction. It may be due to a variety of agents and mechanisms including allergies, exercise, infection, psychological stimuli, chemical mediators and drugs.

Knowledge of the pathology of asthma has usually been derived from those dying in status asthmaticus and is identical in intrinsic and extrinsic types. In those dying in status asthmaticus the lungs appear hyperinflated, bulge over the mediastinum and reveal small areas of atelectasis and plugging of the smaller bronchi by viscid mucous plugs (Figure 8.1). Histologically, all levels of the tracheobronchial tree show infiltration of the walls by neutrophils, lymphocytes, plasma cells and prominent numbers of eosinophils. The bronchi show mucosal oedema, basement membrane thickening, muscle hypertrophy, mucus gland hypertrophy and increased numbers of goblet cells in the epithelium (Figures 8.1 and 8.2).

Leopold[1] drew attention to patchy subpleural, interstitial eosinophilic infiltrates, most marked in the upper half of the lungs, in 30 cases of adult chronic asthma, which resulted in fibrosis in some

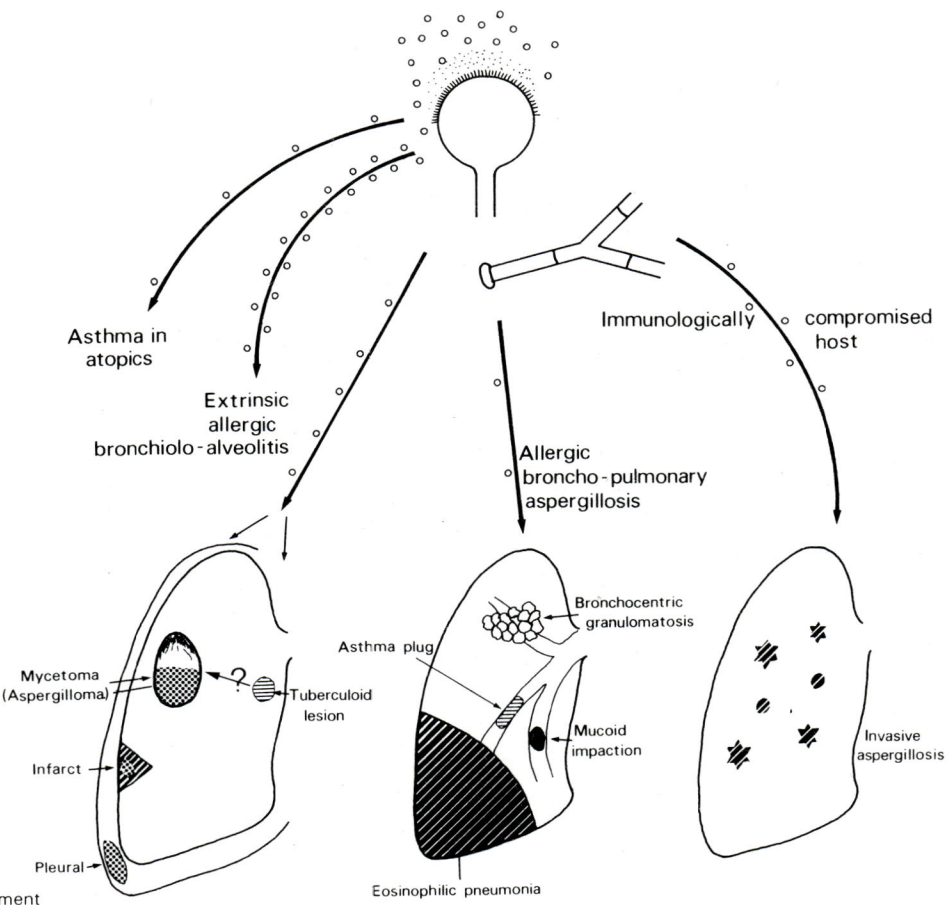

Plate 8.1 Pulmonary aspergillus involvement

ASTHMA AND RELATED CONDITIONS

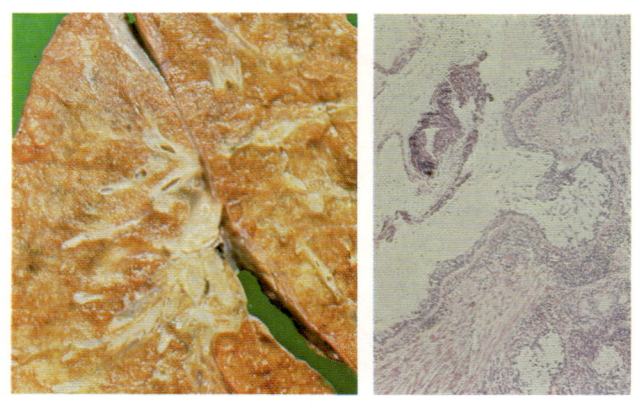

Figure 8.1 *Left:* Patient dying of severe asthma showing mucus plugging or large- and medium-sized bronchi. *Right:* Wall of bronchus shows basement membrane thickening, muscular hypertrophy and eosinophilic infiltration. The lumen contains a mucus plug and desquamated epithelium. H&E × 38.4.

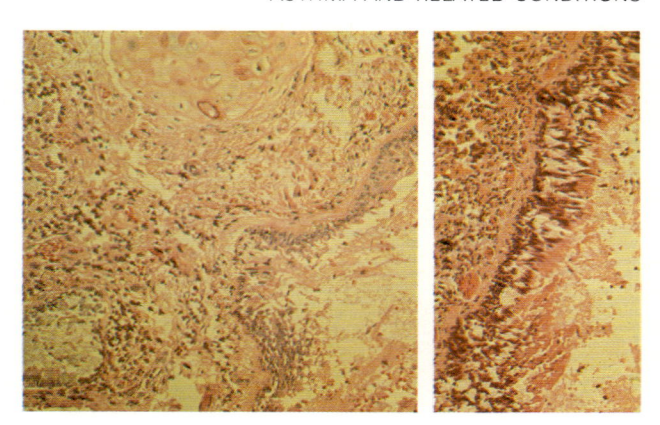

Figure 8.2 *Left:* Bronchial wall of an asthmatic showing prominent 'basement membrane' thickening, submucosal and intraluminal eosinophilic infiltration. The epithelium is being shed at one point. H&E × 96. *Right:* An asthmatic showing prominent goblet cell hyperplasia. H&E × 96.

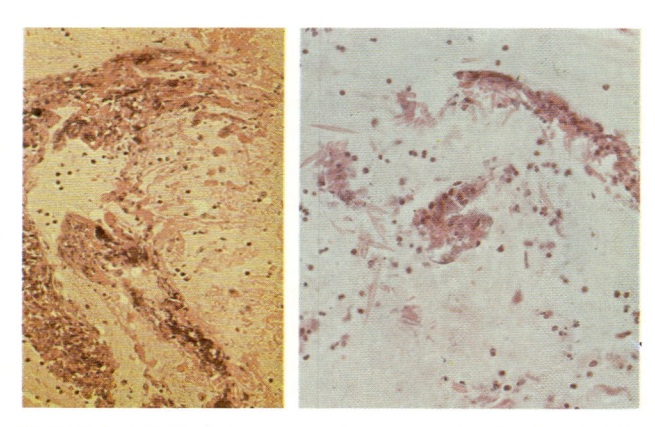

Figure 8.3 *Left:* Sputum from an asthmatic revealing the characteristic pattern of part eosinophilic, part basophilic, curvilinear, material characteristic of asthma. H&E × 240. *Right:* Similar eosinophilic material with sparse eosinophils and spear-head-like eosinophilic Charcot–Leyden crystals. H&E × 384.

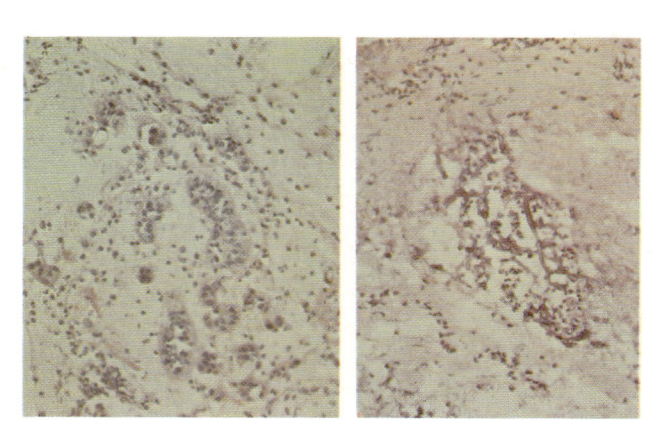

Figure 8.4 *Left:* Asthmatic sputum with small groups of partly rolled up respiratory epithelial cells (Creola bodies). H&E × 240. *Right:* Sputum from an asthmatic with bronchopulmonary aspergillosis; fragments of branching septate mycelium can be seen. H&E × 240.

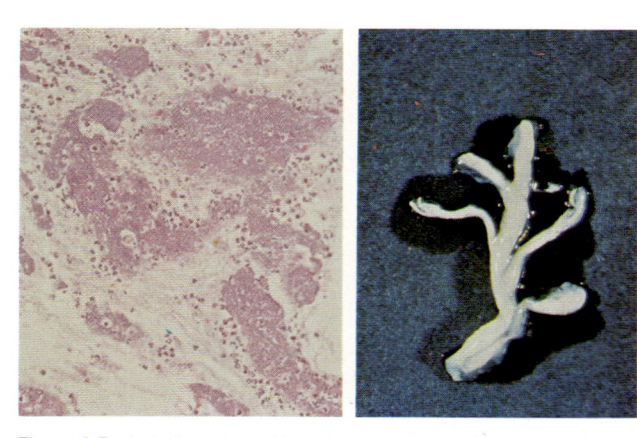

Figure 8.5 *Left:* A patient with asthmatic stigmata in some areas and other areas with neutrophils and basophilic debris; frequently seen in bronchitis with a purulent wheeze and obstruction partially relieved by bronchodilators. H&E × 240. *Right:* A large, hard, laminated bronchial cast which had been coughed up. Histologically, they are identical to ordinary asthmatic plugs.

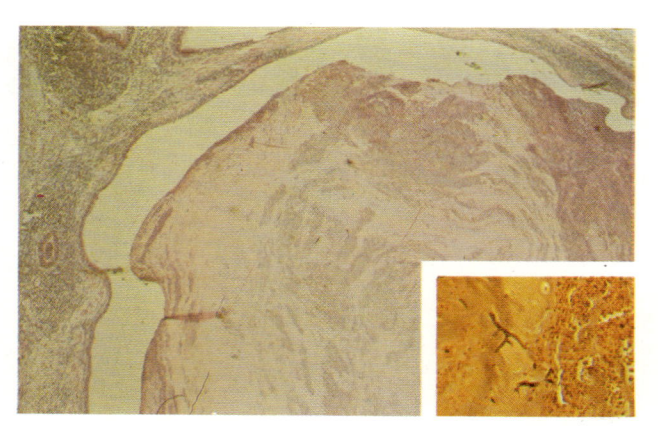

Figure 8.6 A patient with allergic bronchopulmonary aspergillosis, fleeting eosinophilic pneumonia segmental lesions, proximal bronchiectasis. The slide reveals mucoid impaction in a distended segmental bronchus. H&E × 24. *Inset:* Fungal hyphae. Grocott × 150.

ASTHMA AND RELATED CONDITIONS

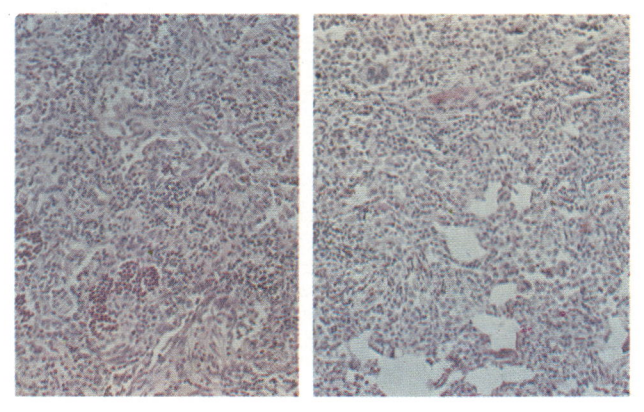

Figure 8.7 *Left:* Biopsy of a consolidated segmental opacity from the previous case shows interstitial pneumonitis with large focal collections of eosinophils. H & E × 96. *Right:* Another area revealing intra-alveolar exudates with an occasional multinucleated giant cell. H & E × 96.

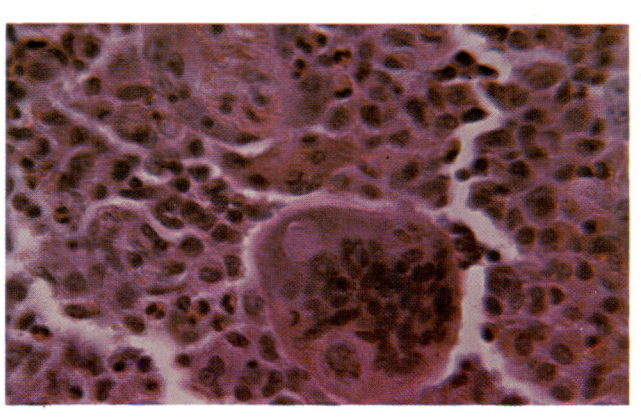

Figure 8.8 Another case of eosinophilic pneumonia showing prominent giant cells, easily confused with giant cell interstitial pneumonia. Both histiocytes and giant cells contain eosinophilic granules and minute Charcot–Leyden crystals. H & E × 384.

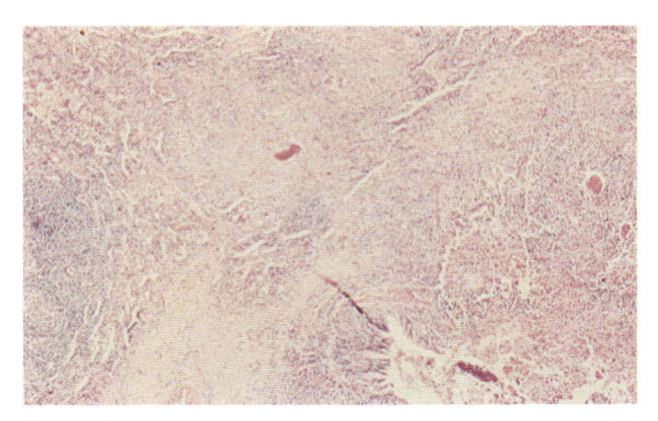

Figure 8.9 A bronchus involved by granulomatous reaction, some of the granulomata showing prominent giant cells and amorphous debris. H & E × 38.4.

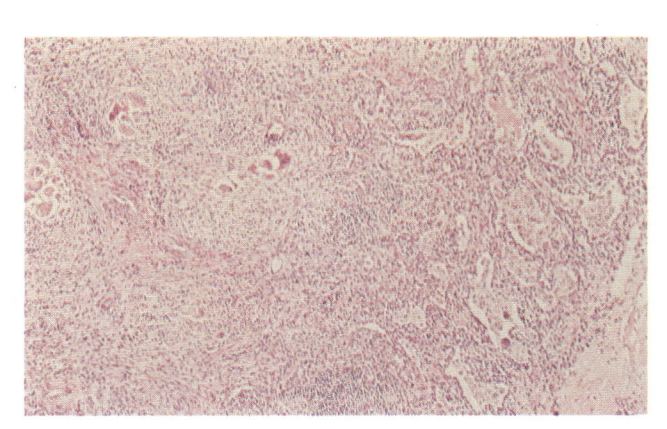

Figure 8.10 Edge of a lobule, interlobular septum (bottom right) with giant cells, amorphous debris, epithelioid cells and eosinophils centrally. The peripheral alveoli contain macrophages, eosinophils and there is cuboidal metaplasia of lining cells. H & E × 38.4.

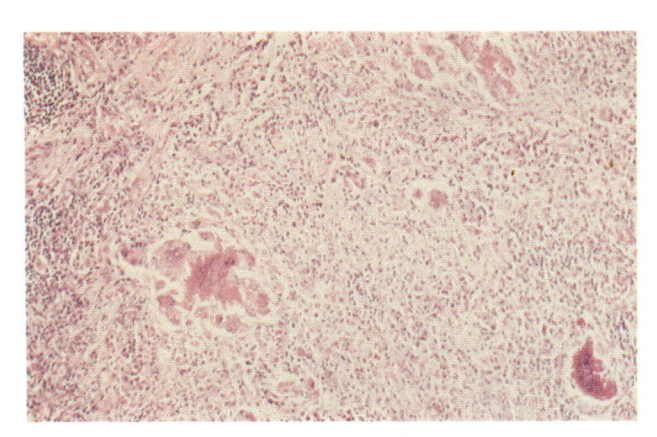

Figure 8.11 Higher power of granulomatous area with giant cells and characteristic debris in which fungal mycelium can not be identified. H & E × 96.

cases. He postulated that this might result in saccular bronchiectasis, an occasional finding in asthmatics.

Bronchial biopsies of asthmatics in remission have usually shown basement thickening and less frequently increase in goblet cells and eosinophilic infiltration[2].

Sputum Examination in Asthma

Histological examination of paraffin sections of sputum is very useful in the diagnosis of asthma since 'asthmatic stigmata' are present in over 90% of patients with severe asthmatic episodes and in approximately 70% of those in a quiescent phase of their illness[3]. This 'asthmatic plug' consists of variable amounts of proteinous fluid, mucus, eosinophils, bronchial epithelium, Charcot–Leyden crystals and Creola bodies. The non-mucoid elements may organize into Curschmann's spirals – these consist of epithelial cells and leukocytes embedded in a matrix of delicate fibres (Figures 8.3 and 8.4). Older plugs show cellular degeneration with eosinophilic debris and complex laminar structures. Infection may result in purulent or mucopurulent clumps in addition to the asthmatic stigmata[3] (Figure 8.5).

Mucoid Impaction of Bronchi

A distinct clinical entity particularized by mucus plugging of segmental bronchi, it may affect one or more lobes of the lung[4]. It occurs in asthma, in cystic fibrosis and in allergic bronchopulmonary aspergillosis. There is often collapse or organizing pneumonia of the obstructed segment of the lung. An unusual variant is so-called 'plastic bronchitis' where the patient intermittently coughs up firm white stringy bronchial casts (Figure 8.5).

Grossly large, laminated mucous plugs, which may be very hard are present in dilated segmental bronchi[4] (Figure 8.6). This entity should be differentiated from the diffuse plugging of smaller airways which occurs in association with eosinophilic pneumonia and bronchocentric granulomatosis.

Eosinophilic Pneumonia

This is characterized by wandering eosinophilic pulmonary infiltrates which may or may not be accompanied by a peripheral blood eosinophilia. It ranges from mild cases, spontaneously remitting within a month of onset (Löffler's syndrome) to persistent, severe cases which may ultimately be life threatening[6]. Many cases occur in association with asthma; in all, an underlying cause should be searched for (Table 8.1), but in many the cause is not identified. In Great Britain the most common cause of eosinophilic pneumonia and asthma is *Aspergillus* infection.

Table 8.1 Some causes of eosinophilic pneumonia

Fungi	Especially *Aspergillus* species but also others, including *Candida*
Helminths	*Ascaris, Toxocara, Schistosoma, Microfilaria*
Drugs	Nitrofurantoin, para-aminosalicylic acid, penicillin, sulphonamides

The pathology is similar in all cases, except for the additional finding of fungal hyphae in those cases due to *Aspergillus* infection. There is interstitial oedema and an infiltrate composed of lymphocytes, plasma cells and numerous eosinophils (Figure 8.7). Alveoli contain eosinophils, histiocytes and multinucleated giant cells, some of 'Touton' type[7] (Figure 8.7). Eosinophilic abscesses are frequently present in distal air spaces. Organization of exudates and the interstitium may occur but is usually sparse and focal. Typical sarcoid-like granulomata may also be present[6]. Features of bronchiolitis obliterans may be observed but the 'polyps' are infiltrated by eosinophils.

A mild eosinophilis vasculitis may be present but if this is severe or necrotizing a diagnosis of Churg--Strauss syndrome must be considered.

The mononuclear cells in the alveoli in eosinophilic pneumonia may cause confusion with desquamative interstitial pneumonia, but in the latter there is usually a minimal interstitial infiltrate and eosinophils are not conspicuous. Sometimes giant cells may be conspicuous in EP mimicking giant cell interstitial pneumonia but in the latter they are very large and bizarre and eosinophils are inconspicuous (Figure 8.8).

Histiocytosis X involving the lung also has to be differentiated from eosinophilic pneumonia. In histiocytosis X the infiltrate is predominantly interstitial and contains the characteristic 'histiocyte' (Figures 9.8 and 9.9).

Bronchocentric Granulomatosis

In this condition lesions resembling necrotic granulomata are distributed predominantly around bronchi and bronchioles[8]. The necrotic lesions, containing variable numbers of neutrophils and eosinophils, are surrounded by pallisaded, radially arranged epithelioid cells (Figures 8.9–8.11). Accompanying vessels may be involved but this appears incidental to the primary bronchial or bronchiolar lesions.

In this condition changes of mucoid impaction and eosinophilic pneumonia may be also seen in varying combinations. *Aspergillus* has been implicated in a number of these cases.

Rheumatoid disease affecting bronchioles may give a similar appearance to bronchocentric granulomatosis.

References

1. Leopold, J. G. (1961). Allergic pneumonia in chronic asthmatics. *Thorax,* **16,** 400 (abstr.)
2. Andersson, E., Smidt, C. M., Sikjaer, B., Ainge, G. and Poynter, D. (1977). Bronchial biopsies after beclomethasone dipropionate aerosol. *Brit. J. Dis. Chest,* **77,** 35
3. Sanerkin, N. G., and Evans, D. M. D. (1965). The sputum in bronchial asthma: pathognomonic patterns. *J. Pathol. Bacteriol.,* **89,** 535
4. Sanerkin, N. G. Seal, R. M. E. and Leopold, J. G. (1966). Plastic bronchitis, mucoid impaction of the bronchi and allergic bronchopulmonary aspergillosis, and their relationship to bronchial asthma. *Ann. Allergy,* **24,** 586
5. Katzenstein, A.-L., Liebow, A. A. and Friedman, P. J. (1975). Bronchocentric granulomatosis, mucoid impaction and hypersensitivity reactions to fungi. *Am. Rev. Resp. Dis.,* **111,** 497
6. Carrington, C. B., Addington, W. W., Goff, A. M., Madoff, I. M., Marks, A., Schwaber, J. R. and Gaensler, E. A. (1969). Chronic eosinophilic pneumonia. *N. Eng. J. Med.,* **280,** 787
7. Liebow, A. A. and Carrington, C. B. (1969). Eosinophilic pneumonia. *Medicine,* **48,** 251
8. Liebow, A. A. (1973). The J. Burns Amberson Lecture – Pulmonary angiitis and granulomatosis. *Am. Rev. Resp. Dis.,* **108,** 1

Systemic Diseases Affecting the Lung

Rheumatoid Arthritis (RA)

There appears to be a genuine association between a variety of pulmonary conditions and rheumatoid arthritis (Plate 9.1). Most of these pulmonary conditions may precede, occur at the onset or develop later in the course of rheumatoid arthritis.

Pleurisy

Pleurisy with or without effusion is the most commonly associated condition, occurring in up to half the patients with rheumatoid arthritis[1]. Pleural biopsy, in our experience, usually shows non-specific chronic inflammatory changes, but occasionally there is pallisading of fibroblasts and histiocytes with overlying fibrin (Figure 9.1). Rarely there are definitive rheumatoid nodules. We have seen one case in which there were numerous pleural rheumatoid nodules and marked atypical mesothelial proliferation which was virtually indistinguishable from malignant mesothelioma. However, the person is still alive many years later, without any progression of the lesion (Chapter 21, Figure 21.11. Walker and Wright[1] have shown a higher incidence of *chronic bronchitis* and *bronchiectasis* in patients with rheumatoid arthritis compared to subjects with non-rheumatoid joint disease.

Obliterative Bronchitis

Recently, Geddes et al.[2] have drawn attention to an association between obliterative bronchitis, resulting in respiratory insufficiency from airways obstruction, and rheumatoid arthritis. None of the six patients whom they reported showed any evidence of chronic bronchitis or emphysema. The main feature of these cases was the presence of narrowing and obliteration of airways measuring 1–6 mm in diameter by mural scar tissue. This scar tissue predominantly affected the mucosa but also involved the muscle coat and peribronchial tissues. Granulation tissue polyps were not observed, but in two cases there was necrotizing ulceration of the bronchial mucosa and severe active chronic inflammatory changes (Figure 9.2). Three examples we have seen were also characterized by a particularly dense round-cell infiltrate. Geddes et al.[2] emphasized that the morphological changes can easily be missed unless careful post-mortem examination is performed.

Necrobiotic nodules

These are rare manifestations of RA and occur predominantly in males. They may be single or multiple, are usually pleural based, vary from a few millimetres in diameter up to 7 cm, and may cavitate. Histologically, they consist of a central zone of fibrinoid necrosis; an intermediate zone of histiocytes and fibroblasts, radially disposed in a pallisaded arrangement where they abut on the central necrotic zone; and a peripheral zone of connective tissue interspersed with lymphocytes and plasma cells.

Rheumatoid Pneumoconiosis (Caplan's syndrome)

This is discussed in Chapter 13.

Diffuse interstitial Fibrosis

Diffuse interstitial fibrosis with honeycombing occurs in the lower lobes of approximatly 1–2% of patients with rheumatoid arthritis[1]. In the majority of cases it is clinically and pathologically indistinguishable from idiopathic chronic interstitial pneumonia (cryptogenic fibrosing alveolitis) in the absence of any specific rheumatoid features[3] (Figure 9.3).

Pulmonary Hypertension in association with Rheumatoid Arthritis

Rare cases have been described of patients with rheumatoid arthritis developing pulmonary hypertension in the absense of interstitial fibrosis. The pulmonary arterioles and small muscular arteries have shown concentric intimal fibroelastic proliferation[4].

Systemic Lupus Erythematosus

Pleural and pulmonary involvement is more frequent in systemic lupus erythematosus (SLE) than in any other collagen disease, the incidence varying from 50–70%. Infections appear to be the most frequent cause of pulmonary infiltrates in SLE and careful search must be made for opportunistic organisms. A variety of acute and chronic changes unrelated to infection do, however, occur in SLE, but the majority of pathological changes that have been described are non-specific. These include non-specific pleural changes, focal atelectasis and diffuse alveolar damage[5]. Haemotoxylin bodies, which are diagnostic of SLE, have been reported rarely in the lung[6] (Figure 9.4). In a post-mortem study, Gross et al[7]. found foci of pulmonary interstitial fibrosis in 70% of subjects with SLE but this was neither severe nor generalized. However, in some cases of SLE end-stage honeycomb lung has developed, indistinguishable from idiopathic chronic interstitial pneumonia. Gross et al.[7] also found distal airway alterations, including focal panacinar emphysema and bronchiolar dilation in 100% cases. They found lesions of the pulmonary vasculature much less frequently than in the systemic vasculature. There was only an acute inflammatory infiltrate in small

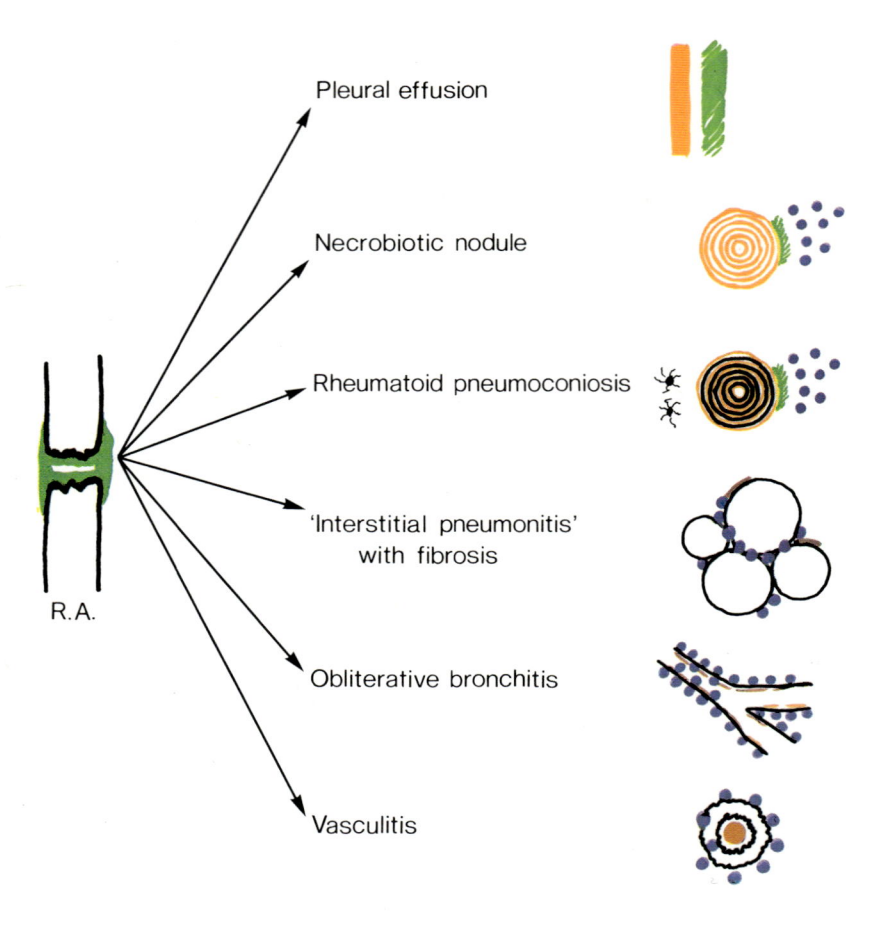

Plate 9.1 Pulmonary conditions associated with rheumatoid arthritis

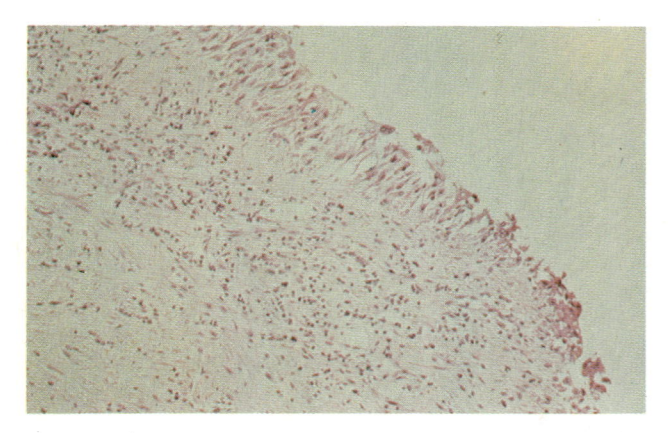

Figure 9.1 Pleuritis with histiocytes arranged at right angles to the pleural surface, typical of rheumatoid pleuritis. H&E × 96.

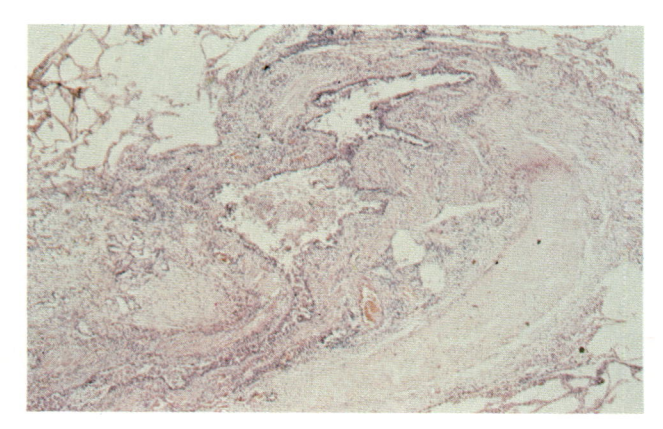

Figure 9.2 Long-standing severe rheumatoid arthritic patient developed severe obstructive airways disease with hypoxic pulmonary hypertension. Medium and small bronchi revealed obliteration of lumen by submucosal fibrosis and a small round cell infiltrate. H&E × 24.

SYSTEMIC DISEASES AFFECTING THE LUNG 65

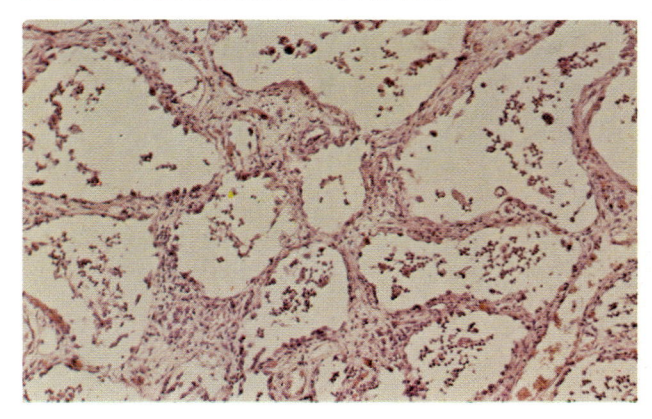

Figure 9.3 A patient with rheumatoid arthritis who developed interstitial disease. Microscopy reveals an interstitial pneumonitis with moderate collagenous thickening of interalveolar septa. The interalveolar cellular infiltrate is a result of terminal pyogenic infection. H&E × 240.

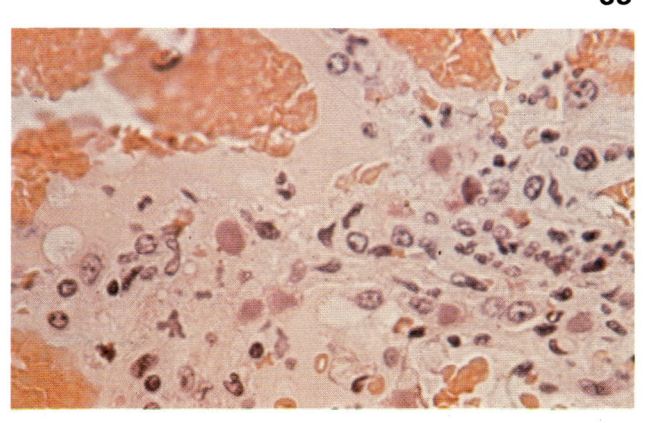

Figure 9.4 Lung from a patient who died from systemic lupus erythematosis revealed haematoxyphil bodies in addition to features of diffuse alveolar damage. H&E × 384.

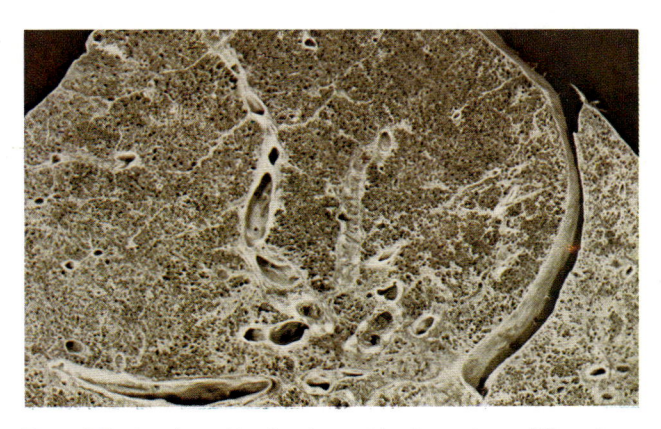

Figure 9.5 A patient with scleroderma dying in respiratory failure shows interstitial fibrosis and fine honeycombing (Barium sulphate impregnation).

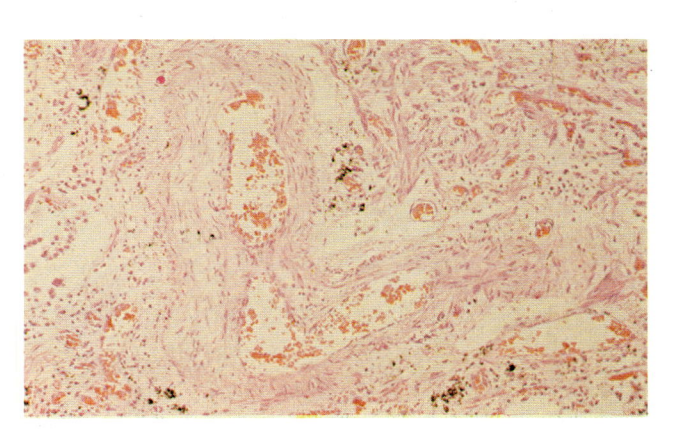

Figure 9.6 Microscopy revealed intimal fibrosis and medial hypertrophy in muscular pulmonary arteries and interstitial fibrosis. H&E × 96.

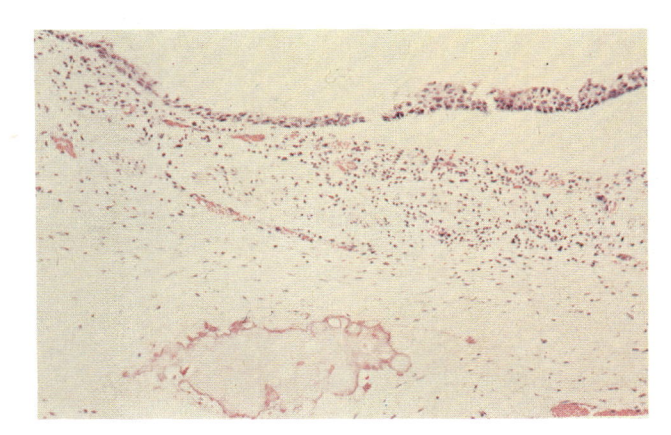

Figure 9.7 The wall of a bronchus from a patient with Sjögren's syndrome showing squamous metaplasia, mucus gland atrophy with lymphocytic infiltration and fibrosis. H&E × 96.

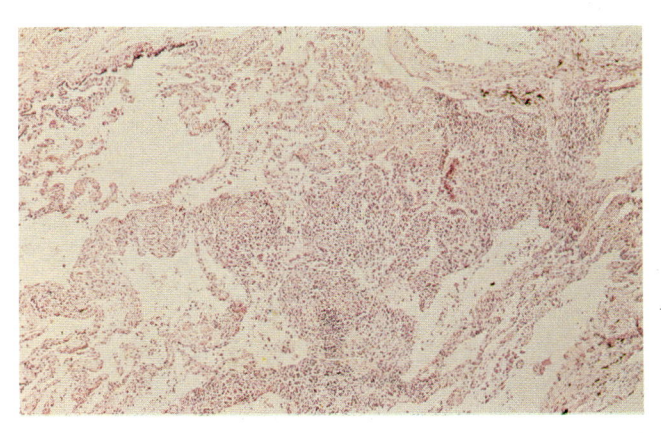

Figure 9.8 A case of histiocytosis X showing the interstitial distribution of the infiltrate. H&E × 38.4.

arteries and arterioles in 19% of the specimens; fibrinoid necrosis was inconspicuous and in no instance were the 'onion-skin' lesions identified.

There is a possible association between SLE (in the absence of Sjögren's syndrome) and the pulmonary lymphoproliferative disorders. Mathay et al.[5] described LIP in one patient with SLE, although their illustrations are unconvincing. We have encountered a middle-aged female who developed a primary pulmonary malignant lymphoma several years after the onset of SLE[8].

Systemic Sclerosis (Scleroderma)

Aspiration pneumonia, a consequence of impairment of oesphageal motility, is frequent in this disease.

However, the dominant lung pathology in this condition is diffuse interstitial pneumonia, similar to idiopathic chronic interstitial fibrosis, which occurs more often in this collagen disease than any other (Figure 9.5). It has been found in 67–100% of autopsy cases[9]. Vascular changes have been said to occur in 29% of cases[10], and affect the muscular pulmonary arteries and arterioles (Figure 9.6). At first there is medial muscular hypertrophy and the development of longitudinal muscle in the intima. This is followed by intimal fibroelastosis, medial fibrous atrophy and finally obliteration of affected vessels. These changes were ar first regarded as specific, but Harris and Heath[11] believe that they are only characteristic of honeycomb lung and not related to the underlying primary disease. Trell and Lindström[9], however, regarded the vascular changes and pulmonary fibrosis as separate and independant manifestations of the disorder.

There appears to be a greater tendency to the development of carcinoma, usually of glandular type, in honeycomb lungs related to scleroderma, which is over and above the increased incidence seen in idiopathic chronic interstitial pneumonia per se.

Polymyositis-Dermatomyositis (PM–DM)

Since 1956 over 30 cases of interstitial pneumonitis occurring in association with PM–DM have been described[12]. The majority respond to treatment with corticosteroids, but a small proportion go on to develop end-stage honeycomb disease which is indistinguishable from idiopathic chronic interstitial pneumonia.

There is a well-known association between PM–DM and neoplasia, in patients over 50 years old. This includes pulmonary tumours.

Sjögren's Syndrome

A recent review of 343 patients with typical Sjögren's syndrome revealed pulmonary changes in 9%[13]. Table 9.1 lists the various types of lung pathology seen in Sjögren's syndrome.

There is an increased likelihood of lower respiratory-tract infections such as bronchitis, bronchiectasis and pneumonitis which has been attributed to the bronchial submucosal gland atrophy that occurs in this syndrome. Histologically, the submucosal gland atrophy is accompanied by a lymphocytic plasma-cell infiltrate and fibrosis (Figure 9.7).

Although Sjögren's syndrome is often accompanied by other collagen disease, it appears to be asociated with diffuse interstitial pulmonary fibrosis in its own right. The pathology is indistinguishable from chronic interstitial fibrosis. It occurred in 4% of Strimlan et al.'s series[13].

Among the connective tissue disorders, Sjögren's syndrome exhibits the strongest association with pulmonary lymphoproliferative disorders. These range from the benign end of the spectrum – lymphoid interstitial pneumonia and pseudolymphoma – to the more malignant end of the spectrum – lymphomatoid granulomatosis and malignant lymphoma.

Ankylosing Spondylitis

In ankylosing spondylitis pulmonary manifestations may occur several years after the onset of joint symptoms. The disease affects the upper lobes and is characterized by fibrosis and the formation of bullae and cavities. It resembles healed post-primary tuberculosis, but there is no evidence that it is caused by tubercle bacilli, since neither granulomata nor bacilli can be identified. As in other disease there is a tendency to colonization by *Aspergillus* to form aspergillomas[14].

Histiocytosis X

This is a condition which occurs at any age and is particularized by a proliferation of histiocytic-like cells, shown by electron microscopy to be similar to the Langerhan's cells of the skin[15]. There are three variants: Hand – Schuller – Christian disease – the chronic generalized form; Letterer – Silve disease – the acute generalized form; and eosinophilic granuloma – the localized form. The lung may be the only site of involvement, but a considerable proportion show disseminated lesions. It is often called eosinophilic granuloma of the lung when the lungs alone are involved. The disease runs an unpredictable course.

Macroscopically, the lungs show small, irregular, often cavitated nodules in the early stages, but later there is honeycombing with cyst formation. The changes are most severe in the upper and middle lobes[15].

Microscopically, the interstitium contains focal infiltrates of mononuclear cells and eosinophils, most marked around centriacinar bronchioles and arteries and small veins in the interlobular septa (Figures 9.8 and 9.9). The characteristic histiocytic cells have a kidney-shaped nucleus with one or two nucleoli, fairly eosinophillic cytoplasm but lack

Table 9.1 Pulmonary conditions associated with Sjögren's syndrome

Pleurisy with or without effusion
Bronchial-gland atrophy
Chronic interstitial pneumonia
Lymphoproliferative conditions:
    Pseudolymphoma, lymphoid interstitial pneumonia, malignant lymphoma, lymphomatoid granulomatosis

pigment. Eosinophils, giant cells, lymphocytes, plasma cells, neutrophils and foamy macrophages are also present in the infiltrate. Although mainly interstitial, the infiltrate often extends into alveoli.

Increasing fibrosis and gradual disappearance of the histiocytes and other cells occurs later, resulting in a hyaline fibrous stellate scar. As the disease progresses, cystic change and honeycombing occurs. In the acute form (Letterer–Siwe disease) the infiltrate tends to be more diffuse than in the chronic form (Hand–Schuller–Christian disease), which exhibits focal and well-circumscribed lesions. A definitive diagnosis may be very difficult at the stage of widespread honeycombing and careful search must be made for the more active cellular lesions.

In the early stages, histiocytosis X must be distinguished from eosinophilic pneumonia. The latter is characterized by a predominantly intraalveolar infiltrate, eosinophilic abscesses and often blood eosinophilia.

However, an occasional case is encountered which shows severe interstitial inflammation with an infiltrate very similar to that seen in histiocytosis X, and marked intraalveolar collections of mononuclear cells (Figures 9.10 and 9.11). The problem is whether to designate it histiocytosis X with an unusual desquamative component, eosinophilic pneumonia with an unusual degree of interstitial change, or idiopathic chronic interstitial pneumonia with an undue prominent component of eosinophils.

Electron microscopy may be of benefit in identifying the histiocytosis X cells, since they have characteristic cytoplasmic organelles[15].

(Figures 9.9–9.11 will be found overleaf)

References

1. Walker, W. C. and Wright, V. (1968). Pulmonary lesions and rheumatoid arthritis. *Medicine*, **47,** 501
2. Geddes, D. M., Corrin, B., Breverton, D. A., Davies, R. J. and Turner-Warrick, M. (1977). Progressive airway obliteration in adults and its association with rheumatoid disease. *Q. J. Med.*, **46,** 427
3. Scadding, J. G. (1969). Philip Ellman Lecture. The lungs in rheumatoid arthritis. *Proc. R. Soc. Med.*, **66,** 227
4. Gardner, D. L., Duthie, J. J. R., Macleod, J. and Allan, W. S. A. (1957). Pulmonary hypertension in rheumatoid arthritis. *Scott. J. Med.*, **2,** 183
5. Matthay, R. A., Schwarz, M. I., Petty,, T. L., Stanford, R. E., Gupta, R. C., Sahn, S. A. and Steigerwald, J. D. (1974). Pulmonary manifestations of systemic lupus erythematosus: Review of twelve cases of acute lupus pneumonitis. *Medicine*, **54,** 397
6. Olsen, E. G. and Lever, J. V. (1972). Pulmonary changes in systemic lupus erythematosus. *Br. J. Dis. Chest*, **66,** 71
7. Gross, M., Esterly, J. R. and Earle, R. H. (1972). Pulmonary alterations in systemic lupus erythematosus. *Am. Rev. Resp. Dis.*, **105,** 572
8. Gibbs, A. R. and Seal, R. M. E. (1978). Primary lymphoproliferative conditions of lung. *Thorax*, **33,** 140
9. Trell, E. and Linstrom, C. (1971). Pulmonary hypertension in systemic sclerosis. *Ann. Rheum. Dis.*, **30,** 390
10. D'Angelo, W. A., Fries, J. F., Masi, A. T. and Shulman, L. E. (1968). Pathologic observations on systemic sclerosis (Scleroderma). *Am. J. Med.*, **46,** 428
11. Harris, P. and Heath, D. (1977). *The Human Pulmonary Circulation* 2nd Edition, p.629 (Edinburgh: Churchill Livingstone)
12. Schwarz, M. I., Matthay, R. A., Kahn, S. A., Stanford, R. E., Marmorstein, B. L. and Scheinhorn, D. J. (1976). Interstitial lung disease in polymyositis and dermatomyositis. *Medicine*, **55,** 89
13. Strimlan, C. V., Rosenow, E. C., Divertic, M. B. and Harrison, E. G. (1976). Pulmonary manifestations of Sjögren's syndrome. *Chest*, **70,** 354
14. Davies, D. (1972). Ankylosing spondylitis and lung fibrosis. *Q. J. Med.*, **41,** 395
15. Basset, F., Corrin, B., Spencer, H., Lacronique, J., Roth, C., Soler, P., Battesti, J., Georges, R. and Chrëtien, J. (1978). Pulmonary histiocytosis X. *Am. Rev. Resp. Dis.*, **118,** 811

SYSTEMIC DISEASES AFFECTING THE LUNG

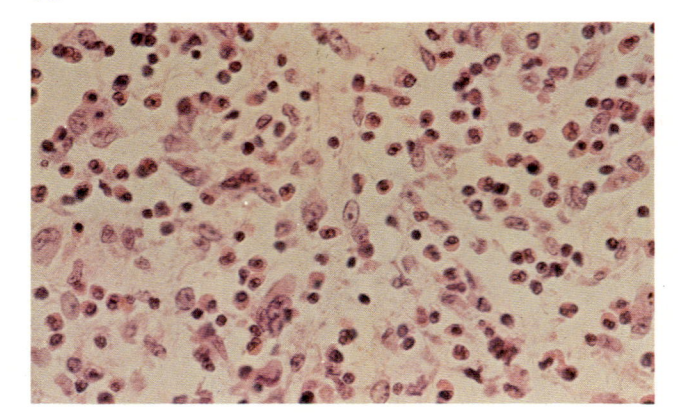

Figure 9.9 The cellular infiltrate consists of typical histiocytes, numerous eosinophils, lymphocytes and plasma cells. H&E × 384.

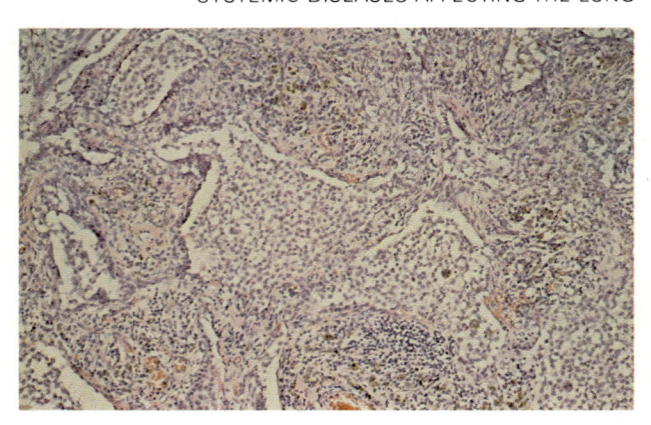

Figure 9.10 A problem case. A 22-year-old male was noted to have 'honeycomb lungs' on mass miniature radiography and enquiry revealed 6-month history of dyspnoea and weight loss. Biopsy revealed marked insterstitial pneumonitis and fibrosis with numerous interalveolar mononuclear cells. H&E × 240.

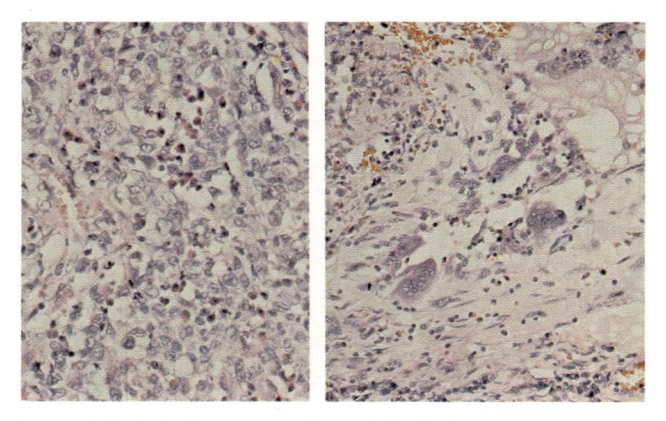

Figure 9.11 *Left:* (Same case as Figure 9.10). The interstitium contained eosinophils, histiocytes and lymphoid cells. H&E × 384. *Right:* Occasional giant cells were also present. The patient was put on steroids but showed no improvement clinically or radiologically and was taken off. His condition remains static.

Pathology of the Pulmonary Vasculature

10

Good detailed accounts of the different conditions associated with pulmonary hypertension and their effects are given by Harris and Heath[1], Edwards and Edwards[2] and Wagenvoort and Wagenvoort[3]. In this chapter we consider the basic pulmonary vascular lesions that occur in association with the various types of pulmonary hypertension and the various combinations and patterns which will enable a correct diagnosis to be made. Pulmonary hypertension is arbitrarily defined as a resting pulmonary

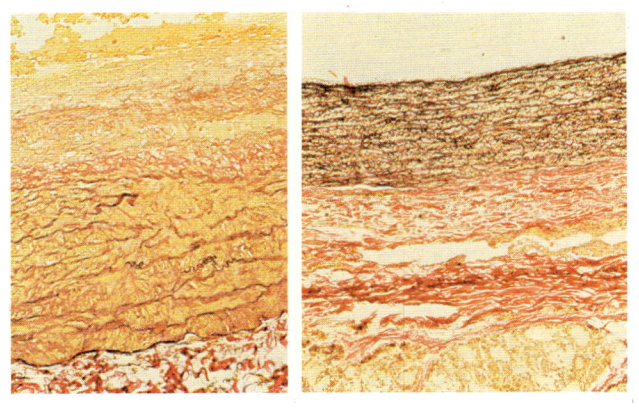

Figure 10.1 *Left:* An elastic pulmonary artery of a 45-year-old male showing short, branched irregular elastic fibrils in the media. EVG × 240. *Right:* The fine, paralleled arrangement of elastic fibres (fetal pattern) seen in the pulmonary trunk of a 7-year-old male, who had had pulmonary hypertension since birth. EVG × 96.

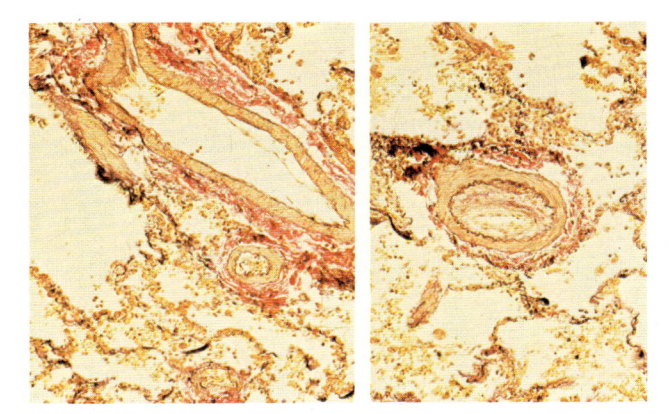

Figure 10.2 *Left:* Medial hypertrophy of an arteriole and small muscular pulmonary artery of an adult female with plexogenic pulmonary hypertension. EVG × 96. *Right:* Medial hypertrophy with eccentric cellular and collagenous intimal proliferation of a small muscular artery. EVG × 96.

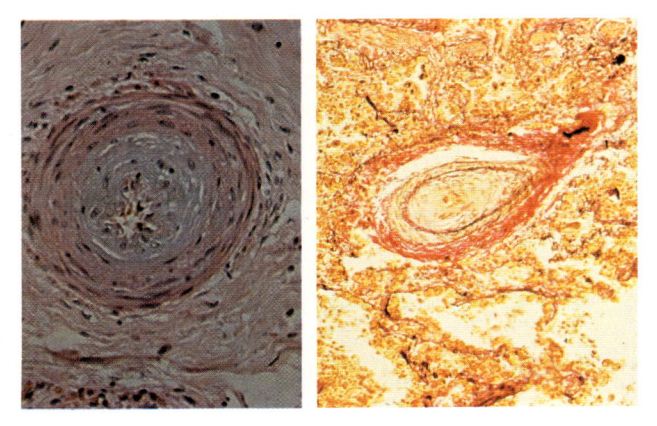

Figure 10.3 *Left:* Concentric laminar intimal fibrosis and medial hypertrophy of a muscular pulmonary artery, from a case of plexogenic pulmonary hypertension. Trichrome × 240. *Right:* Intimal proliferation of a hypertrophied muscular pulmonary artery with complete occlusion. EVG × 96.

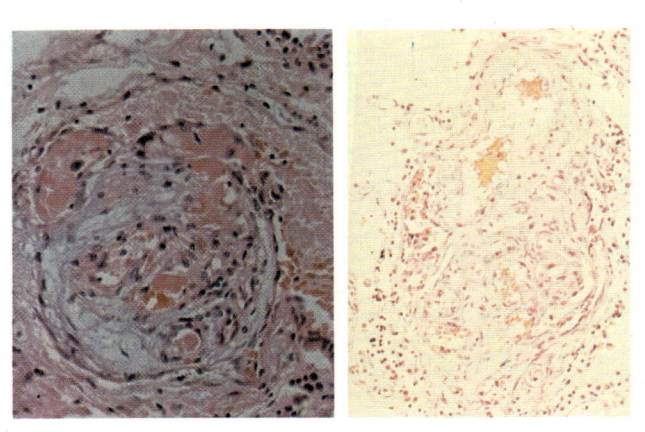

Figure 10.4 *Left:* Plexogenic pulmonary hypertension. Plexiform lesion of a muscular pulmonary artery containing fibrin. H & E × 96. *Right:* Another plexiform lesion from a 34-year-old female dying from plexogenic pulmonary arteriopathy. H & E × 96.

artery systolic–diastolic pressure of above 30/13 mmHg. Pulmonary arterial pressure is governed by the volume of pulmonary blood flow per unit time and the resistance of this flow. Certain features are common to all types of chronic pulmonary hypertension, namely right ventricular hypertrophy, prominence of major pulmonary arteries and the presence of atheroma in the elastic pulmonary arteries[4]. Other features reflect the different causes and sites of involvement of the pulmonary vascular tree.

Before going on to describe the pathological changes that occur within the vessels, a brief summary of the anatomy of the pulmonary vascular bed is given.

The *elastic* pulmonary arteries include the main pulmonary artery, its branches outside the lung, and those within the lung with an external diameter greater than 1000 μm. The media of these vessels consists predominantly of short, branched and irregular elastic fibrils (adult pattern) (Figure 10.1, left.).

The *muscular* pulmonary arteries (external diameters between 1000 and 100 μm) have a thin media of circular muscle separated from a thin intima and adventitia by an internal and external elastic lamina, respectively. The percentage medial thickness (i.e. width of media compared to diameter between the external elastic lamina) of arteries between 100 and 300 μm external diameter in the upper and lower lobes of the lung is approximately 2.8–3.1%. The muscular arteries lie in close relation to bronchioles, respiratory bronchioles and alveolar ducts.

The *arterioles* (external diameter less than 100 μm) resemble the parent muscular artery proximally, but more distally have an endothelial lining resting on a small quantity of connective tissue. The arterioles arise as terminations (related to alveolar ducts) or side branches (related to small bronchi) of muscular pulmonary arteries.

The *capillaries* lie within the alveolar wall.

The *venules* are identical structurally to arterioles and are formed within the alveolar walls and pass into connective tissue septa between secondary lobules. Serial sections may be necessary to distinguish them from arterioles by tracing them to the interlobular septa where they can be confidently identified.

The pulmonary *veins* (external diameter greater than 100 μm) lie within interlobular septa and have irregularly arranged elastic fibrils interspersed with small bundles of smooth muscle and varying amounts of collagen in the media, and an intima consisting of an endothelial layer lying on an internal elastic lamina.

A thin layer of eccentric and diffuse intimal fibrosis may occur in the pulmonary arteries and veins in normal individuals as an age-related phenomenon. It is not normally seen before the age of 20 years and may be hyaline in appearance.

Pathological Changes

The following pathological changes may be seen in the muscular pulmonary arteries in association with pulmonary hypertension.

(i) *Medial Hypertrophy* (Figure 10.2, left)

The earliest response to pulmonary hypertension, occurring firstly within arterioles, then, small muscular arteries (less than 300 μm external diameter) and later larger muscular arteries.

(ii) *Intimal Proliferation*

Cellular intimal proliferation, either eccentric (Figure 10.2, right) or concentric (Figure 10.3, left) may follow medial hypertrophy, and is observed firstly within the arterioles and smaller muscular arteries and later within the medium-sized muscular arteries (300–500 μm). The intimal fibrotic lesions may also show fine or coarse elastic fibrils and there may be elastosis of the elastic laminae. Complete occlusion may result (Figure 10.3, right).

(iii) *Plexiform Lesions* (Figure 10.4)

These are associated with severe pulmonary hypertension and they consist of a thin-walled sac, derived from a small muscular artery, which contains a plexus of channels separated by proliferating endothelial cells. The parent artery shows medial hypertrophy and often concentric laminar intimal fibrosis.

(iv) *Dilatation Lesions*

Sustained pulmonary arterial hypertention may result in thinning and generalized dilatation of the walls of arterioles and muscular arteries. Two types of lesion may develop:

(a) *Vein-like branches of hypertrophied pulmonary muscular arteries* may suddenly emerge from a hypertrophied muscular artery, sometimes forming clusters (Figure 10.5).

(b) *Angiomatoid lesions,* which are uncommon and essentially post-stenotic dilatation lesions. They consist of an angioma-like mass of dilated and tortuous channels.

(v) *Necrotizing Arteritis* (Figure 10.6)

Associated usually with very severe pulmonary hypertension, the muscular arteries undergo fibrinoid necrosis with or without a concomitant neutrophilic infiltrate. Thrombosis may also occur.

Healing results in replacement of the dead muscle by granulation tissue and collagen, and this may lead to vascular occlusion.

Grading

A grading system can be utilized for the lesions of muscular arteries occurring in primary pulmonary hypertension or pulmonary hypertension secondary to congenital heart disease[1]. The grades are in order of increasing severity.

Grade 1 – Medial hypertrophy.
Grade 2 – Medial hypertrophy with cellular intimal proliferation.
Grade 3 – Progressive fibrous vascular occlusion.
Grade 4 – Progressive generalized arterial dilatation, with the formation of complex dilatation lesions.
Grade 5 – Chronic dilatation with formation of numerous dilatation lesions and pulmonary haemosiderosis.
Grade 6 – Necrotizing arteritis.

Grades 4–6 are often seen together when there is severe pulmonary hypertension.

Changes may also occur within *elastic pulmonary arteries*. These include an increase in thickness of the media due to muscle hypertrophy which parallels the degree of right ventricular hypertrophy and medial thickness of the small muscular pulmonary arteries. There may also be an increase in the ground substance of the media (which stains metachromatically with toluidine blue) in pulmonary hypertension.

The 'adult pattern' of the elastic pulmonary arteries consists of a loose arrangement of branched, fragmented elastic fibrils, with club-like terminal expansions (Figure 10.1, left) whereas the 'fetal pattern' shows a medial elastic pattern like that of the aorta (Figure 10.1, right). The 'adult pattern' is usually achieved by the age of 2 years, but the fetal pattern persists in those who have pulmonary hypertension from birth (Figure 10.1, right).

Pulmonary atherosclerosis is characteristic of all conditions associated with pulmomary arterial hypertension, but is not specific and is commonly found in the middle aged and elderly.

Certain changes may be found in the pulmonary veins in association with elevated pulmonary venous pressure. Thickening of the media due to an increase of muscular, collagenous and elastic fibrils is common. Although intimal fibrosis is common above the age of 20 years, it may occur at an earlier age or be more severe in pulmonary venous hypertension. Other changes include arterialization and adventitial thickening.

Classification of Changes

A good working classification of changes that occur in the different forms of pulmonary hypertension is that of Wagenvoort[5]. He proposed five main categories (Plate 10.1).

(i) *Vasoconstrictive Group*

This group includes plexogenic pulmonary arteriopathy (primary pulmonary hypertension) and pulmonary hypertension associated with left to right congenital cardiac shunts. The latter may be of pre-tricuspid type (atrial septal defect and anomalous pulmonary venous drainage) or post-tricuspid type (ventricular septal defect, patent ductus arteriosus, aortopulmonary shunts, transposition of vessels). When complicated by pulmonary vascular hypertension, equalization or reversal in blood flow may occur in these defects – so-called Eisenmenger syndrome.

Unless pulmonary hypertension has developed within the first year of life, the elastic pulmonary arteries show an adult elastic pattern.

The vascular changes are seen evenly throughout the lungs, the earliest change being medial hypertrophy of arterioles and small muscular arteries. The changes then may progress to concentric laminar-intimal fibrosis, then plexiform and other local dilatation lesions, and finally to fibrinoid necrosis with or without leukocytic infiltration. Pulmonary haemosiderosis, if present, is mild and venous changes absent or minimal (Figures 10.2–10.6).

The majority of cases of plexogenic pulmonary arteriopathy have been idiopathic, but it has been linked with autoimmune diseases of other organs, hepatic cirrhosis, and an appetite suppressant (aminorex fumarate).

(ii) *Thromboembolic Pulmonary Hypertension*

Multiple recurrent thromboemboli may lead to high levels of pulmonary hypertension with normal or subnormal pulmonary blood flow.

The obstructive lesions usually involve muscular arteries and arterioles more frequently than the elastic pulmonary arteries, and are more prevalant in the lower lobes.

Histologically, the thrombi show a variety of appearances, ranging from organized and recanalized thrombus, eccentric intimal fibrous thickening, intimal fibroelastic pads from old organized thrombi, fibrous luminal septa and recent thrombi undergoing organization. In occasional cases, intimal fibrosis may be concentric but not laminar (cf. Group i). Muscle hypertrophy is less pronounced than in the plexogenic type. This group does not commonly manifest dilatation or arteritic lesions (Figure 10.7).

(iii) *Pulmonary Venous Hypertension*

In this group there is obstruction to pulmonary venous outflow, either at the venules (venocclusive disease), mitral valve (incompetence and/or stenosis), or left ventricle (left ventricular failure).

The muscular arteries show severe medial hypertrophy and eccentric and/or concentric but not laminar intimal fibrosis.

The characteristic features are located in the veins (Figures 10.8–10.10), namely medial hypertrophy, intimal fibrosis and 'arterialization'. The latter is characterized by a change from the normal haphazard medial arrangement of elastic fibrils to the formation of distinct internal and external elastic laminae.

Other changes include interstitial fibrosis and pulmonary haemosiderosis – more marked in the lower lobes – tortuosity and dilatation of capillaries, dilatation of lymphatics and occasionally the formation of intraalveolar spicules of bone.

In pulmonary veno-occlusive disease, a disease of unknown aetiology occurring mainly in children and young adults, 30–95% of the intrapulmonary venules and veins may be partially occluded by intimal fibrous lesions, which are often loose and oedematous. The veins and venules may also reveal what appear to be recanalized channels suggestive of previous thrombosis. Haemosiderosis is frequently very striking in this condition, mimicking idiopathic pulmonary haemosiderosis (Figures 10.9 and 10.10). Foci of interstitial pneumonia may also be evident.

The duration of symptoms usually varies between a few months and two years before the demise of the patient.

(iv) *Chronic Hypoxia (Hypoxic Pulmonary Hypertension)*

This category includes a wide varity of conditions, including high altitude, kyphoscoliosis, chronic airways obstruction, bronchiectasis, interstitial pulmonary fibrosis and the pneumoconioses.

'Emphysema' may also be associated with this variety of pulmonary hypertension and here, as in some of the other conditions, where there is destructive obliteration of the pulmonary vascular bed, it is difficult to evaluate the precise contribution of this to the pulmonary hypertension.

72 PATHOLOGY OF THE PULMONARY VASCULATURE

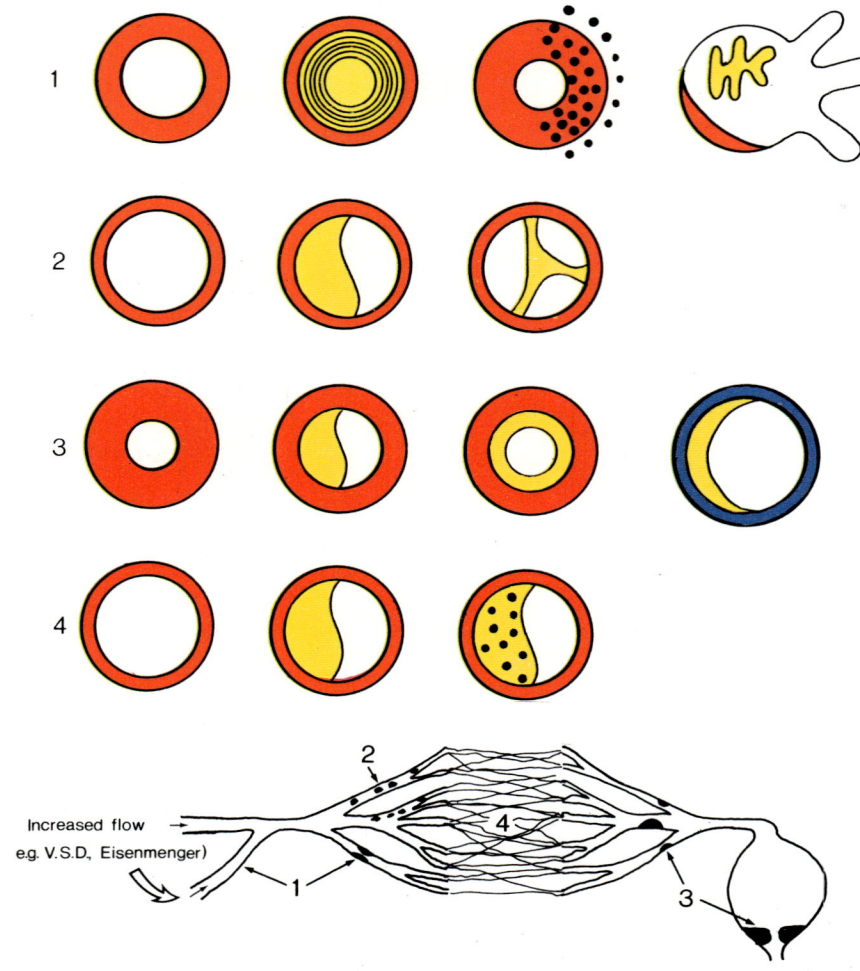

1. VASOCONSTRICTIVE GROUP (including plexogenic pulmonary arteriopathy)
2. THROMBOEMBOLIC HYPERTENSION
3. PULMONARY VENOUS HYPERTENSION (e.g. venocclusive & mitral stenosis)
4. CHRONIC HYPOXIC GROUP

(After C.A.Wagenvoort)

Plate 10.1 Morphological changes in pulmonary hypertension and anatomical site.

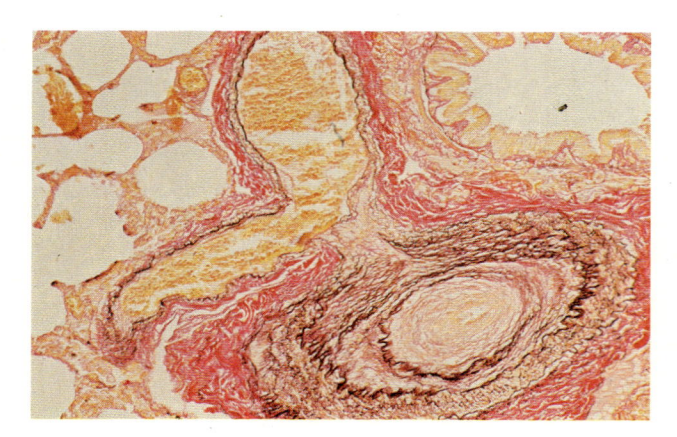

Figure 10.5 Plexogenic pulmonary hypertension. There is a completely occluded muscular artery due to intimal fibroelastosis (bottom right) with dilatation lesions of the branches (left and middle of the picture). EVG × 96.

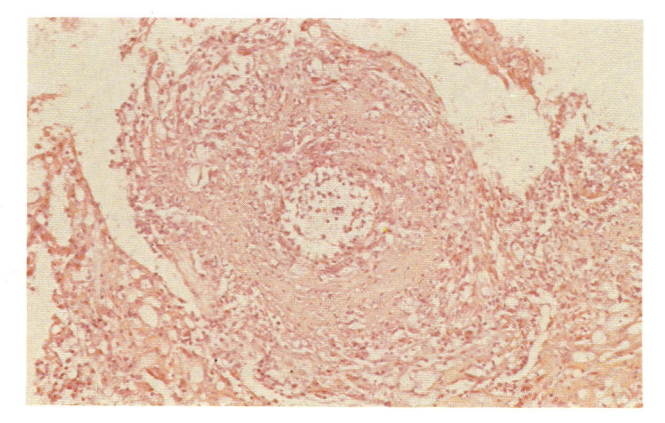

Figure 10.6 A muscular pulmonary artery, showing fibrinoid necrosis and an inflammatory infiltrate of its wall, from a 7-year-old female dying from pulmonary hypertension, which complicated a congenital ventricular septal defect. H&E × 96.

PATHOLOGY OF THE PULMONARY VASCULATURE

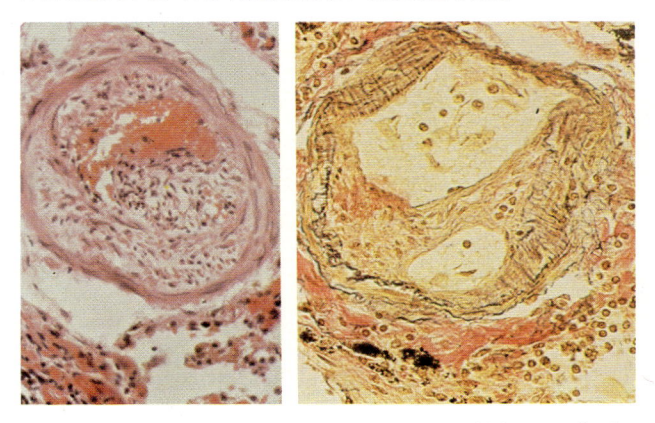

Figure 10.7 *Left:* Muscular pulmonary artery with multiple recanalization channels. H & E × 192. *Right:* Muscular pulmonary artery with fibrous septa traversing the lumen. EVG × 240.

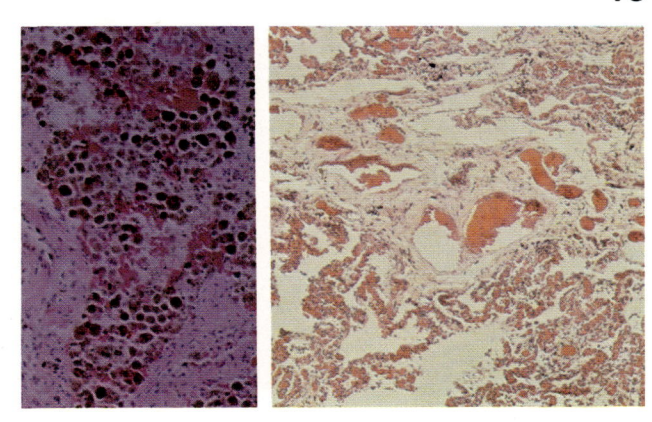

Figure 10.8 *Left:* Severe mitral stenosis producing haemosiderosis H & E × 96, and *Right:* Intimal fibrosis of pulmonary veins which are confidently identified within interlobular septa. H & E × 192.

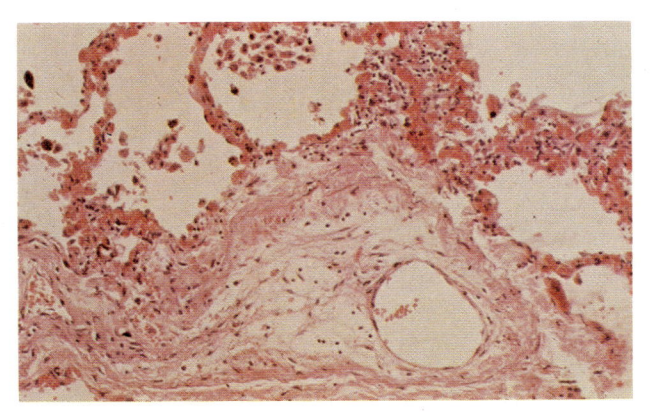

Figure 10.9 Veno-occlusive disease. The interlobular septa should be examined carefully, since these contain the venules and veins which evince the characteristic morphology. This shows an interlobular septum containing a vein which exhibits marked, rather oedematous, intimal fibrosis. H & E × 240.

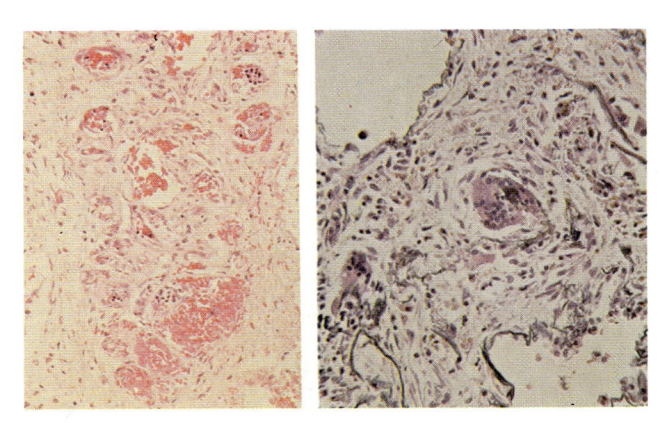

Figure 10.10 *Left:* Veno-occlusive disease. This shows an obliterated vein with multiple recanalization channels within an interlobular septum. H & E × 96. *Right:* Haemosiderosis with elastosis and giant-cell formation is often pronounced in this condition. It often brings to mind idiopathic pulmonary haemosiderosis. H & E × 192.

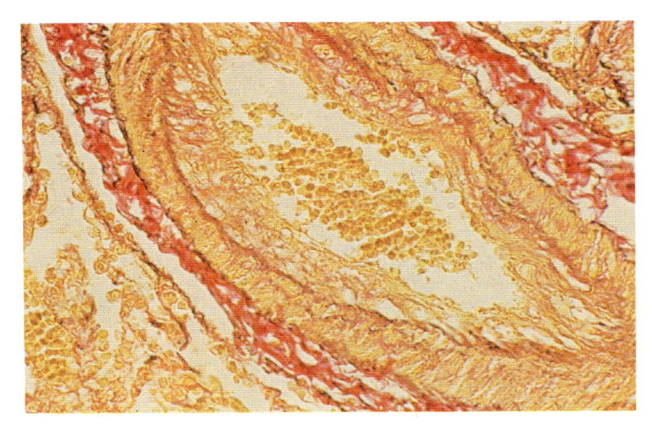

Figure 10.11 A muscular pulmonary artery showing medial hypertrophy with intimal longitudinal muscle bundles in a patient dying from obstructive airways disease. EVG × 240.

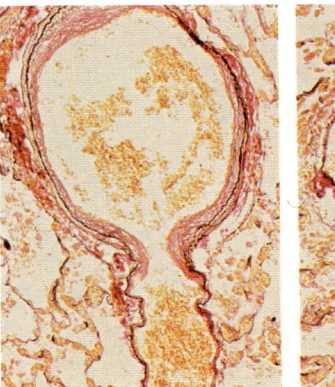

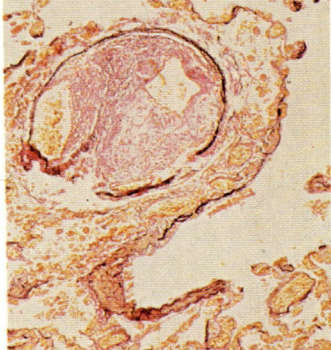

Figure 10.12 4-year-old male with Fallot's tetralogy showing: *Left:* A muscular pulmonary artery with medial atrophy and intimal fibrosis EVG × 240. *Right:* Muscular artery with intraluminal fibrous septa suggestive of previous thrombosis. EVG × 240.

In addition to medial hypertrophy of arterioles and small muscular arteries, a frequent distinctive feature is the presence of intimal longitudinal smooth muscle bundles (Figure 10.11).

Pulmonary veins and venules may exhibit medial hypertrophy, intimal fibrosis and intimal longitudinal smooth muscle bundles.

There may also be bronchopulmonary arterial and venous anastomoses in this group.

(v) Decreased Pulmonary Blood Flow (Lesions Without Hypertension)

This group includes patients with decreased pulmonary blood flow who do not have pulmonary hypertension, e.g. Fallot's tetralogy. There is dilatation of the small muscular arteries and a propensity to develop *in-situ* thrombi due to polycythaemia. The thrombi may show various stages of organization, recanalization, focal mural thickening and luminal fibrous septa (Figure 10.12).

It is important to realize that changes of more than one group may be present in the same lung, e.g. changes of pulmonary venous obstruction may complicate the vasoconstrictive changes seen in cardiac left to right shunts which develop left ventricular strain and heart failure.

All varieties of pulmonary hypertension may be complicated by extensive autochthonous thrombosis, rapidly leading to low output cardiac failure.

References

1. Harris, P. and Heath, D. (1977). *The Human Pulmonary Circulation. Its Form and Function in Health and Disease.* 2nd. Edn. (Edinburgh: Churchill Livingstone)
2. Edwards, W. D. and Edwards, J.E. (1978). Recent advances in the pathology of the pulmonary vasculature. In Thurlbeck, E. (Ed.), *The Lung-Structure, Function and Disease,* pp.235–261 (IAP Monograph No. 19) (Balitmore: Williams and Wilkins)
3. Wagenvoort, C. A. and Wagenvoort, N. (1977). *Pathology of Pulmonary Hypertension.* (New York: Wiley)
4. Edwards, J. E. (1974). Pathology of chronic pulmonary hypertension. *Pathol. Annu.,* **1**
5. Wagenvoort, C. A. (1973). Classifying pulmonary vascular disease. *Chest,* **64,** 503

Pulmonary Angiitides

11

Pulmonary angiitis may accompany severe pulmonary hypertension and this is discussed in Chapter 10. Pulmonary angiitis may also occur as a local complication of infections due to bacteria or fungi, e.g. pseudomonas and aspergillus. It may also be a consequence of septic emboli. Another form of local pulmonary vasculitis which we recognize is that seen as a component of rheumatoid pneumoconiosis (Chapter 9). Pulmonary angiitis may also rarely occur as a complication of systemic disease, such as rheumatoid arthritis and SLE. All of these conditions affect pulmonary parenchymal vessels, but occasionally primary arteritis of the main pulmonary artery and its branches may occur. Takayasu's arteritis may extend to involve the main pulmonary artery.

However, in this chapter we concentrate on several forms of systemic vasculitis which show a striking tendency to involve the lung, and present as a pulmonary problem. Pulmonary manifestations in these conditons frequently overshadow those due to involvement of other organs. The conditions which show certain affinities to each other are:

(1) Wegener's granulomatosis (WG), including the local form.
(2) Necrotizing sarcoid granulomatosis (NSG).
(3) Allergic granulomatosis and angiitis of Churg and Strauss (CSS).
(4) Polyarteritis nodosa (PN).
(5) Lymphomatoid granulomatosis, which is discussed in Chapter 19, on lymphoproliferative conditions.

Angiitis implies inflammation, with varying degrees of necrosis, of blood vessels. In some, the inflammation may be principally acute and in others, a chronic inflammatory process with or without giant cells. The consequence of the vascular changes is differing amounts of ischaemic change and inflammation in the lung parenchyma. It is likely that many of these conditions are a result of immune-complex deposition in vessel walls.

Wegener's Granulomatosis (WG)

Classical WG comprises a triad of necrotizing granulomatous vasculitis of the upper and lower respiratory tract and focal glomerulonephritis. The term limited WG was coined by Carrington and Liebow[1] for pulmonary lesions similar to those of the classical type, occurring in the absence of the two other elements of the triad. However, since the advent of cytotoxic therapy and clinicopathological studies which suggest that the respiratory tract is the initial site of the hypersensitivity reaction which later affects the kidney[2], it is better to regard them as aspects of one disease.

In a recent series of patients with Wegener's granulomatosis, respiratory tract involvement occurred in 100%, renal involvement in 83%, joint involvement in 56% and skin involvement in 44%[2]. Upper respiratory tract lesions included mucosal ulcerations, septal perforations, saddle deformities and paranasal sinusitis. Renal involvement included glomerulonephritis and granulomatous necrotic lesions similar to those found in other organs.

The upper respiratory tract may show diffuse membranous inflammation or focal areas of ulceration (Figure 11.1). Biopsy of either may only reveal non-specific chronic inflammatory changes, the vasculitic component not being apparent.

The pulmonary lesions show a variety of appearances. They may be located in any area of the lung, although we have noted a predilection for the upper lobes. They are usually multiple, bilateral and vary from a few millimetres to several centimetres in diameter. They are usually yellowish-grey, but may be haemorrhagic, irregularly shaped and merge with the background lung. Sometimes they are rather friable, at other times firm. They may cavitate. They can resemble tubercle or metastatic carcinoma. Occasionally, WG is misdiagnosed as a primary lung carcinoma[3] when it presents as a solitary, circumscribed lesion, and rarely as a segmental lesion (Figures 11.2 and 11.3).

Microscopically, the lesions are seen to be mainly centred around vessels, but parenchymal and bronchial lesions also occur. Bronchial biopsy material may sometimes reveal the typical appearances, but often the chronic inflammation is diffuse and non-specific. The lesions consist of confluent or isolated basophilic necrotic areas containing granular material and disintegrating neutrophils. Necrotic vessels may be revealed within the lesions by elastic staining. Histiocytes, fibroblasts, fibrous tissue, lymphocytes and variable numbers of eosinophils are located around and in the central necrotic area. Giant cells of many types may be seen, but frequently they are difficult to classify into the recognized Langhans, foreign body and Touton type, having rather characteristic appearances. Discrete, sarcoid-like granulomata, which include asteroid bodies within giant cells, may be evident in about one fifth of cases[4] (Figures 11.4–11.7).

Small arteries and veins show infiltration of their walls by mononuclear cells and polymorph neutrophils, with variable destruction of their elastic tissue and luminal occlusion. Less frequently the vessels evince granulomatous involvement, which includes giant cells (Figure 11.8).

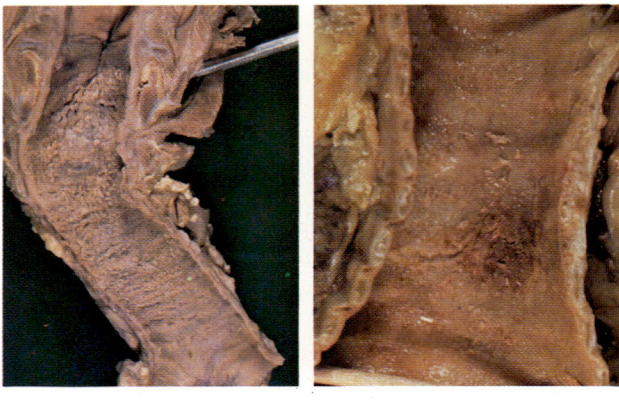

Figure 11.1 *Left:* The granular membranous 'bronchitis' typically seen in Wegener's granulomatosis. *Right:* A less diffuse, ulcerated area, sometimes seen in the upper respiratory tract of patients with Wegener's granulomatosis.

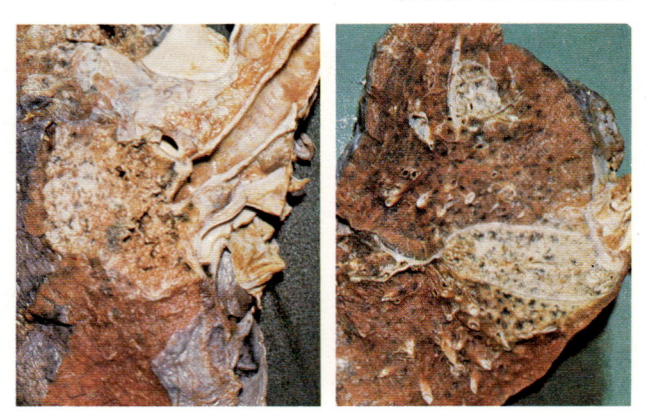

Figure 11.2 *Left:* A segmental pneumonia-like lesion which extended proximally to involve the bronchus at the level of bronchoscopic examination. The proximal bronchus and trachea appeared normal. *Right:* The upper lobe contains the common focal ill-defined area of necrosis whilst the middle lobe is involved in its entirety and had produced a 'segmental' radiological opacity.

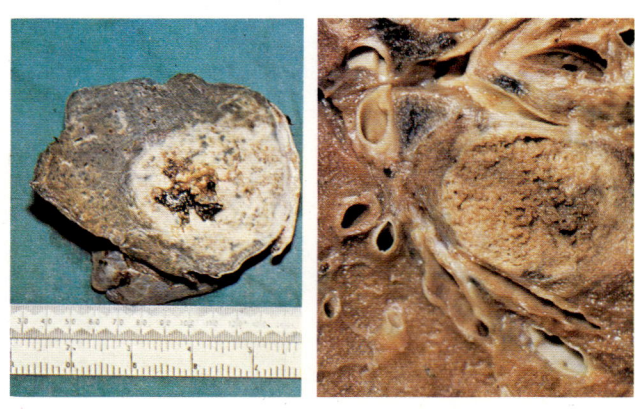

Figure 11.3 *Left:* A similar characteristic necrotic area now cavitating. *Right:* A more circumscribed grey-brown infarct-like area.

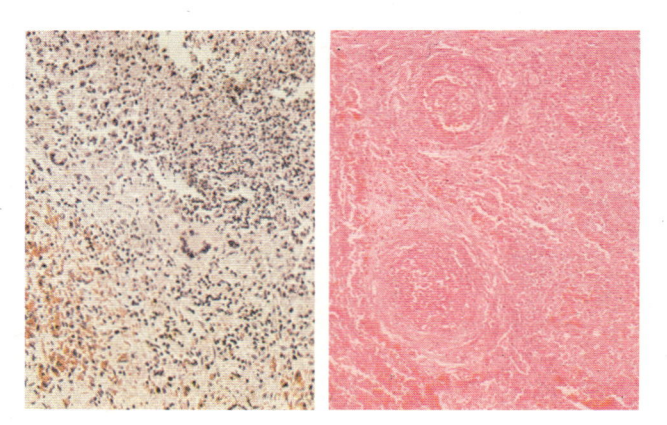

Figure 11.4 *Left:* Characteristic field of necrosis, inflammation, haemorrhage and scattered giant cells H&E × 96. *Right:* A haemorrhagic infarct-like area with outlines of the vasculitis visible. H&E × 38.4.

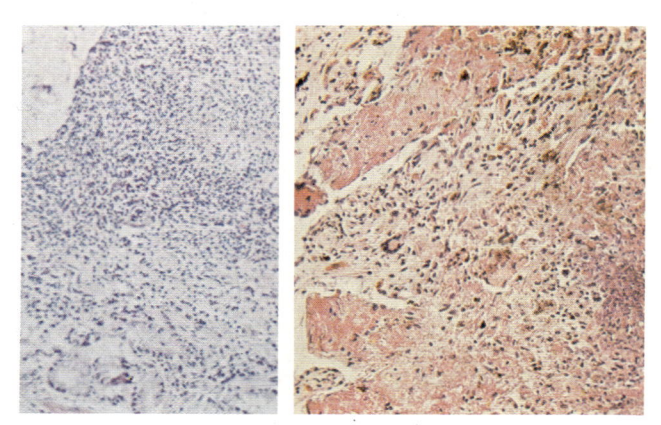

Figure 11.5 *Left:* Superficial non-specific inflammatory changes in a bronchus of a patient with Wegener's granulomatosis. H&E × 48. *Right:* A more characteristic appearance with chromatin-rich necrosis, scattered giant cells and a fibrinous intraalveolar exudate. H&E × 96.

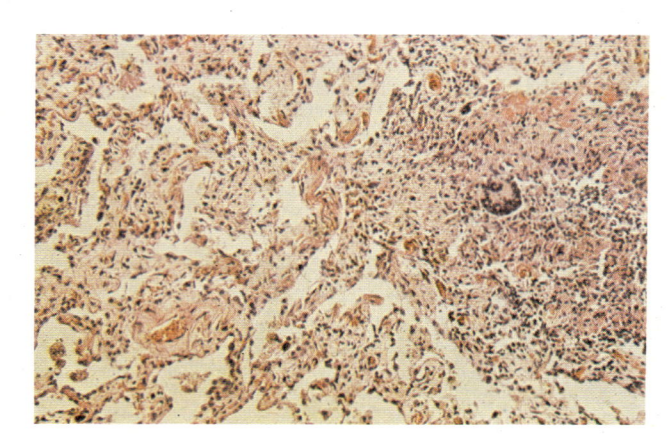

Figure 11.6 This reveals an accompanying non-specific interstitial pneumonitis (left) and a small necrotic focus with giant cells. H&E × 96.

PULMONARY ANGIITIDES

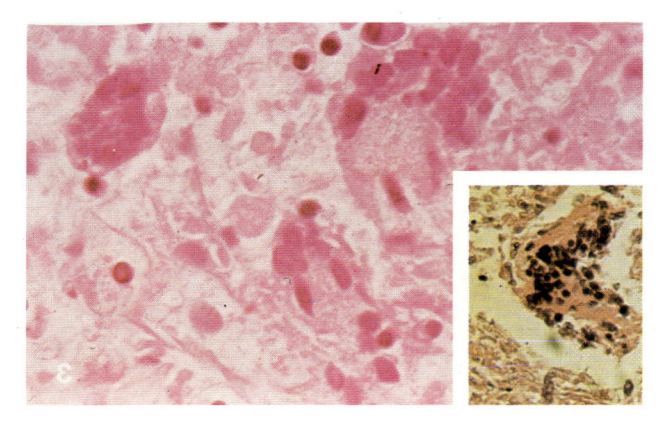

Figure 11.7 A selection of giant cells seen in Wegener's granulomatosis. H&E × 384. *Inset:* × 153.5.

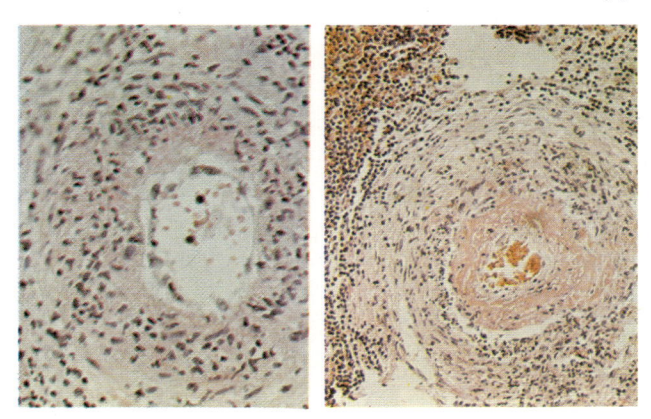

Figure 11.8 *Left:* An acute arteritis with fibrinoid necrosis and polymorphonuclear infiltrate. H&E × 153.6. *Right:* An arterial lesion with more extensive fibrinoid necrosis and a lighter cellular infiltrate. H&E × 48.

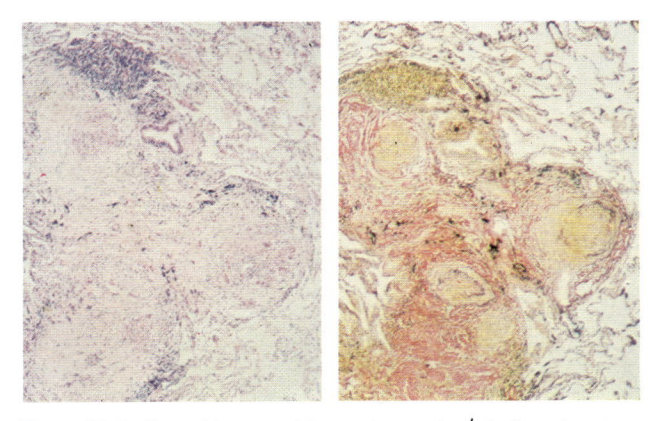

Figure 11.9 Necrotizing sarcoid granulomatosis. *Left:* Granulomatous lesions, apparently peribronchial. H&E × 24. *Right:* EVG demonstrates their vascular origin. EVG × 24.

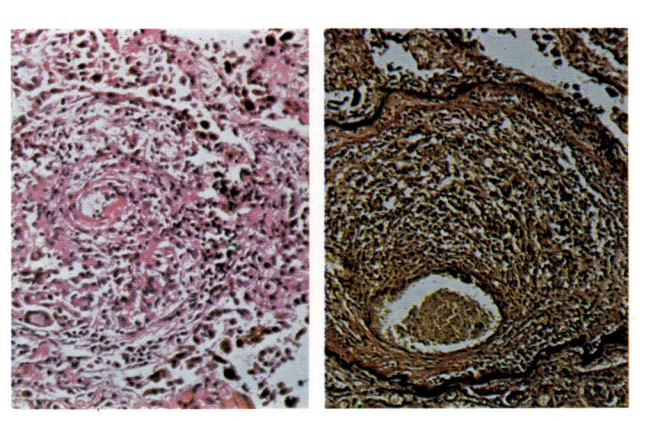

Figure 11.10 Necrotizing sarcoid granulomatosis. A pulmonary artery showing giant cell vasculitis with disorganization of the architecture and luminal narrowing. *Left:* H&E × 38.4. *Right:* EVG × 38.4.

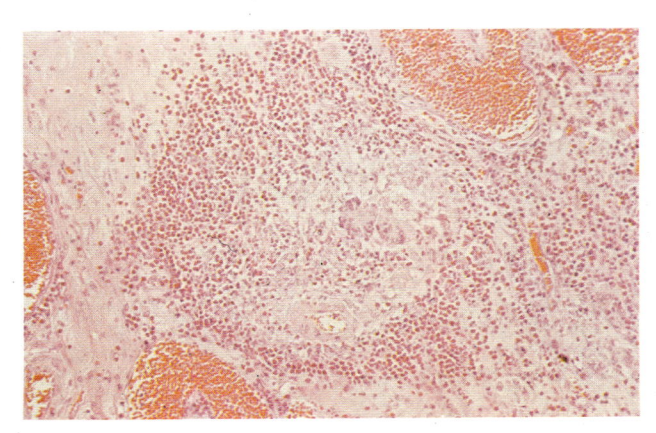

Figure 11.11 A patient with asthma and blood eosinophilia showing eosinophilic and granulomatous vasculitis – Churg Strauss Syndrome. H&E × 96.

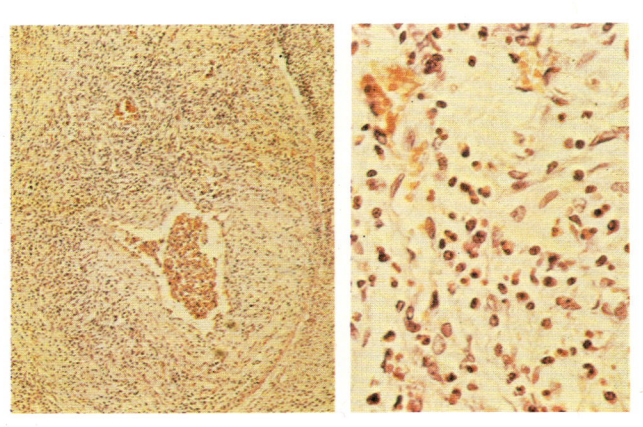

Figure 11.12 A 50-year-old male presenting to the respiratory unit with 'flu-like' illness who developed hypertension, proteinuria, haematuria and oedema. He died in renal failure. A systemic vasculitis was present. *Left:* A polymorphonuclear arteritis. H&E × 38.4. *Right:* Neutrophils and eosinophils mainly – overlap syndrome. H&E × 240.

Necrotizing Sarcoid Granulomatosis (NSG)

Liebow conceived this name for an ill-understood, rare, pulmonary condition of unknown aetiology, characterized by granulomatous vasculitis, sarcoid-like granulomata and parenchymal necrosis[4]. It shows certain similaritis to both sarcoidosis and Wegener's granulomatosis. In the original 11 cases described by Liebow the lesions appeared confined to lung, and there was a benign course responding to steroids. In a more recent study of 12 cases, six showed hilar node enlargement[5].

The lungs may show solitary or multiple bilateral nodules in this condition. The nodules range from a few millimetres to 4–5 cm in diameter, are grey and often appear necrotic[5].

The nodules consist of a central mass of confluent sarcoid-like granulomata, with discrete granulomata scattered around the periphery and in between the main masses. The granulomata are composed of epithelioid cells, Langhans giant cells and foreign body giant cells admixed with lymphocytes, histiocytes and fibroblasts. Necrosis, in contrast to typical sarcoidosis, is conspicuous even in small isolated granulomata. The necrosis varies from the entire central portion of a nodule to small single or multiple foci. Not infrequently, the central areas of the masses are hyalinized[5] (Figure 11.9).

Another striking feature of the condition is the marked vessel involvement by three types of inflammatory lesion[4]. The most characteristic is the presence of compact, structured, sarcoid-like granulomata related to both arteries and veins, with resultant part or total disorganization of their architecture (Figure 11.9). A second type consists of a looser collection of lymphoid cells and giant cell arteritis (Figure 11.10). The third type consists of a diffuse lymphocytic-plasma cell infiltrate affecting large and small arteries and veins with concomitant destruction of their walls.

Whenever this diagnosis is considered, appropriate stains and microbiological investigations should be conducted in order to exclude tuberculous and fungal infections. Allergic angiitis of Churg and Strauss can be ruled out by the relative paucity of eosinophils.

Churg et al.[5], based upon clinicopathological features of 12 cases, concluded that NSG was a variant of sarcoidosis. Two systematic studies of sarcoidosis revealed pulmonary vessel involvement in a considerable proportion of cases, but it was less extensive and much less severe than in NSG[6,7].

Allergic Granulomatosis and Angiitis of Churg and Strauss (CSS) and Polyarteritis Nodosa (PN)

Although closely related, these two disorders manifest several important differences (Table 11.1)[8]. CSS is rare and characterized by asthma, systemic necrotizing vasculitis and tissue eosinophilia with or without blood eosinophilia. The typical pathology consists of fibrinoid necrosis and eosinophilic infiltration of small arteries and veins. Epithelioid cell granulomata admixed with eosinophils may be located in the walls of vessels and in the extravascular tissue. In the lung, the appearance simulates eosinophilic pneumonia but with an additional prominent necrotizing vasculitic component (Figure 11.11).

Table 11.1 Major differentiating features between CSS and PN[8]

	Churg–Strauss Syndrome	Polyarteritis Nodosa
Allergic history (Asthma)	Usually present	Usually absent
Blood eosinophilia	Usually present	Usually absent
Pulmonary involvement	Common	Uncommon
Site of vessel involvement	Small and medium-sized muscular arteries, arterioles, capillaries and venules	Small and medium-sized muscular arteries
Aneurysms	Usually absent	Typically present
Histology	Eosinophils and granulomata	Polymorph neutrophils predominate. Eosinophils and granulomata inconspicuous or absent

By contrast, classic PN does not involve the lung and allergic histories are infrequent. PN characteristically exhibits aneurysms in medium-sized arteries. Microscopically the vessels show a polymorph neutrophil infiltrate in the acute stages, with varying degrees of fibrinoid necrosis. Eosinophils and granulomata are not usually evident.

Rose and Spencer[9], when describing PN with pulmonary involvement, were probably referring to CSS. However, occasionally cases manifest features of both disorders and are then best referred to as 'overlap syndrome'[8] (Figure 11.12).

References

1. Carrington, C. B., and Liebow, A. A. (1966). Limited forms of angiitis and granulomatosis of Wegener's type. *Am. J. Med.*, **41**, 497
2. Fauci, A. S., and Wolff, S. M. (1973). Wegener's granulomatosis: studies in eighteen patients and a review of the literature. *Medicine*, **52**, 535
3. Blennerhassett, J., Barrie, J., Lichter, I. and Taylor, A. J. (1976). Localised pulmonary Wegener's granuloma simulating lung cancer: a report of four cases. *Thorax*. **31**, 576
4. Liebow. A. A. (1973). The J. Burns Amberson Lecture – Pulmonary angiitis and granulomatosis. *Am. Rev. Resp. Dis.*, **108**, 1
5. Churg, A., Carrington, C. B. and Gupta, R. (1979). Necrotizing sarcoid granulomatosis. *Chest*, **76**, 406
6. Carrington, C. B., Gaensler, E. A., Mikens, J. P., Schachter, A. W., Burke, G. W. and Boff, A. M. (1976). Structure and function in sarcoidosis. *Ann. N.Y. Acad. Sci.*, **278**, 265
7. Rosen, Y., Moon, S., Huang, C., Gorrin, A. and Lyons, H. A. (1977). Granulomatous pulmonary angiitis in sarcoidosis. *Arch. Pathol. Med. Lab.*, **101**, 170
8. Fauci, A. S., Haynes, B. F. and Katz, P. (1978). The spectrum of vasculitis, clinical, pathological, immunologic and therapeutic considerations. *Ann. Intern. Med.*, **89**, 660
9. Rose, G. A. and Spencer, H. (1977). Polyarteritis nodosa. *Q. J. Med.*, **26**, 43

Diseases of Uncertain Aetiology 12

Pulmonary Amyloidosis

Amyloidosis involving the pulmonary system may be classified into three types: (a) tracheobronchial amyloidosis; (b) nodular parenchymal amyloidosis and (c) diffuse alveolar-septal amyloidosis. The tinctorial characteristics of the amyloid are the same in all types. It is amorphous, eosinophilic material which stains metachromatically with crystal violet and it fluoresces brightly with thioflavin T. Congo red stains it orange red, with apple green birefringence in polarized light. A peculiar tendency of all types of pulmonary amyloid is to form calcium, cartilage and bone and to excite a giant-cell reaction.

(a) *Tracheobronchial Amyloidosis*

Rarely amyloid may be deposited focally within the tracheobronchial tree to form a tumour, with consequent obstruction, or diffusely which may result in stenosis of the smaller bronchi[1]. The amyloid is laid down in the submucosa with resultant atrophy of bronchial mucous glands and cartilage[2]. In this type, amyloid is restricted to the lung (Figures 12.1 and 12.2).

(b) *Nodular Parenchymal Amyloidosis*

This occurs in the older age group, has a good prognosis and there is no underlying systemic disease[3].
Macroscopically, single or multiple, discrete, homogenous, waxy, grey nodules, composed of amyloid and measuring up to 8 cm in diameter, are located, usually in the subpleural region (Figure 12.3).

(c) *Diffuse Alveolar-Septal Amyloidosis*

This is the rarest type and is often associated with primary systemic amyloidosis, multiple myeloma, senescent cardiac amyloidosis and, very rarely, secondary amyloidosis. The severity of amyloid in the lung parallels that in the heart in these conditions[4]. This form has a very poor prognosis.
Macroscopically, the lungs appear heavy, bulky and have a rubber-sponge like appearance due to the amyloid deposited along alveolar septa and within vessels[5]. (Figure 12.4).

Pulmonary Corpora Amylacea

Discovered incidentally at autopsy, corpora amylacea are rounded, eosinophilic, acellular, lamellar, non-calcified structures usually lying free within the alveoli[2]. They excite little inflammatory reaction. They can usually be related to previous episodes of pulmonary oedema (Figure 12.5).

Pulmonary Alveolar Microlithiasis

A rare condition, usually manifesting in the fourth to sixth decades, a family history being obtained in approximately half the cases[6].
The lungs appear hard, incompressible, heavy (as much as 1500 g each) and are very difficult to cut.
Histologically, numerous concentrically laminate, calcified bodies (calcospherites) are evident within the alveoli. The alveolar walls show little fibrosis usually, but occasionally marked fibrosis and or chronic inflammatory infiltrate may be observed around the calcospherites (Figure 12.6). Groups of calcified bodies may sometimes be seen in the submucosa of bronchi[7].

Pulmonary Calcinosis

This is seen in association with disorders causing abnormalities in serum calcium and phosphorous levels, e.g. chronic renal disease, hyperparathyroidism and widespread skeletal metastases[2].
The lungs are heavy, gritty, rigid and cut section may reveal scattered nodules up to 0.5 cm diameter.
Calcification first occurs along the alveolar and bronchiolar basement membranes, and then within vessels, particularly pulmonary veins and venules (Figure 12.7). Further progression results in calcific masses distorting and thickening alveolar walls. These calcific masses may be surrounded by giant cells and fibrous tissue[8]. These calcific masses lack the concentric laminar structure of those in pulmonary alveolar microlithiasis.

Dystrophic Pulmonary Calcification

This is calcification occurring within already damaged lung tissue, in the absence of disorders of calcium and phosphorous metabolism. It may progress to bone formation. One of the most common causes is tubercle. An unusual form is the calcification which sometimes occurs within the exudate due to pneumocystis infection (Figure 12.8).

Pulmonary Ossification Associated With Mitral Stenosis

Bony masses, measuring up to 2 mm in diameter are seen frequently within the alveoli of patients with mitral stenosis. Attributed usually to organization of intra-alveolar oedema, it has never been explained satisfactorily why this particularly occurs in relationship to mitral stenosis (Figure 12.9).

DISEASES OF UNCERTAIN AETIOLOGY

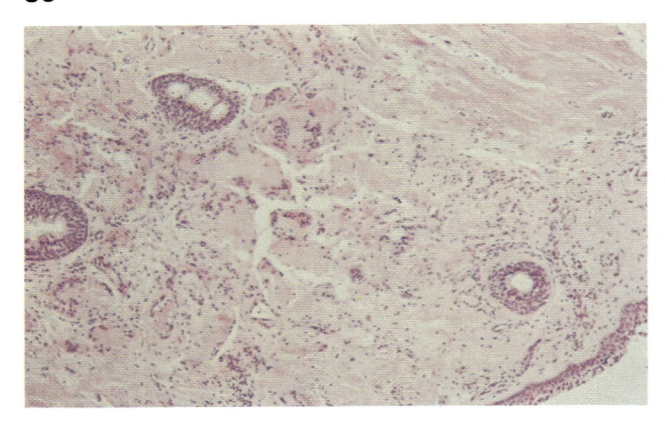

Figure 12.1 Amyloid deposited in the submucosa of a bronchus which has resulted in mucous-gland atrophy. There are giant cells present. H & E × 78.

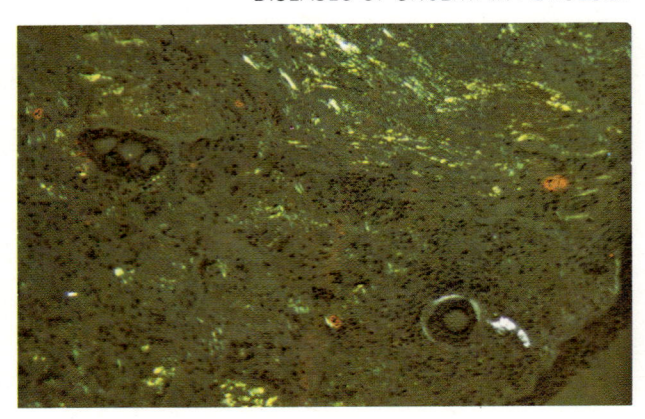

Figure 12.2 The same case as Figure 12.1 showing the apple green birefringence on Congo Red staining. Congo Red × 78.

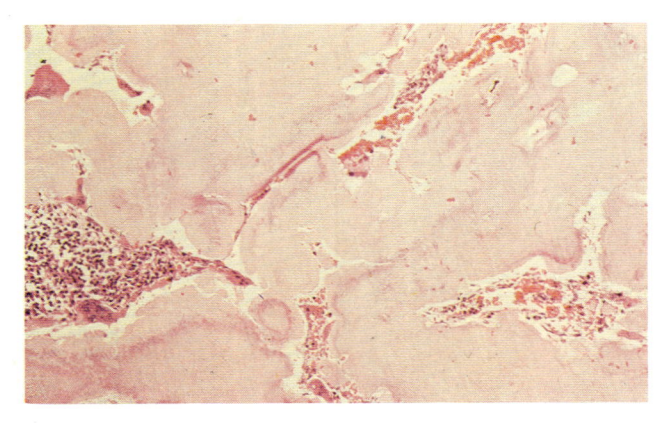

Figure 12.3 An elderly male found to have a pulmonary tumour at autopsy. Microscopy reveals amyloid in which calcification and ossification had occurred. There is an associated plasma cell infiltrate. H & E × 96.

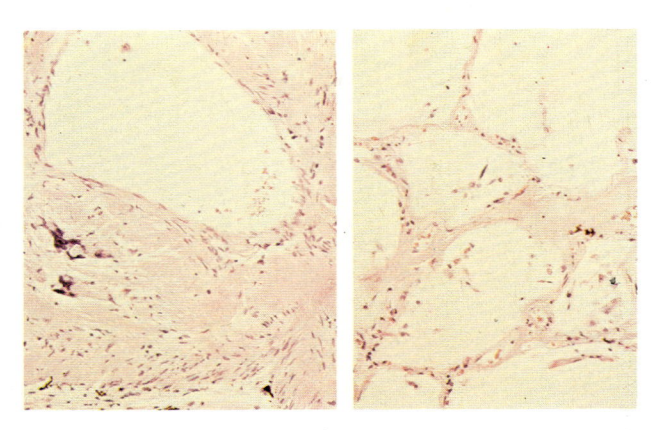

Figure 12.4 A patient with multiple myeloma who developed systemic amyloidosis. In the lung the amyloid is deposited *(left)* in the walls of vessels and *(right)* along the alveolar septa. H & E × 96.

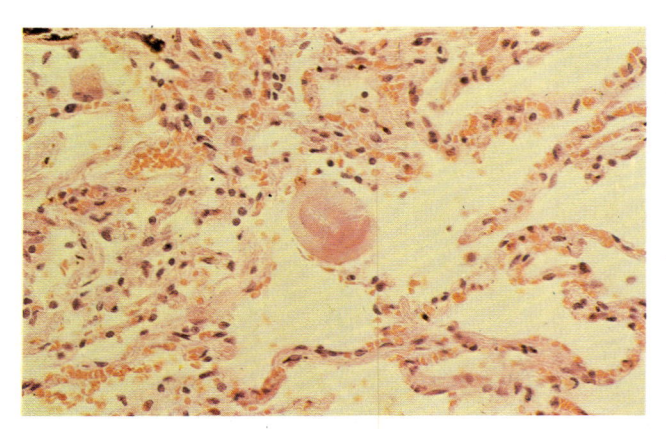

Figure 12.5 Patient dying in congestive cardiac failure. In the centre there is a rounded eosinophilic body – corpora amylacea – one of the many found incidentally on microscopy. H & E × 96.

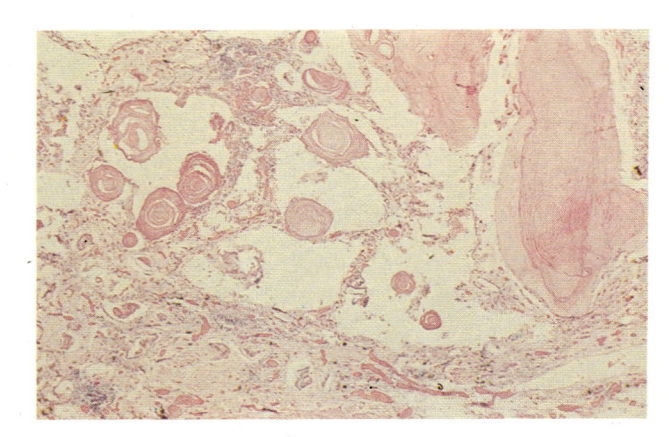

Figure 12.6 In this case of pulmonary alveolar microlithiasis there was considerable fibrosis in relation to the calcospherites, and bone formation in some of the subpleural regions. H & E × 96.

DISEASES OF UNCERTAIN AETIOLOGY

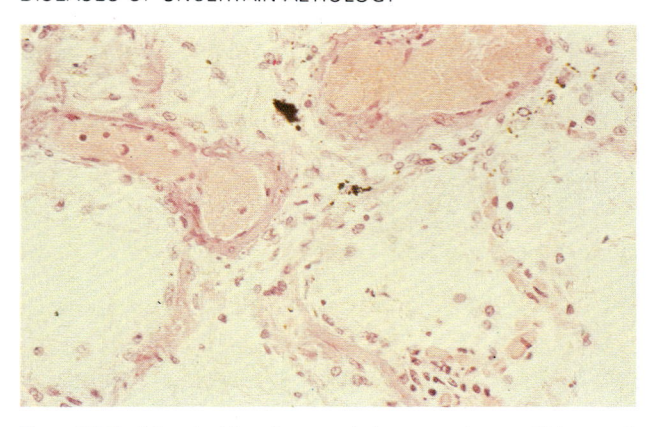

Figure 12.7 A female dying of metastatic breast carcinoma with hypercalcaemia showed pulmonary calcification in vessels and along alveolar walls. H&E × 240.

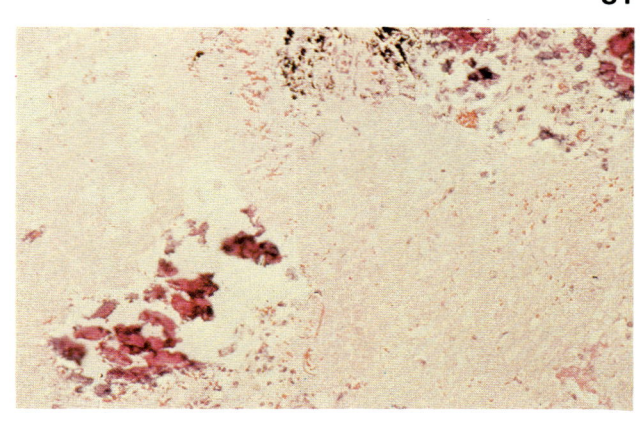

Figure 12.8 A renal transplant patient who died of pulmonary infection due to pneumocystis, cytomegalovirus and aspergillus. Foci of calcification were seen in the areas infected by pneumocystis. H&E × 96.

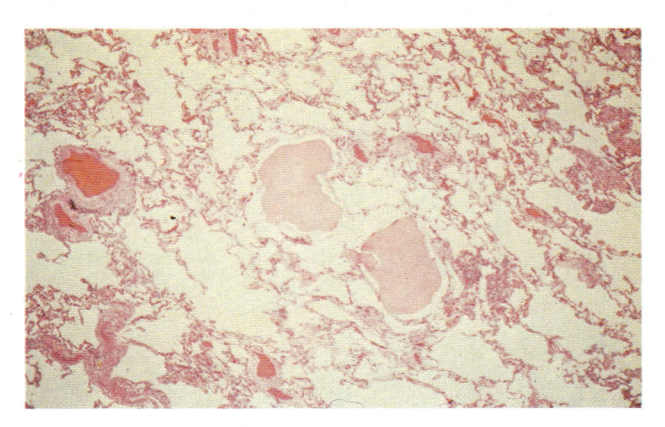

Figure 12.9 A patient with mitral stenosis. The lung shows congestion and intraalvaolar bone masses. H&E × 24.

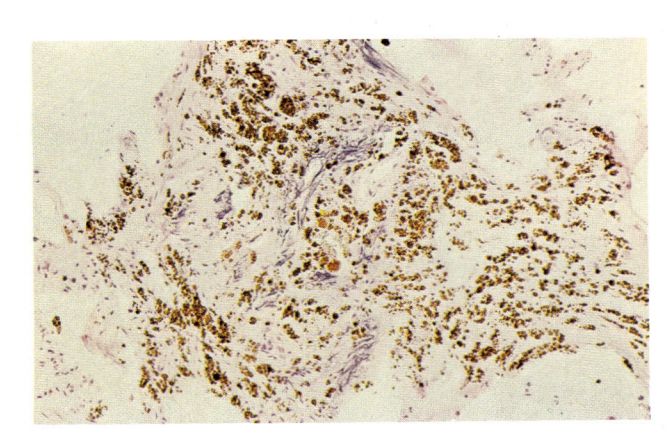

Figure 12.10 Patient with idiopathic pulmonary haemosiderosis, showing haemosiderin laden macrophages with iron encrustation and fragmentation of elastic. H&E × 240.

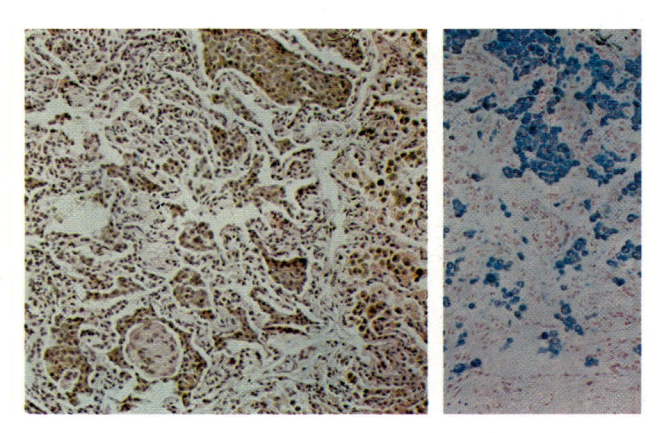

Figure 12.11 Patient with Goodpasture's Syndrome showing numerous haemosiderin laden macrophages. *Left:* H&E × 96. *Right:* Perl's × 24.

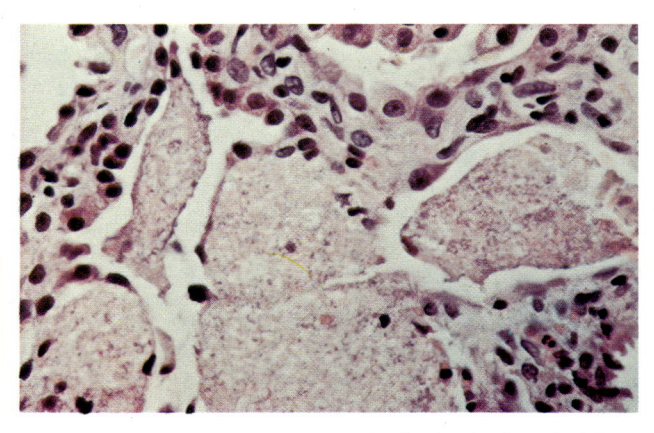

Figure 12.12 Patient with alveolar proteinosis, showing the typical alveolar exudate but more interstitial infiltrate than normal. H&E × 384.

Diffuse Intrapulmonary Haemorrhage

Excluding secondary causes such as chronic mitral stenosis and pulmonary veno-occlusive disease, idiopathic pulmonary haemosiderosis (IHP) and Goodpasture's Syndrome (GS) were the two main categories of primary diffuse intrapulmonary haemorrhage, formerly recognized according to clinicopathological criteria.

IHP usually affects children and young adults and is characterized by recurrent haemoptysis, progressive dyspnoea and pulmonary hypertension. Death follows within a few years of onset. The lung shows tortuosity and dilatation of alveolar capillaries, numerous haemorrhages and haemosiderin-containing macrophages within alveoli and bronchioles, and variable degrees of interstitial fibrosis. A considerable degree of fragmentation, thickening and encrustation of elastic fibrils by iron and calcium is normally present[9] (Figure 12.10). No renal involvement is present.

By contrast, GS refers to episodes of pulmonary haemorrhage accompanied by glomerulonephritis. In this condition the lung shows numerous haemorrhages and haemosiderin-containing macrophages within the alveoli and interstitium, but encrustation of elastic fibres by iron and calcium is seldom found (Figure 12.11).

It has been established that in practically all cases of GS an antibody to basement membrane of both lung and kidney is present. It is seen as a diffuse line along the basement membrane by immunofluorescence. By contrast, no immune mechanism has been demonstrated in IPH. Due to the immunopathological differences and the fact that lung haemorrhage can precede renal manifestations in GS by as much as one year[10], Thomas and Irwin[11] proposed that diffuse pulmonary haemorrhage should be classified according to immunopathological criteria into three types:

(a) One in which antibasement membrane antibody to lung and kidney is present. This corresponds to GS.
(b) One in which immune complexes can be demonstrated in the lung. This has been reported rarely in systemic lupus erythematosus.
(c) A type in which neither mechanism can be demonstrated. This corresponds to IPH.

This should enable a more precise diagnosis to be made, since clinicopathological features often overlap.

Alveolar Proteinosis

Alveolar proteinosis is characterized by filling of alveoli with amorphous, eosinophilic, proteinaceous material, which is strongly positive with periodic-acid–Schiff stain, and rich in lipid[12]. Interstitial infiltration by lymphoid cells, if present, is mild (Figure 12.12).

Diagnosis often has to be achieved by lung biopsy since the clinical features are often vague. Examination of sputum may be of help, since amorphous, eosinophilic, periodic-acid–Schiff-positive material may be present in this condition. Further, electron microscopic examination of sputum may reveal extracellular lamellar bodies, which are said to be highly characteristic of this disorder[13].

Corrin and King[14] have suggested that it is due to inadequate removal of surfactant, produced excessively in response to a variety of agents, e.g. silica and certain drugs. Human cases of acute silicosis have shown a similar histological picture to alveolar proteinosis, but there is in addition a severe interstitial chronic inflammatory infiltrate.

Alveolar proteinosis can be distinguished from pneumocystis infection by the foamy nature of the latter and the demonstration of the sickle shaped cysts by Gomori's methenamine silver stain.

References

1. Attwood, H. D., Price, C. G. and Riddell, R. J. (1972). Primary diffuse tracheobronchial amyloidosis. *Thorax*, **27**, 620
2. Spencer, H. (1977). *Pathology of the Lung*. 3rd. Edn. (Oxford: Pergamon Press)
3. Lee, S. and Johnson, H. A. (1975). Multiple nodular pulmonary amyloidosis. A case report and comparison with diffuse alveolar-septal pulmonary amyloidosis. *Thorax*, **30**, 178
14. Corrin, B. and King, E. (1970). Pathogenesis of experimental pulmonary alveolar proteinosis. *Thorax*, **25**, 230
4. Smith, R. R. C., Hutchins, G. M., Moore, G. W. and Humphrey, R. L. (1979). Type and distribution of pulmonary parenchymal and vascular amyloid. Correlation with cardiac amyloidosis. *Am. J. Med.*, **66**, 96
5. Poh, S. C., Tjia, T. S. and Seah, H. C. (1975). Primary diffuse alveolar septal amyloidosis. *Thorax*, **30**, 186
6. Thind, G. S. and Bhatia, J. L. (1978). Pulmonary alveolar microlithiasis. *Brit. J. Dis. Chest*, **72**, 151
7. Sears, M. R., Chang, A. R. and Taylor, A. J. (1971). Pulmonary alveolar microlithiasis. *Thorax*, **26**, 704
8. Heath, D. and Robertson, A. J. (1977). Pulmonary calcinosis. *Thorax*, **32**, 606
9. Soergel, K. H. and Sommers, S. C. (1962). The alveolar epithelial lesion of idiopathic pulmonary haemosiderosis. *Am. Rev. Resp. Dis.*, **85**, 540
10. Abboud, R. T., Chase, W. H., Ballon, H. S., Crzybowski, S. and Magil, A. (1978). Goodpasture's Syndrome: diagnosis by transbronchial lung biopsy. *Ann. Intern. Med.*, **89**, 635
11. Thomas, H. M. and Irwin, R. S. (1975). Classification of diffuse intrapulmonary haemorrhage. *Chest*, **68**, 483
12. Rosen, S. H., Castleman, B. and Liebow, A. A. (1958). Pulmonary alveolar proteinosis. *N. Engl. J. Med.*, **258**, 1123
13. Costello, J. F., Moriarty, D. C., Branthwaite, M. A., Turner-Warwick, M. and Corrin, B. (1975). Diagnosis and management of alveolar proteinosis: the role of electron microscopy. *Thorax*, **30**, 121

Occupational Lung Disorders – I. Coal and Silica

Occupational lung disease may be a consequence of inhalation of fumes, gases, dusts or infectious agents at the place of work. By convention, pneumoconiosis implies fibrosis of the lungs due to the inhalation of a variety of dusts. (Fumes consist of metal oxides ranging in size from 0.1 to 1 μm; dust refers to solid particles dispersed in a gaseous medium such as air.) Most particles of larger size are eliminated from the lungs by the mucociliary apparatus, but particles of 2 μm or less reach the alveoli where they may remain, particularly when the macrophage clearance mechanisms are overwhelmed. The dust particles tend to collect in the alveoli around fixed points, such as around vessels, septa, respiratory bronchioles and beneath the pleura. Some may accumulate in the alveoli of the respiratory bronchioles.

The consequences of this particle accumulation can involve a wide range of pathological responses: fibrogenesis with crystaline silica, granulomatous reactions with beryllium, purely destructive with cadmium and occasionally, as with asbestos, neoplasia (Table 13.1). Factors which influence the reaction are the physiochemical characteristics of the material, concentration and duration of exposure, immunological factors and the co-existence of other pulmonary diseases. An accurate diagnosis can be inferred from the pathological appearances sometimes, but more often the pathologist can only suggest the agent(s) which are the likely cause of the response. Often the pathologist is the first to suggest the possibility of an occupational disease. A history of exposure to specific agents or further analytical procedures, e.g. energy-dispersive X-ray analysis, may be of benefit in rendering a specific diagnosis. Exposures to multiple agents are not infrequent and mixed tissue reactions may occur. The pathologist may be the final arbiter in determining whether a disease is occupational in origin and compensation paid.

No attempt will be made to provide a fully comprehensive description of the pathological changes caused by the vast number of agents capable of producing environmental lung disease. Exposure to coal dust will be dealt with in detail as it is common and interpretation still somewhat controversial, and it serves as a model for examination of occupational lung disease. Silicosis- and asbestosis-related disease will be dealt with in detail as they represent important and different pulmonary responses.

Coal Workers' Pneumoconiosis

The composition of the dust which accumulates in coal miner's lung is complex and is determined by a variety of factors, including the nature of the coal mined, often referred to as its rank, and the type of mining job executed. There also appears to be considerable individual variation in ability to clear dust from the lungs. A high silica content in mine dust (greater than 18%) results in the pathological picture of silicosis[1] rather than conventional coal worker's pneumoconiosis.

One would have surmised that with the vast volume of literature on the subject, the clinical–radiological–pathological relationships would have been well understood and no controversial issues remain. This is far from being the case. In this account the authors will indicate those factors generally accepted, and their own experience and views on the more controversial issues.

Examination of the Lung

First of all, we suggest a plan for systematically examining the lung in coal workers' pneumoconiosis which can also be utilized for other pneumoconioses. It can equally apply to an ordinary fixed section of whole lung or to a Gough–Wentworth whole lung section[2]. However, it must be stressed that the lung should be well inflated for accurate assessment. Table 13.2 illustrates the form which we use to record the pulmonary pathological findings in cases

Table 13.1 Types of reaction to occupational hazards

Type of reaction	Example
Dust accumulation with minimal reaction	Tin, titanium
Stellate nodules with mild collagenization	Coal worker's pneumoconiosis
Discrete circumscribed nodules with marked collagenization	Silicosis
Interstitial fibrosis	Asbestosis
Extrinsic allergic bronchiolo-alveolitis	Farmer's lung, bird fancier's lung
Diffuse alveolar damage	Fumes of nitrogen, cadmium and sulphur
Sarcoid-like reaction	Berylliosis
Bronchiolitis obliterans	Silofillers disease
Desquamative interstitial pneumonia	Asbestos, tungsten carbide
Emphysema	Cadmium
Obstructive airways disease	Toluene diisocyanate
Infections	Tubercle in silicosis
Neoplasia	Carcinoma related to nickel and arsenic exposure; mesothelioma related to asbestos exposure

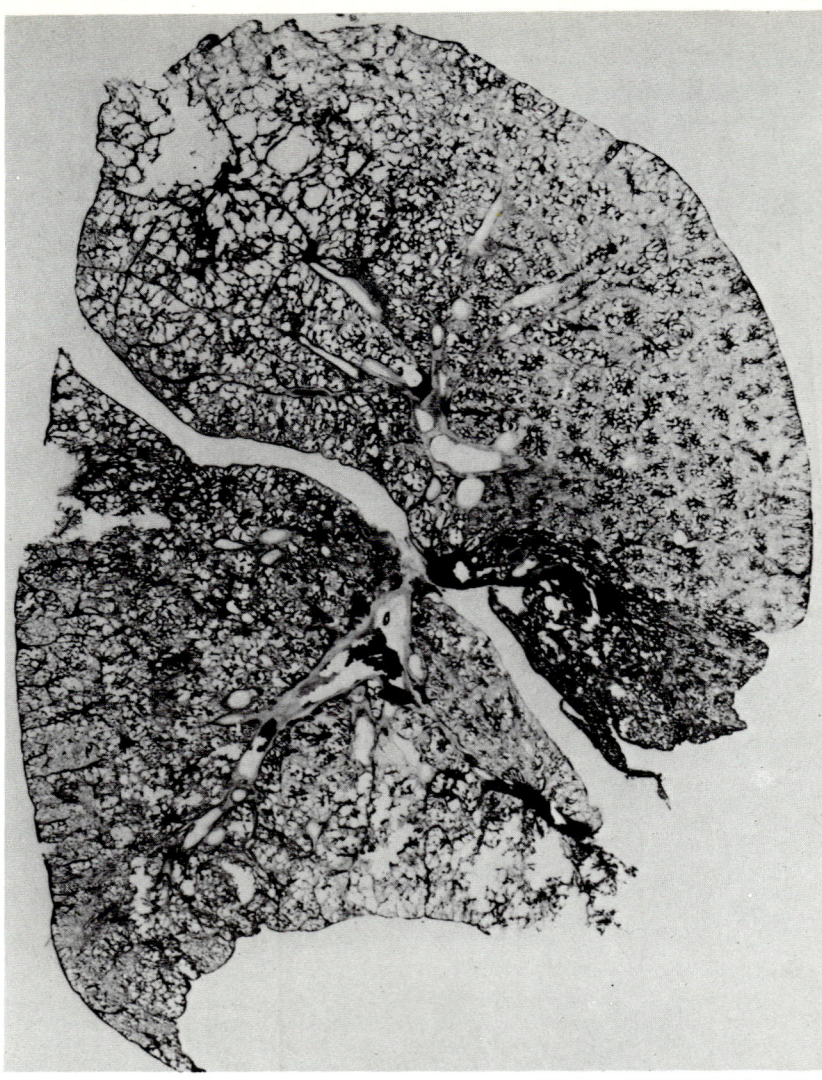

Figure 13.1 A 'Gough–Wentworth' whole lung section taken from a 72-year-old male, who had worked underground for 24 years (assistant collier, conveyor operator, underground labourer for different periods) up until 1964. He had been a light to moderate cigarette smoker. Assessment of chest radiographs by the Pneumoconiosis Panel was given as category 2 simple pneumoconiosis in 1956, category 1/2 simple pneumoconiosis in 1963, category 1 simple pneumoconiosis in 1976. He was assessed at 5% disability in 1976. Serial spirometry tests over the period showed an obstructive profile; the last results (1973) were FEV_1 of 1.5 l and an FVC of 2.0 l. His demise was considered to be due to bronchopneumonia, cor pulmonale and chronic obstructive airways disease.

Pathologically the lung was assessed at: primary dust foci – Grade 2, extent 3; secondary foci (stellate) – 3 less than 0.5 cm, 3 between 0.5 and 2 cm; centrilobular emphysema – Grade 2/3, extent 3.

This case questions the current view that emphysema in simple pneumoconiosis is non-occupational and illustrates that on occasion radiology varies inversely with pulmonary damage and disability.

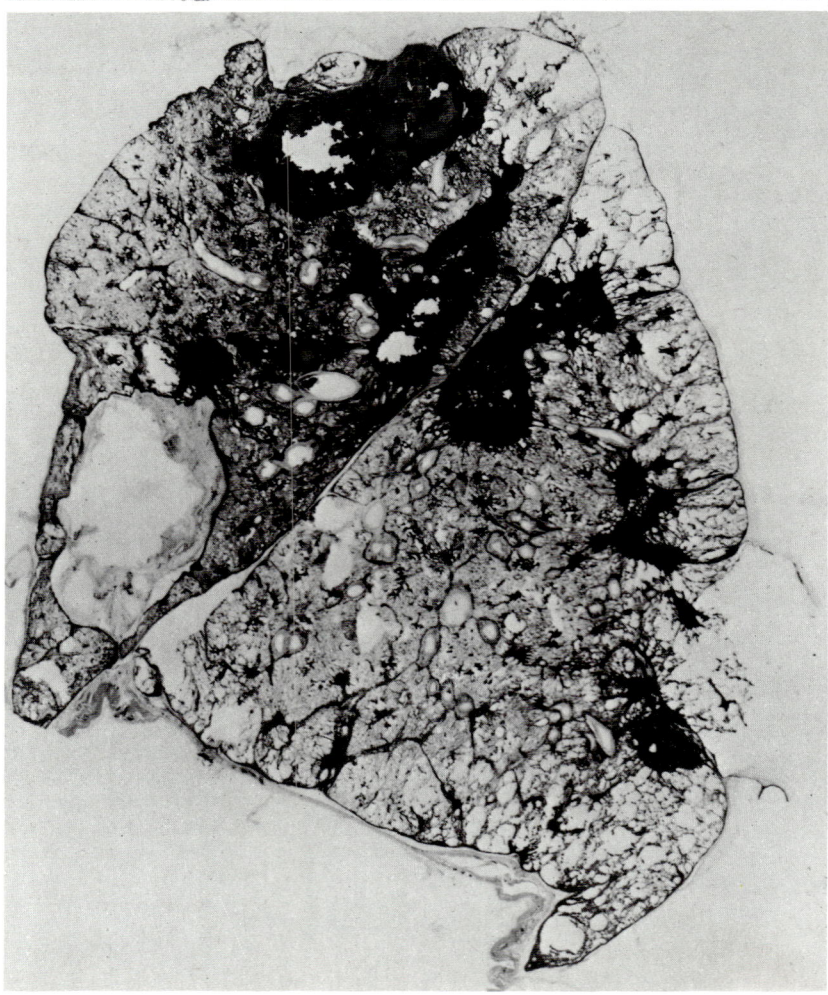

Figure 13.5 A 'Gough–Wentworth' whole lung section from an 86-year-old coal miner who had worked underground, including at the coal face, for 47 years (collier, fireman and deputy) up to 1960. He had not smoked since 1962. Assessment of chest radiographs by the Pneumoconiosis Panel was given as category 3 simple pneumoconiosis in 1954, category 3 simple with an A shadow (complicated pneumoconiosis) in 1961, category 3 simple with B shadow (complicated pneumoconiosis) in 1969, and category 3 simple with C shadows (complicated pneumoconiosis) in 1975. In 1979 he was assessed at 80% disability. Serial spirometry tests over the period showed an obstructive profile – FEV_1 of 1.5 l and FVC of 2.6 l in 1969. Death was considered to be a result of cor pulmonale secondary to complicated pneumoconiosis.

Pathologically, the lung was assessed: primary dust foci – Grade 2, extent 2; secondary dust foci (stellate) – 6 less than 0.5 cm, 5 between 0.5 and 2.0 cm, 3 greater than 2 cm; no circumscribed secondary dust foci; centrilobular emphysema – Grade 1, extent 2/3; ?? irregular emphysema and fine honeycombing in the posterior basal segment of the lower lobe.

This illustrates progression of complicated pneumoconiosis after cessation of exposure and that disability in complicated pneumoconiosis is a summation of the extent of the complicated pneumoconiosis and degree of emphysema; the lesser degree of epmhysema in this case probably accounting for longevity.

OCCUPATIONAL LUNG DISORDERS – I. COAL AND SILICA

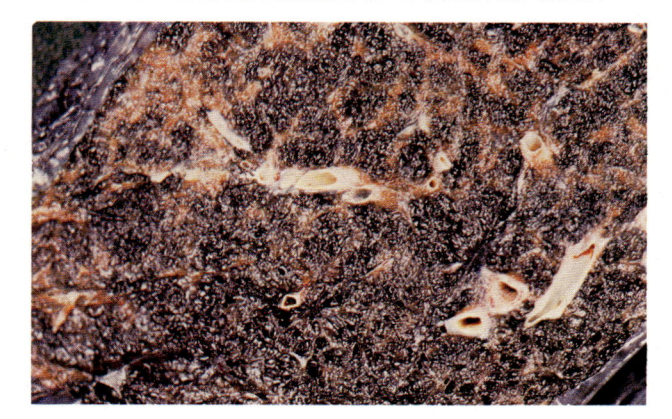

Figure 13.2 Close-up of the slice taken for Gough–Wentworth section in Figure 13.1 after alcohol immersion, illustrating the combination of moderate-sized dust foci with both moderate (top) and severe emphysema (bottom).

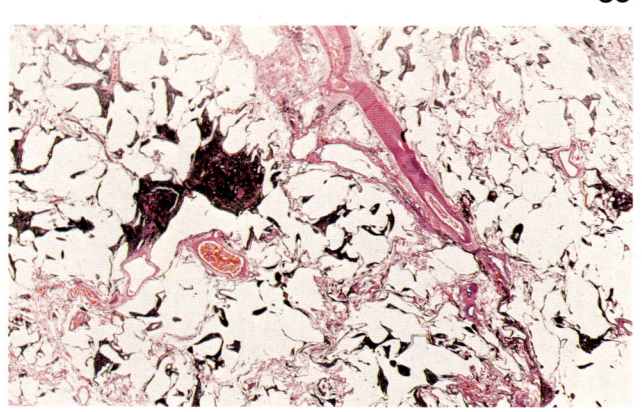

Figure 13.3 Taken from the RUL of Figure 13.1 where there were moderate-sized dust foci and moderate to severe emphysema. The slide illustrates a slightly collagenous central dust focus, destructive emphysema, designated centrilobular, in that several normal-sized alveolar sacs can be seen at the periphery of the lobule (bottom left). There is extension of the central dust focus irregularly along the interstitium.

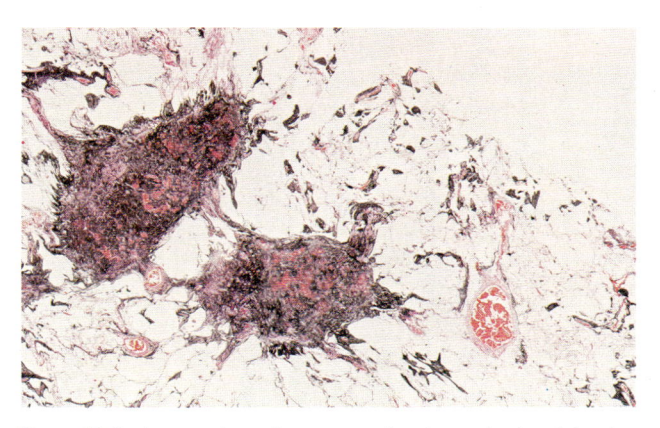

Figure 13.4 A somewhat collagenous stellate 'secondary' nodule taken from the middle lobe of Figure 13.1.

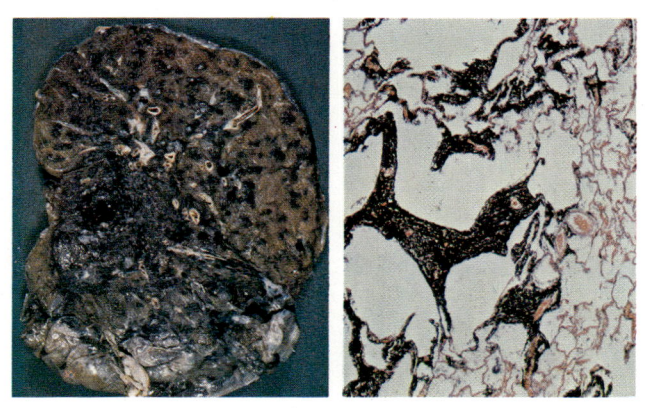

Figure 13.6 *Left:* The centrolateral lung showed PMF in the apical lower segment (a common site) with moderate-sized primary dust foci in the background. There is a small emphysematous bulla in the posterior basal segment. There is much non-emphysematous functional lung tissue, particularly in the upper lobe. *Right:* A non-collagenous primary dust focus, from the same lung, with the distended respiratory bronchioles (focal emphysema). The surrounding alveolar sacs appear relatively normal.

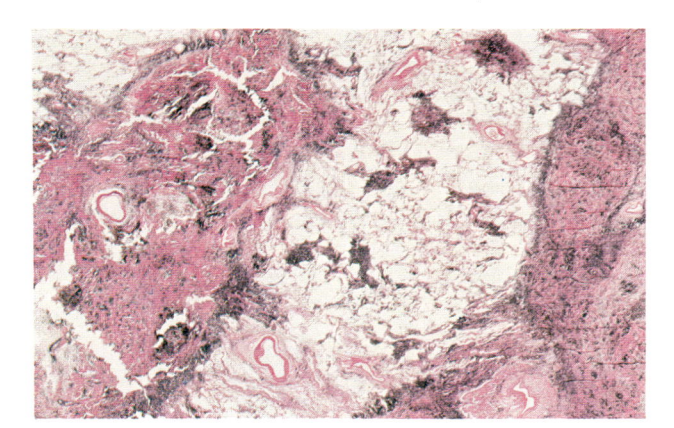

Figure 13.7 Edge of the massive lesion from the upper lobe showing collagen, dust-laden macrophages, some amorphous material and thickening of pulmonary vessels.

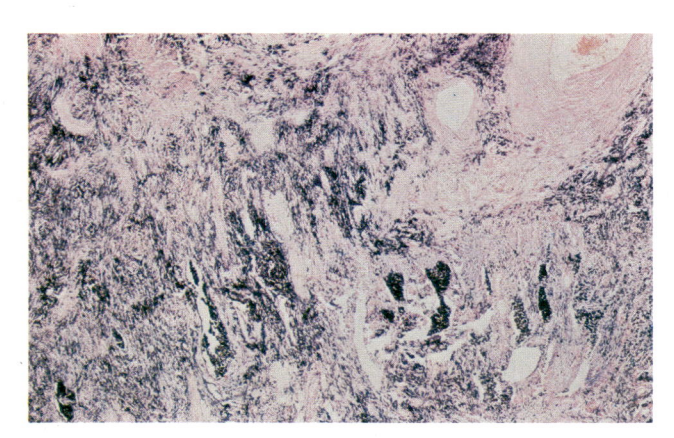

Figure 13.8 This is taken from a massive fibrotic lesion and reveals a random admixture of anthracotic pigment, some still within macrophages, collagen, chronic inflammatory cells, a thickened pulmonary artery (top right) and coal-dust pigmentation extending through the nearby bronchi.

Table 13.2 Macroscopical assessment of the lungs of miners

Primary dust foci (soft stellate)

Average size (1-3 scale)	Proportions of lobules involved
0	0
1	1 (< 33%)
2	2 (33-66%)
3	3 (66-100%)

Secondary dust foci

Stellate	Circumscribed
Absent	Absent
No. - (< 0.5 cm)	No. - (< 0.5 cm)
No. - (0.5-2.0 cm)	No. - (0.5-2.0 cm)
No. - (> 2.0 cm)	No. - (> 2.0 cm)

Dust impregnated interlobular septa	Generalized pleural thickening
0	0
1	1
2	2
3	3

Emphysema
Type: centrilobular, panacinar, irregular plus fine honeycombing.

Severity in average affected lobules	Proportion of lobules involved		
	Whole lung	Upper lobes	Lower lobes
0	0	0	0
1	1	1	1
2	2	2	2
3	3	3	3

of pneumoconiosis. The lesions which occur in 'simple pneumoconiosis' can be divided into two main types:

(a) *Primary (macular) coal dust foci* are widely distributed, focal, impalpable, stellate lesions centrilobularly located, often with a cluster of dilated respiratory bronchioles (focal emphysema).

(b) *Secondary (nodular) coal dust foci* are larger, few in number, irregularly distributed, palpable lesions which can be subdivided into (i) stellate and (ii) circumscribed nodules. They contain an increased amount of collagen, accounting for their palpability. Their pathogenesis is uncertain but the presence of higher silica content in the mine dust, a rheumatoid diathesis or mycobacterial infection are factors which have been considered.

The whole of a lung slice is examined macroscopically and the average size of primary dust foci (recorded on a 0-3 scale) and the proportion of involved lobules (0-3 scale - 1, up to 33%; 2, up to 66%; 3, more than 60%) are recorded. Emphysema is similarly assessed and recorded and categorized as to whether it is centrilobular (including focal emphysema), panacinar, or irregular. No attempt is made to distinguish between focal emphysema and the so-called centrilobular emphysema of Gough and Leopold[3]. This may require additional examination, including conventional histological sections and 5 × 5 cm sections from large blocks. The latter are particularly useful since they can be projected and the relationship of the changes to the lobule more readily appreciated.

The number of stellate and rounded secondary dust foci are recorded within different size ranges (less than 5 mm, 5-20 mm, over 20 mm).

Other features recorded on a semiquantitative basis include dust-impregnated interlobular septa and pleural thickening. Central lymph nodes are also assessed according to the degree of pigmentation, whether the capsule is breached by the dust-laden macrophages, or whether there is concomitant involvement of the related bronchus or pulmonary artery. Figures 13.1-13.11 illustrate the way in which we assess the lungs in pneumoconiosis.

It is hoped that recording the results in this way will eventually solve the problem of whether and how emphysema is related to coal worker's pneumoconiosis, whether there is association with interstitial fibrosis, and provide more meaningful correlations between pathological, radiological, physiological and clinical features.

When a pathologist is required to determine whether pneumoconiosis is a causative factor in the death of a patient, no argument will ensue if complicated pneumoconiosis is stated to be a factor. However, simple pneumoconiosis, regardless of the profusion of dust lesions, is not thought to cause any significant clinical disability and therefore cannot be regarded as a factor in causing death. However, when a coal miner dies from emphysema, the role of coal dust in its causation is controversial *(vide infra)*.

Pathologists are expected to retain the heart and both lungs, at least one of which should be properly inflated, for inspection by the Pneumoconiosis Medical Panel. They advise the insurance officer as to whether pneumoconiosis materially influenced the cause of death. It is prudent for the histopathologist to be sure of his ground, as disagreement with the panel can result in long, drawn out procedures, involving a local appeals tribunal (predominantly medical), and then a national insurance commissioner (a lawyer).

Simple Pneumoconiosis

In this type no dust lesion measuring greater than 2 cm diameter is present by definition. As stated above, the essential lesion is the primary coal-dust focus - a collection of coal dust containing macrophages admixed with reticulin and minimal collagen. The lesions show a predilection for the upper lobes; free silica appears unnecessary for their development[4,5].

Often present around these dust foci are enlarged respiratory bronchioles - focal emphysema, which as Heppleston has shown is non-destructive of the acinar anatomy, except possibly in the very largest lesions[6].

The presence of focal emphysema and marked pigmentation relative to the small amount of collagen production distinguishes the simple dust lesion of coal workers from the silicotic nodule.

Complicated Pneumoconiosis (Pulmonary Massive Fibrosis)

Pulmonary massive fibrosis (PMF) is arbitrarily defined as pneumoconiosis with dust lesions greater than 2 cm in diameter. The degree of background simple pneumoconiosis is usually marked.

The lesions are solid or cavitated, black, homogenous, may cut easily with a knife and generally are well demarcated. The massive lesions are usually situated in proximity to the fissure in the posterior segment of the upper lobes and upper portions of the lower lobes. Cavitation may be the result of ischaemic necrosis or tubercle. A black inky fluid, containing cholesterol, lies within the cavity. Infiltration of the adventitia and media of muscular arteries by dust-laden cells, often with endarteritis, is frequently seen in tissue at the margins of complicated pneumoconiosis.

Histologically, the massive lesions consist of a haphazard arrangement (cf. silicosis) of reticulin fibres, collagen fibres, coal dust, proteinous material and scattered lymphocytes and plasma cells. A small quantity of crystaline silica may be seen at the periphery of the lesion by polarized light.

PMF lesions, particularly the more severe ones, are associated with respiratory difficulties and premature death and therefore can be considered the major or a contributing factor to death in appropriate circumstances.

PMF lesions may continue to enlarge after the person has left the mine. Factors which hve been implicated in its pathogenesis include mycobacterial infection, immunological factors, silica and individual idiosyncrasy.

Caplan Lesions (Rheumatoid Pneumoconiosis)[7]

Caplan lesions are usually multiple, round, necrobiotic nodules occurring in a background of pneumoconiosis, due to a variety of dusts, and often of no more than slight degree (Figures 13.12 and 13.13). Macroscopically, they are difficult to distinguish from silicotic nodules, in some instances, and caseous tuberculous foci. As in tuberculous lesions, careful inspection will reveal concentric dust laminations suggesting episodes of inflammatory activity followed by quiescence. Central liquefaction and calcification may occur. The rheumatoid nature of these Caplan lesions, in most instances, is charactrized by overt inflammatory activity, often around basophilic necrotic zones with neutrophils and macrophages, and often a pallisaded layer of fibroblasts with a small round cell infiltrate rich in plasma cells (Figure 13.14). This appearance is readily distinguished from tuberculosis.

In some lesions, however, the external capsule is entirely collagenous when it is impossible to decide between 'burnt-out' Caplan lesions and well-encapsulated tuberculosis (Figure 13.15).

Apart from endarteritic lesions of vessels in the centre and periphery of the lesions a frequent feature is infiltration of the walls of pulmonary arteries by lymphocytes and plasma cells (Figure 13.15).

Caplan nodules may occur in other pneumoconioses, e.g. asbestosis, silicosis, and china-clay workers.

Relationship of Emphysema to CWP

It is generally accepted that focal (anatomically non-destructive) emphysema is related to coal workers' pneumoconiosis, but it results in no clinical disability. The controversial issue is whether the centrilobular emphysema of Leopold and Gough[3] is related to CWP. Several authors maintain that this pattern of emphysema is related to smoking rather than to coal dust exposure[8]. However, it must be realized that those who deny a relationship between CWP and the non-focal types of emphysema have based their findings on epidemiological and radiological studies, whereas the consensus of pathological opinion would regard non-focal types of emphysema as not uncommon with coal miners pneumoconiosis. A recent study in South Wales has shown that the degree of emphysema central in the lobules increases with the degree of primary dust foci and that this could occur in non-smoking subjects with simple and early complicated pneumoconiosis[2].

Interstitial Fibrosis in Coal Workers

We have been surprised at the number of coal workers' lungs which have exhibited interstitial fibrosis (pigmented and/or unpigmented). This has sometimes been recognized macroscopically as overt honeycombing, but in many cases only by projection of 5 × 5 cm sections or microscopy[9] (Figure 13.16). Only a small proportion could be explained by the presence of other diseases, such as extrinsic allergic bronchioloalveolitis and cryptogenic fibrosing alveolitis (Figure 13.16). The precise significance of this finding and its pathogenesis requires further study.

Graphite Pneumoconiosis

Workers exposed to carbon may develop simple or complicated pneumoconiosis which is indistinguishable from coal worker's pneumoconiosis.

Pneumoconiosis Due to Silica

Particles of silicon dioxide (silica) dust measuring between $0.5\,\mu m$ and $5.0\,\mu m$ are most likely to cause silicosis. However, the physical nature of silica determines, to a great extent, its fibrogenic quality – amorphous silica being least and crystalline tridymite the most fibrogenic. Acute silicosis results from inhalation of large quantities of finely particulate silica (e.g. in sandblasting).

Four forms of lung disease may result from free silica:

(1) Acute silicosis
(2) Nodular silicosis
(3) Mixed dust fibrosis
(4) Interstitial fibrosis.

Acute Silicosis

Inhalation of a high concentration of finely particulate crystalline silica results in a pathological picture similar to that of alveolar proteinosis. The alveoli are filled by eosinophilic, amorphous exudate which is PAS positive and the interstitium shows a prominent lymphoid infiltrate with a variable amount of fibrosis. (The interstitial element is usually absent in alveolar proteiniosis). Energy dispersive X-ray analysis reveals a large amount of silica within the lung tissue, but this may not be identified on conventional polarization. Granulomata, resembling those of sarcoid, have occasionally been described in these cases[10].

OCCUPATIONAL LUNG DISORDERS – I. COAL AND SILICA

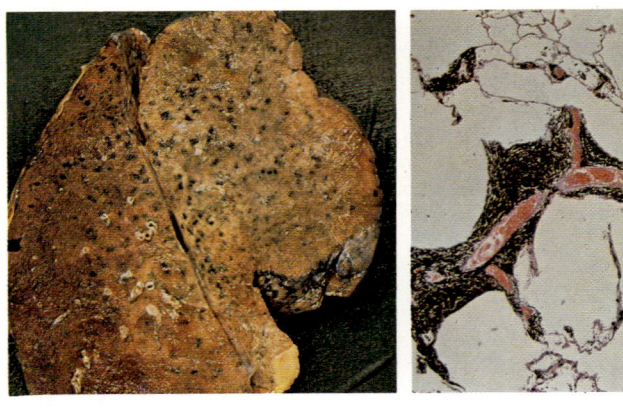

Figure 13.9 *Left:* Part of a lung slice from a 56-year-old man with less than 10 years mining history, showing Grade 1 central dust foci occupying one third of the lung lobules, with minimal related emphysema. *Right:* Part of a central dust focus with presumed non-destructive (focal) emphysema. H&E × 16.8.

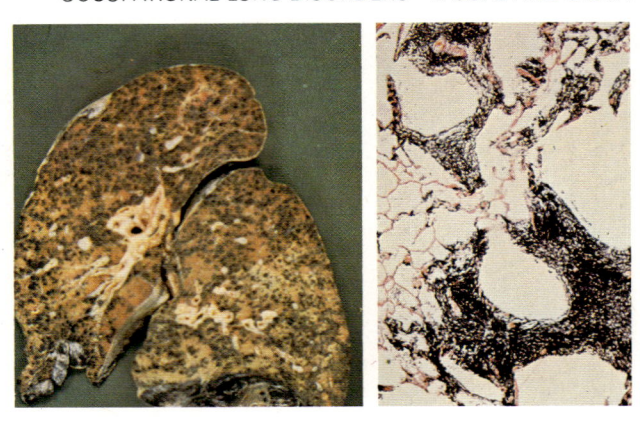

Figure 13.10 *Left:* Moderate-size (Grade 2) central dust foci occupying over two thirds (Grade 3) of the lung lobules. Emphysema was assessed as moderate (Grade 2). *Right:* a non-collagenous soft central dust focus; the emphysematous spaces probably represent dilated respiratory bronchioles. Adjacent alveolar sacs are normal. H&E × 16.8.

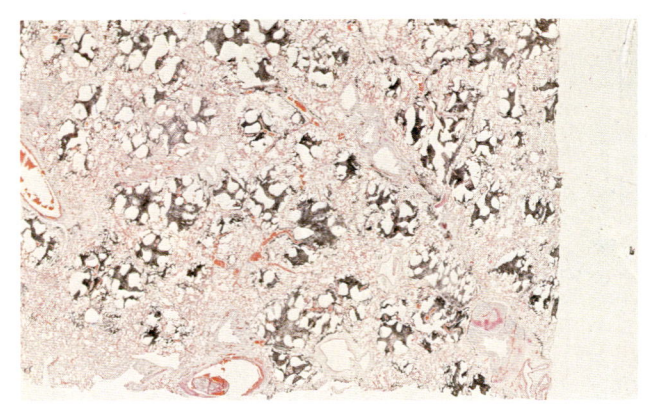

Figure 13.11 A 5 × 5 cm block taken from the right upper lobe of Figure 13.10 showing the appearance of Grade 2 in 20 μm sections. The degree of emphysema is now more easily assessible.

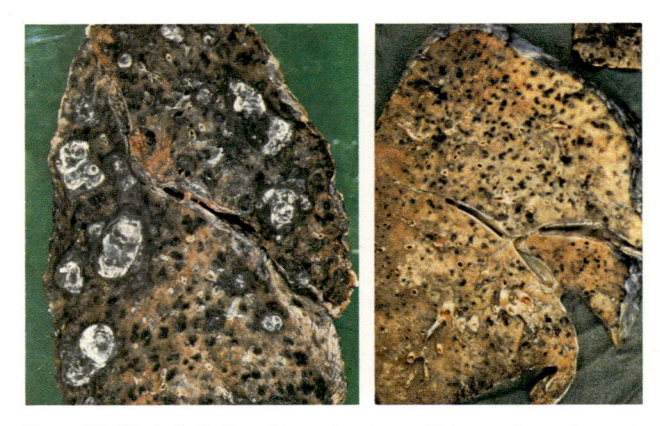

Figure 13.12 *Left:* Portion of lung showing multiple conglomerate, partly calcified Caplan lesions. The dust foci are larger and more numerous than is usual. *Right:* Portion of a lung with sparse dust foci, but several small circumscribed nodules. Alongside is a characteristic subpleural Caplan lesion.

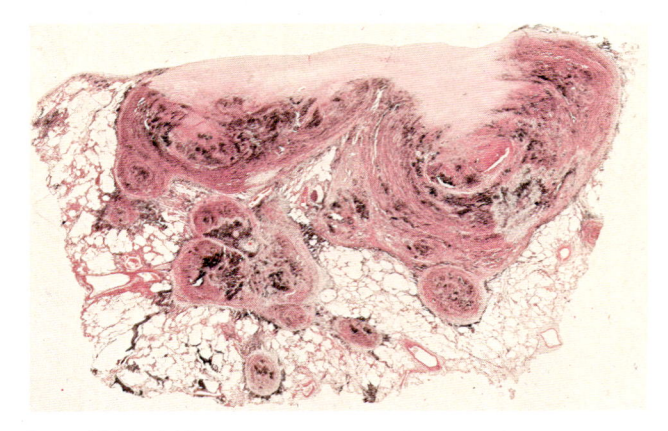

Figure 13.13 A 20 μm section of the latter (Figure 13.12, right) revealing the characteristic pleural thickening and the coalescence of the laminated lesions.

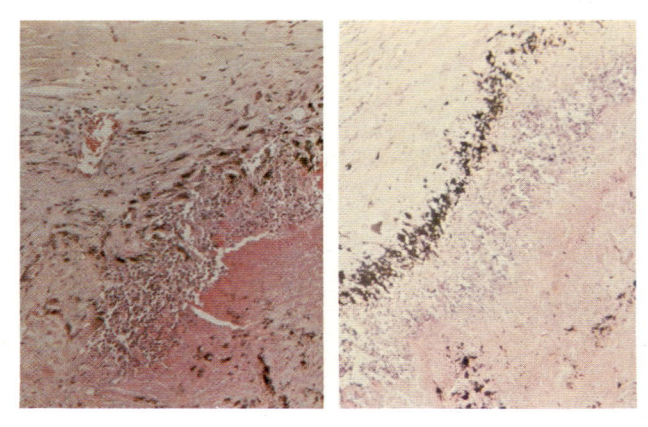

Figure 13.14 *Left:* Characteristic edge of necrotic area with non-tuberculous inflammatory activity where neutrophils, lymphocytes and plasma cells predominate. *Right:* A similar area also showing somewhat radially arranged effete dust-laden macrophages, resulting in a lamination.

OCCUPATIONAL LUNG DISORDERS – I. COAL AND SILICA

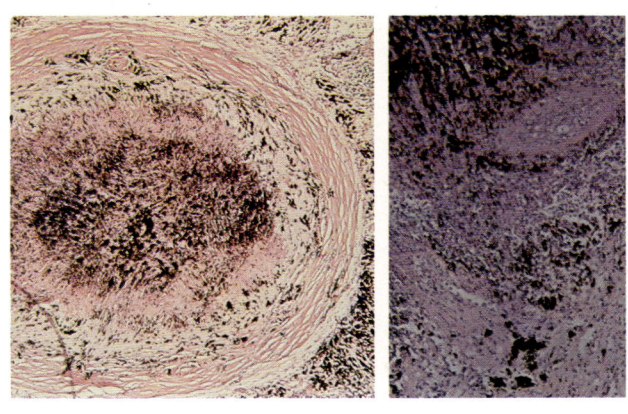

Figure 13.15 *Left:* A 'burnt out' Caplan lesion showing several laminae; difficult to distinguish from tuberculosis. *Right:* Edge of a Caplan lesion showing lympho-plasmocytic infiltrate in a thickened pulmonary artery.

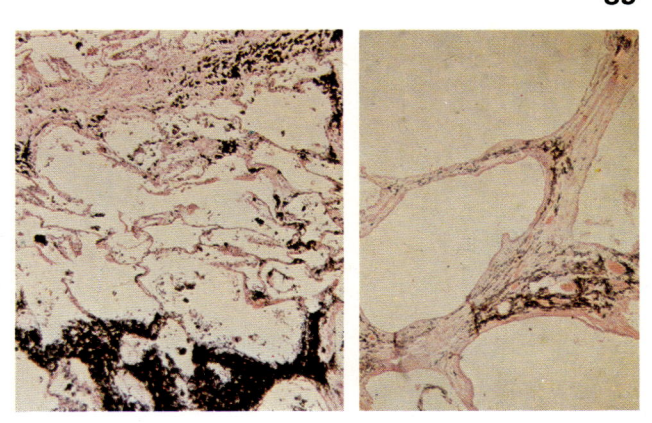

Figure 13.16 *Left:* A coal miner more disabled than the radiographic category would suggest. Though no fibrosis was discernible on macroscopic evaluation, microscopy shows collagenous thickening of septa, part dust-pigmented, extending from the central focus (below) to the interlobular septum (above). *Right:* A coal miner with clubbing, diagnosed as 'cryptogenic fibrosing alveolitis'. Microscopy reveals coal dust-impregnated honeycomb lung.

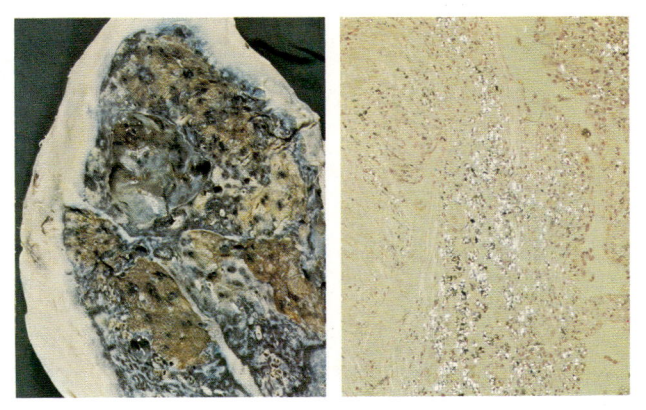

Figure 13.17 *Left:* a slate-quarry worker effectively treated for tuberculosis during life, showing dense collagenous pleural thickening, a large glistening lined, healed tuberculous cavity, several discrete grey/bluish silicotic nodules, best seen in upper lobes, with much basal and middle lobe dust-pigmented fibrosis. *Right:* Polarization of Figure 13.18 revealing doubly refractile silica particles at the edge of a silicotic nodule.

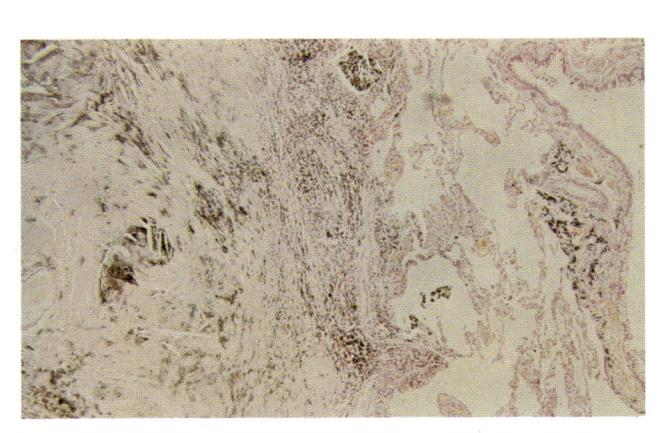

Figure 13.18 A silicotic nodule showing dense, part whorled, collagen bounded by dust-laden macrophages.

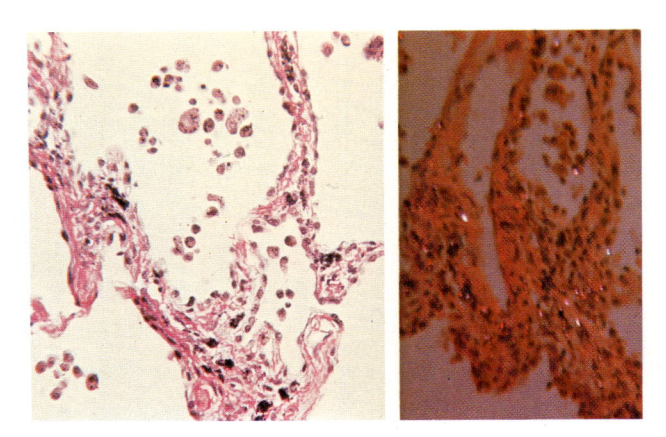

Figure 13.19 *Left:* A tin miner with interstitial, rather than nodular disease, on drill biopsy reveals dust-impregnated interstitial fibrosis. *Right:* This demonstrates much darkly refractile material within the interstitium.

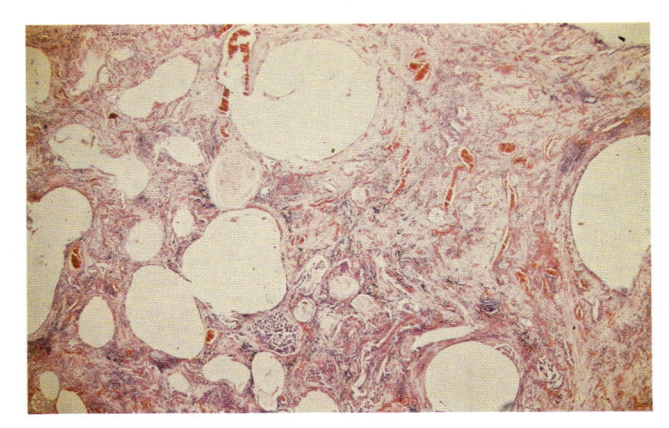

Figure 13.20 A slate-quarry worker, later a farm labourer, developed progressive interstitial disease. Microscopy shows dense interstitial fibrosis with honeycombing, a residual collagenous nodule (top left). Polarized light revealed quartz in the interstitium.

Nodular (Classical) Silicosis

Two forms exist, simple and complicated (PMF). In both there is usually marked pleural thickening (Figure 13.17). In the simple type there are firm, hard, isolated nodules composed of concentric layers of collagen which are sometimes calcified, present mostly in the upper lobes and hilar nodes. PMF lesions can form by conglomeration of nodules over 2 cm diameter and similar aggregation can occur in the Caplan pneumoconiosis. Both Caplan and silica massive fibrosis may cavitate. The lesions of silicosis are prone to show active tuberculous infection. Focal emphysema is not a characteristic of the silicotic nodule (Figures 13.17 and 13.18).

Microscopically, the silicotic nodule is composed of a core of concentrically arranged collagen fibres, which show hyalinization. Macrophages may or may not be present (Figure 13.18). Under polarized light, doubly refractile silica particles can usually be found in the outer part of the nodule (Figure 13.17). The edges of the nodules extend into the surrounding interstitial tissue. During the evolution of the nodule the structure of respiratory bronchiole and small pulmonary vessels is obliterated by fibrosis.

The lesions of PMF due to silicosis are aggregates, as has been described, of dense hyalinized collagen, some silica demonstrable by polarized light, a small amount of anthracotic pigment and scattered lymphocytes. The whorled appearance typical of silicotic nodules may be partly lost.

Tuberculous infection in silicotic lesions is common, and the usual histology of tubercle which characterizes coal workers' PMF with viable or attenuated tubercle bacilli.

In those cases which progress rapidly the nodules may be numerous, small, and lack a concentric pattern. Rheumatoid silicotic nodules (Caplan lesions) which have light grey necrotic centres, and lack the concentric black rings of rheumatoid coal pneumoconiosis may be seen rarely in patients with a rheumatoid diathesis. The regional lymph nodes are dense, hard and grey with a similar histology to the pulmonary lesion and are more prone to calcification which may often be peripheral (egg-shell calcification on radiology).

Mixed Dust Fibrosis

See Chapter 16.

Interstitial Fibrosis

Silica exposure does not always produce classical nodular disease radiologically; occasionally a predominantly fine interstitial fibrosis results (Figure 13.19). It must be remembered that silicotics may be advised to change their occupation, and in rural communities it is not unusual for exposure to organic dusts to occur later. This modifies the pathology, resulting in extensive quartz laden interstitial fibrosis (Figure 13.20).

References

1. Naeye, R. L. (1973). Black lung disease, the anthracotic pneumoconiosis. Pathology Annual, p.349
2. Lyons, J. P., Ryder, R. C., Seal, R. M. E. and Wagner, J. C. (1981). Emphysema in smoking and non-smoking coal workers with pneumoconiosis. *Bull. Eur. Physiopathol. Resp.*, **17,** 75
3. Leopold, J. G. and Gough, J. (1957). The centrilobular form of hypertrophic emphysema and its relation to chronic bronchitis. *Thorax*, **12,** 219
4. Gough, J. (1940). Pneumoconiosis of coal trimmers. *J. Pathol. Bacteriol.*, **51,** 277
5. Heppleston, A. G. (1947). The essential lesion of pneumoconiosis in Welsh coal workers. *J. Pathol. Bacteriol.*, **59.,** 453
6. Heppleston, A. G. (1953). The pathological anatomy of simple pneumoconiosis in coal workers. *J. Pathol. Bacteriol.*, **66,** 235
7. Gough, J., Rivers, D. and Seal, R. M. E. (1955). Pathological studies of modified pneumoconiosis in coal miners with rheumatoid arthritis (Caplan's syndrome). *Thorax*, **10,** 9
8. Morgan, W. K. C. and Lapp, N. L. (1976). State of the art. Respiratory disease in coal miners. *Am. Rev. Resp. Dis.*, **113,** 531
9. Cockcroft, A. E., Wagner, J. C., Seal, R. M. E., Lyons, J. P. and Campbell, M. J. (1981). Irregular opacities in coal workers' pneumoconiosis – Correlation with pulmonary function and pathology. *Inhaled Particles*, **5,** (In Press)
10. Suratt, P. M., Winn, W. C., Brody, A. R., Bolton, W. K. and Giles, R. D. (1977). Acute silicosis in tombstone sandblasters. *Am. Rev. Resp. Dis.*, **115,** 521

Occupational Lung Disorders – II. Silicate Pneumoconioses

Silicates, which are compounds of silica with calcium, magnesium, aluminium and other bases, occur in fibrous and non-fibrous forms. A fibrous particle has a length : diameter ratio of greater than three to one. Some of the most important fibrous silicates are asbestos and talc, whilst the non-fibrous silicates include kaolin and fuller's earth.

Asbestos-Induced Lung Diseases

The term asbestos includes a number of naturally occurring fibrous silicates of different chemical compositions. Chrysotile, which now accounts for approximately 90% of world asbestos production, has a serpentine form, whilst the amphiboles (crocidolite, amosite, anthophyllite and tremolite) occur as straight, needle-like fibres. Chrysotile fibres tend to be intercepted higher up the small airways than the straight fibres of the other types, which tend to reach the peripheral airways and alveoli. This is put forward as the reason why chrysotile is not often associated with mesothelioma, although often with asbestosis. The world production of asbestos has been rising and although crocidolite has been replaced by substitutes it is anticipated that the incidence of asbestos-induced diseases including mesothelioma, will not peak until the end of the century. Its effects are multiplicative with smoking and it is surmised that it will play an increasing role in the causation of lung cancer in the future.

Exposure to asbestos may result in a variety of pulmonary lesions:

(1) pleural effusions
(2) pleural plaques
(3) diffuse pleural thickening
(4) asbestosis
(5) massive fibrotic lesions
(6) Caplan nodules (see Chapter 13)
(7) DIP-like reaction (see Chapter 14)
(8) asbestosis plus bronchial carcinoma
(9) mesothelioma (see Chapter 21)

See plate 14.1.

Asbestos bodies

These are yellow-brown structures, measuring 20–30 μm in length and 2–5 μm in diameter, consisting of an asbestos fibre core coated with iron-containing protein. They are segmented, have clubbed ends and give a positive Prussian-blue reaction (Figures 14.9 and 14.10). Ultrastructural examination reveals hundreds or thousands of fibres for every fibre visible by light microscopy. Such studies have shown that the large majority of fibres remain uncoated. Presence of asbestos bodies in sputum indicates past exposure, but does not signify asbestos-induced pulmonary disease.

Concentration techniques with amounts of asbestos fibres and bodies expressed per gram of lung-tissue are useful and we utilize the method of Ashcroft and Heppleston[1] (Figure 14.11). As a general guide, we find counts of greater than 1 000 000/g of tissue in asbestosis, approximately 60 000/g in mesothelioma and between 20 000 and 50 000/g in those with pleural plaques, which is in general agreement with Whitwell et al.[2]. However, our experience does differ from these workers, in that we have observed higher counts in lung-cancer patients than controls and also found pleural plaques three times as frequently in lung-cancer patients than controls.

Electron microscopic examination of asbestos fibres in tissue is also useful since it gives information about the types of fibres as well as the quantity and it may reveal fibres which are below the limit of resolution of the light microscope[3]. Asbestos bodies are often referred to as ferruginous bodies since other material may give rise to structures of similar appearance including glass and cotton fibres, talc, graphite, carborundum and other particles[4]. Nevertheless Churg and Warnock[5] have shown that 90% of ferruginous bodies occurring in non-occupationally exposed individuals have, in fact, asbestos cores.

Pleural Effusions in Asbestos Workers

It has been recently recognized that apart from mesotheliomas presenting as pleural effusions, some asbestos workers may develop pleural effusions, earlier in their exposure, which may ultimately resolve. In these, biopsy of the pleura reveals only non-specific chronic inflammatory changes.

Pleural Plaques

These are circumscribed, pearly grey, raised nodular lesions situated in the parietal pleura (Figure 14.1). They are often calcified. They are located most frequently over the postero-lateral and basal parts of the lungs, the central tendon of the diaphragm and beneath the surface of the rib. They are usually bilateral and show a fairly strong correlation with exposure to the majority of asbestos forms, but occasionally they are observed with no known asbestos exposure. They have a covering of mesothelial cells and consist of a basket-weave pattern of collagen fibres (Figure 14.1). The deeper layers contain fibroblasts and a scattering of lymphocytes and plasma cells. Calcification, when present, is situated at the centre of the plaque. Asbestos fibres are not often identified within the plaque. Plaques are not a precursor of mesothelioma.

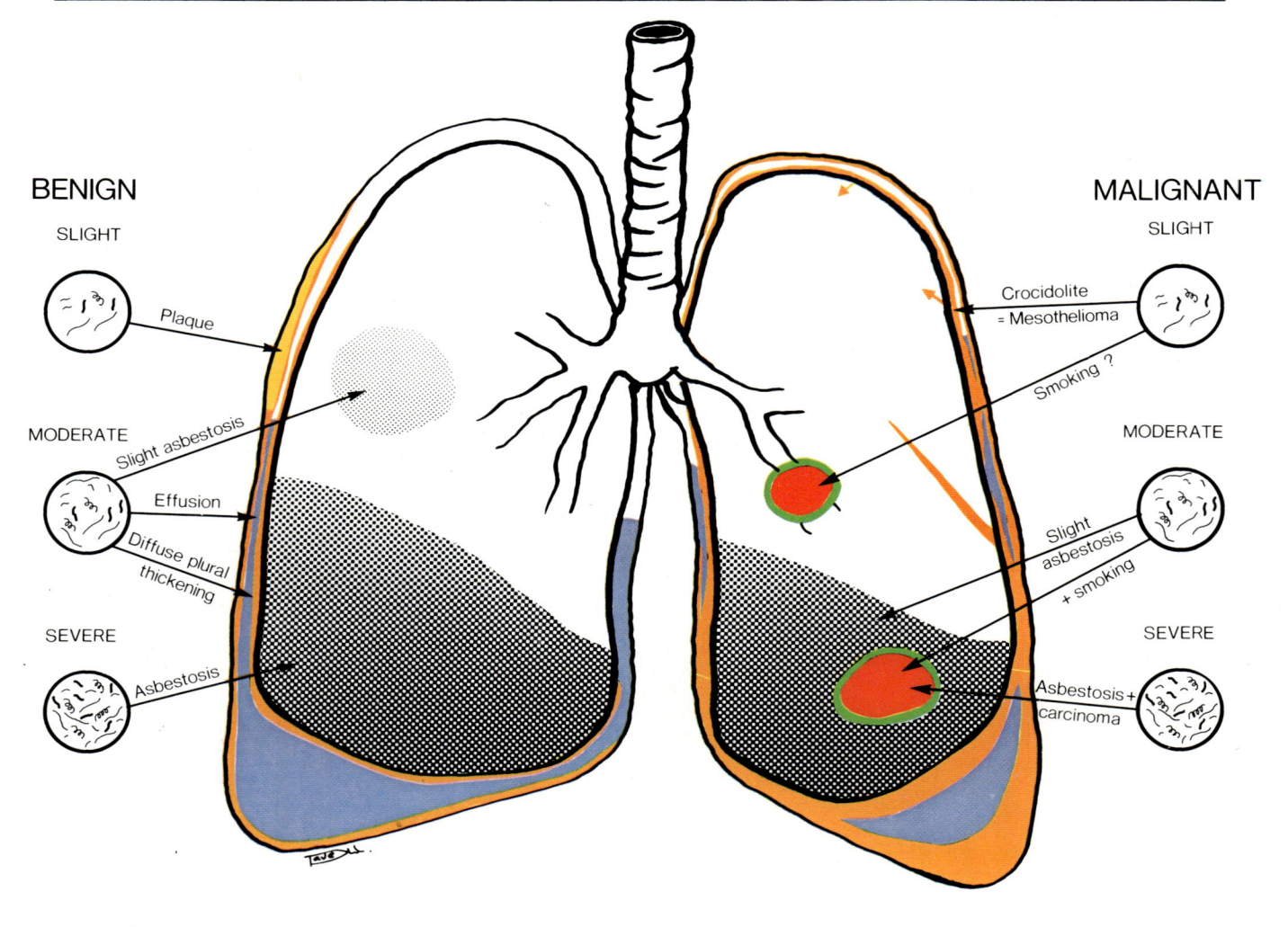

Plate 14.1 Possible results of exposure to asbestos

Diffuse Pleural Thickening

In addition to the common pleural plaques which, even when heavily calcified and extensive, do not cause pulmonary dysfunction, asbestos exposure has recently been recognized as a cause of diffuse fibrosis of the parietal pleura (Figure 14.9). Pleural plaques may be present on one side and diffuse parietal pleural thickening on the other. Recently, cases with pulmonary disability have been ascribed to this diffuse pleural thickening and a case made for regarding the disability as compensatable. On light microscopy, similar appearances to those of plaques are observed.

Asbestosis

This term implies pulmonary fibrosis due to asbestos-dust exposure. The 'barn door' case poses no problem; the subject is dyspnoeic, there is interstitial fibrosis radiologically, and lung function abnormalities. In such cases asbestos counts of well over 1 000 000/g of lung tissue are seen[2]. Macroscopically, these cases reveal parietal pleural plaques, shrinking of the lung and obvious fibrosis and/or induration most marked in lower zones of the lung (cf. extrinsic allergic bronchiolo-alveolitis, sarcoid and tubercle) (Figure 14.2). Cysts may also be present, usually small in relation to the areas of scarring (honeycombing), but occasionally they are large. The more severe the condition, the more likely the mid and upper zones of the lung are to be involved by fibrosis. Rarely the changes may predominate in the upper rather than the lower lobes[6]. Microscopically the degree of fibrosis varies from field to field, but numerous areas will be seen with considerable interstitial fibrosis and marked distortion of the lung architecture. In relation to the areas of fibrosis, asbestos bodies will be found with ease.

Occasionally, massive fibrotic lesions, analogous to the massive coal worker pneumoconiotic lesions, occur in asbestosis. They tend to be situated in the lower lobes in contradistinction to those of the coal worker.

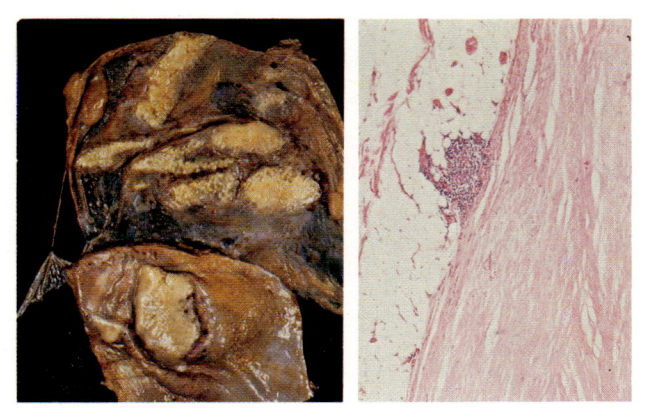

OCCUPATIONAL LUNG DISORDERS – II. SILICATE PNEUMOCONIOSES 93

Figure 14.1 *Left:* The typical raised, white, shiny plaques with serpiginous edges. Careful inspection sometimes reveals small raised nodules. *Right:* A block taken from one of the plaques shows typical basket-weave collagenous tissue with a scattering of lymphocytes.

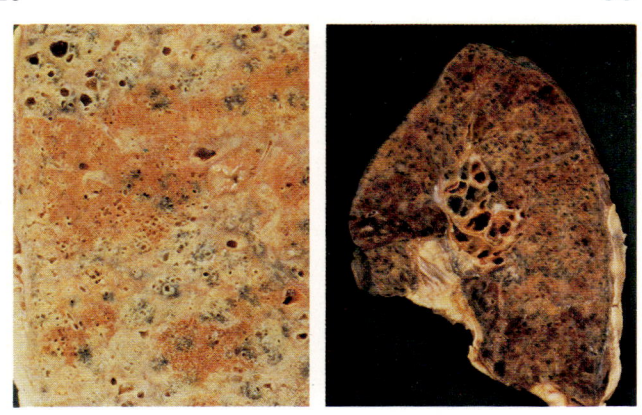

Figure 14.2 *Right:* Typical appearances of asbestosis easily missed on superficial examination of the lung. Fibrosis and fine honeycombing are most marked in the lower zones of the lung – shown in close up on the *left*.

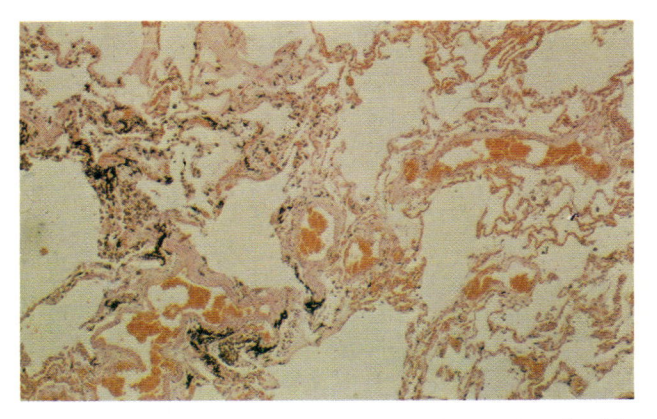

Figure 14.3 Grade 1 asbestosis. Fibrosis is confined to the walls of the alveolar sacs around respiratory bronchioles. H & E × 38.4.

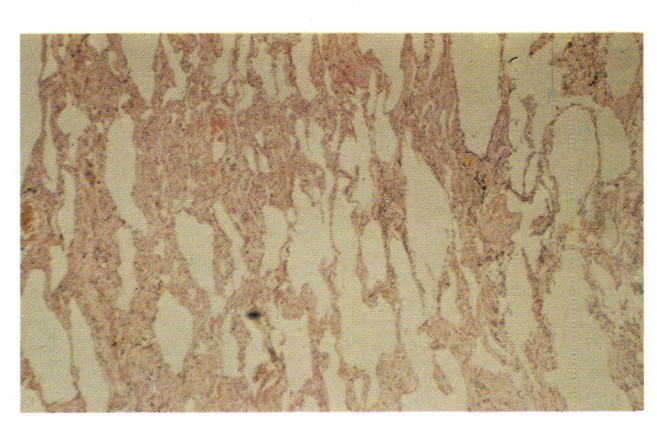

Figure 14.4 Grade 2 asbestosis. Similar to Figure 14.2 but the fibrosis is extending to involve alveolar walls more peripherally in the lobule but with preservation of lung architecture. H & E × 38.4.

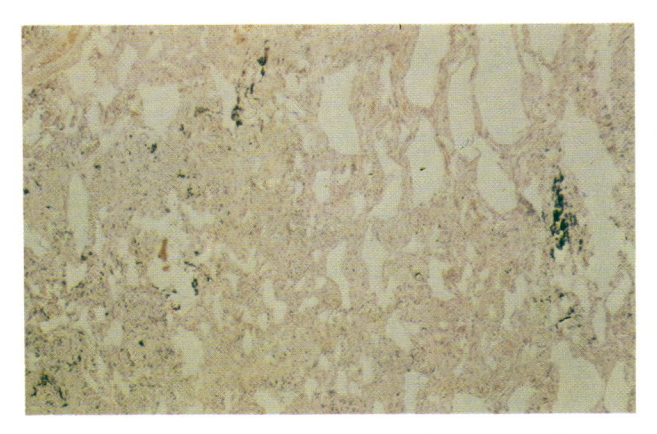

Figure 14.5 Grade 3 asbestosis. The fibrosis is more extensive and is becoming confluent with obliteration of a proportion of alveolar sacs. H & E × 38.4.

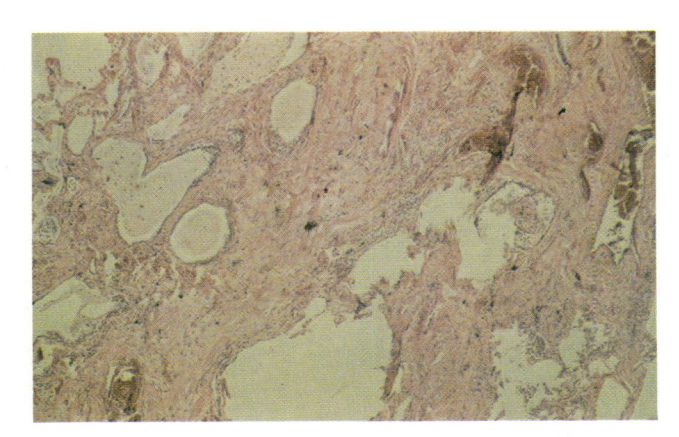

Figure 14.6 Grade 4 asbestosis. Solid areas of fibrosis with loss of pulmonary architecture, the spaces seen being modified respiratory bronchioles ('honeycomb' lung). H & E × 38.4.

Even more uncommon are Caplan lesions, which occur in patients with the rheumatoid diathesis. They show a predilection for the lower lobes.

Having described 'barn door' asbestosis we come to the problem of minimal and intermediate grades of asbestosis. This is particularly important in regard to the question of whether the development of a lung cancer in a subject is a result of asbestosis and thus compensatable. It must be emphasized that careful macroscopic examination of a well-fixed inflated lung, together with examination of 2 × 2 inch and carefully selected conventional sections is necessary to evaluate the extent and grade of fibrotic change. Barium sulphate impregnation[7] is also of value in bringing out the fibrotic changes macroscopically, which may be subtle in some cases.

There is general agreement with regard to the grading of the severity of fibrosis on histological sections, and it reflects that the earliest lesion of asbestosis occurs in relation to the respiratory bronchioles[8]. The fibres impact in alveoli adjacent to respiratory bronchioles and excite a macrophage response. Reticulin is then deposited around the asbestos fibres, followed by collagen. After a time the affected alveoli become obliterated and there is associated hyperplasia of the alveolar lining cells – cytoplasmic hyaline, not specific for asbestosis, may be seen within these cells. After further exposure, more and more respiratory bronchioles become involved in this process and the fibrosis extends down into alveolar ducts, atria and alveoli. The individual lesions then condense, leading to diffuse interstitial fibrosis with or without modification of distal air spaces (honeycombing). Our histological grades of severity of fibrosis are similar to those laid down by the IARC[9] (Figures 14.3–14.6).

Grade 0 – None.

Grade 1 – Lesions consist of slight focal fibrosis around respiratory bronchioles, associated with the presence of asbestos bodies.

Grade 2 – The lesions are confined to respiratory bronchioles of scattered acini. Fibrosis extends to alveolar ducts and atria, as well as to the walls of adjacent air spaces.

Grade 3 – There is a further increase and condensation of the peribronchiolar fibrosis with early widespread interstitial fibrosis.

Grade 4 – Few alveoli are recognizable in the widespread diffuse fibrosis; honeycombing may or may not be present.

It should be realized that Grades 3 and 4 are visible macroscopically, but not Grades 1 and 2. Histological evaluation on its own is of little benefit in asbestosis, since a variety of histological grades may be seen, even in the same area. Therefore, assessment of distribution, macroscopical severity and asbestos counts should be taken into account. This is a suitable point to describe a few cases which highlight the difficulties that are sometimes encountered.

Case 1 – Mr. P. a middle-aged, moderate smoker, died from carcinomatosis due to a central adenocarcinoma in the left upper lobe. He had been moderately exposed to asbestos for 12 years, commencing 20 years previously. There was no longstanding history of dyspnoea, but review of his chest X-rays revealed early interstitial disease compatible with a mild degree of asbestosis.

Macroscopically, his right lung revealed interlobular septal thickening, fine fibrosis posteriorly, several normal-appearing lobules particularly in the upper lobe and other lobules with enlarged spaces easily interpreted as emphysema and others with more recognizable interstitial fibrosis (Figure 14.7). Several sections showed histological severity ranging from 0 to 3 (Figure 14.8). The asbestos count was below the 1 000 000 fibres/g lower level for severe asbestosis[2] at 425 000 fibres/g and 20.7 million/g on electron microscopy quantitation (49.4% amosite, 17.1% chrysotile, 18.5% crocidolite and 8.6% mullite).

This case is considered, on clinical and radiological grounds, to be 'early' asbestosis but on macroscopic and histological examination to be 'moderate' asbestosis, emphasizing the need for careful correlation between clinical, physiological, radiological and pathological findings. This case was accepted as an industrial malignancy.

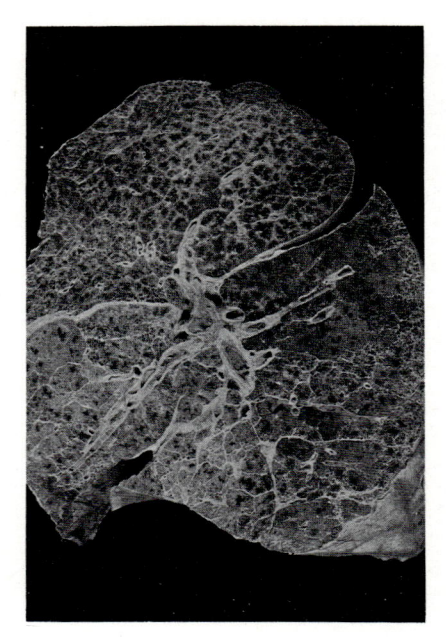

Figure 14.7 Thickening of interlobular septa and fine fibrosis posteriorly. Some lobules appear normal, others have enlarged spaces easily interpreted as ephysema and others show more recognizable interstitial fibrosis (barium sulphate impregnation).

Case 2 – Mr. J., a 58-year-old ex-smoker developed an adenocarcinoma of the lower lobe of the right lung and died of disseminated malignancy. He had been moderately exposed to blue asbestos for 9 years, 20 years previously. He had been declined compensation one year previously on the grounds that his chest radiograph showed pleural plaques, but no parenchymal disease, and his dyspnoea was ascribed to ischaemic heart disease. His left lung and pleura are illustrated in Figure 14.9.

Fibrosis was clearly visible posteriorly in his left lower lobe and moderate numbers of asbestos bodies seen. Histological grading varied from 0 to 3 in different areas and the asbestos count was 387 000 fibres/g by light microscopy and 39 million by electron microscopy (72% crocidolite, 23% chrysotile, 5% rutile).

Although the fibrosis occupied less than 15% of the lung, this borderline case was regarded as an adenocarcinoma arising in a patient with previously undiagnosed mild asbestosis. His diffuse parietal pleural thickening is commented upon above.

Case 3 – Mr. B. illustrates a typical problem encountered when the possibility of asbestos exposure comes to light after surgical resection of a lung cancer, either as a result of the surgeon recognizing pleural plaques or the pathologist seeing asbestos bodies in tumour or parenchyma (Figure 14.10).

In this case asbestos bodies were identified in a peripheral papillary adenocarcinoma. The parenchyma had been interpreted as emphysematous, but on microscopy Grade 1 fibrosis was observed and asbestos bodies were seen in moderate numbers (287 000 fibres/g by light microscopy). This was eventually interpreted as localized emphysematous/fibrotic lung destruction not warranting a designation of asbestosis, it being regarded as a focal area of scarring to which asbestos bodies had been attracted.

Case 4 – Mr. W. had no respiratory disability or chest radiographic abnormality, but died of peritoneal mesothelioma. The lung is of interest in that careful inspection of an inflated lung reveals central dust foci and questionable fine fibrosis easily interpretable as simple coal worker's pneumoconiosis (Figure 14.11). However, on histological examination there was Grade 1 asbestosis – asbestos bodies were seen with ease and readily demonstrated in 'lung juice'. The asbestos fibre count was 7 000 000 fibres/g by light microscopy and 238 000 000 fibres/g by electron microscopy (90.1% amosite, 5.4% chrysotile, 4.5% crocidolite). This change was present throughout most of the lung. Such findings of high counts after being exposed to asbestos are the rule in mesothelioma of the peritoneum, but these pulmonary findings in a patient dying of lung carcinoma would constitute a problem in that, in spite of the high counts, the asbestos is essentially microscopic. It also demonstrates that amosite fibres are readily seen at light microscopy.

The following guidelines, based upon a combination of macroscopic, microscopic – both by conventional and 2 × 2 inch sections – and concentration counts, although arbitary, are given because we find them useful in assessing the degree of asbestosis. They may be modified in time as more detailed studies and knowledge about the relationship of lung cancer and asbestos exposure come to light.

Minimal – Not visible on careful inspection macroscopically, but with histological Grade 1 lesions and supported by asbestos counts well above those normally seen in controls.

Slight – Fibrosis is observed macroscopically or the lung is indurated, but less than 25% of the lung is involved. There are no clinical or radiological manifestations.

Moderate – 25–50% of the lung is abnormal with recognizable fibrosis and induration. Histological grades vary from 2 to 4 and there is usually a count of around 250 000 fibres/g.

Bronchogenic Carcinoma

Sixty per cent of patients with severe asbestosis, i.e. with clinical and radiological manifestations, die of lung cancer. The risks are much higher in those who smoke. Since lung cancer seen in association with asbestosis is compensatable, determination of lesser degrees of asbestosis, as outlined above, is particularly important. All major histological types occur but more frequently it is adenocarcinoma, and it is usually situated in the lower lobe, in proximity to the fibrosis. All types of asbestos are implicated.

Talc Pneumoconiosis

The fibrogenic properties of talc, a hydrated magnesium silicate ($Mg_6Si_8O_{20}(OH)_4$), may be due to impurities such as tremolite, anthophyllite, calcite and quartz. There also apears to be differences in susceptibility amongst similarly exposed workers.

Three types of pulmonary lesion may result from inhalation of talc according to the composition of the dust inhaled:

1. irregular nodular fibrosis
2. diffuse interstitial fibrosis (Figure 14.12)
3. foreign body granulomas.

These lesions may appear singly or in differing combinations in the same individual.

In affected individuals there are usually pleural adhesions and the cut surfaces of the lungs may reveal small, grey nodules, softer than silicotic nodules, which are most prevalent in the lower lobes and/or diffuse interstitial fibrosis predominantly affecting the lower lobes. Occasionally massive fibrotic lesions form; these may undergo cavitation.

Microscopically, there may be ill-defined nodules consisting of irregular, acellular collagenous tissue which sometimes show incomplete whorling and numerous dust-laden macrophages. Interstitial fibrosis, which begins around respiratory bronchioles, may obliterate the lung architecture in areas. 'Talc bodies', similar to asbstos bodies, may be found in the fibrotic areas. Foreign body granulomata consisting of epithelioid cells, foreign body giant cells and a peripheral rim of lymphocytes may be present. Birefringent, needle-shaped talc crystals, are present within and around all these lesions either lying free or within macrophages (Figure 14.12).

Talcosis may occasionally be caused by very fine particles of less than 0.5 μm which cannot be identified by light microscopy; electron microscopy or X-ray diffraction examination of ashed lung sections may be required for identification.

Kaolin (China Clay) Pneumoconiosis

An increasing number of deaths in Cornish china clay workers have been ascribed to kaolin, a hydrated aluminium silicate. The lungs usually reveal greyish nodules, resembling those of talcosis. Well circumscribed, grey and firm, massive lesions may occur in the upper lobes[10]. They are softer than silicotic nodules. Histologically, the lesions consist

OCCUPATIONAL LUNG DISORDERS – II. SILICATE PNEUMOCONIOSES

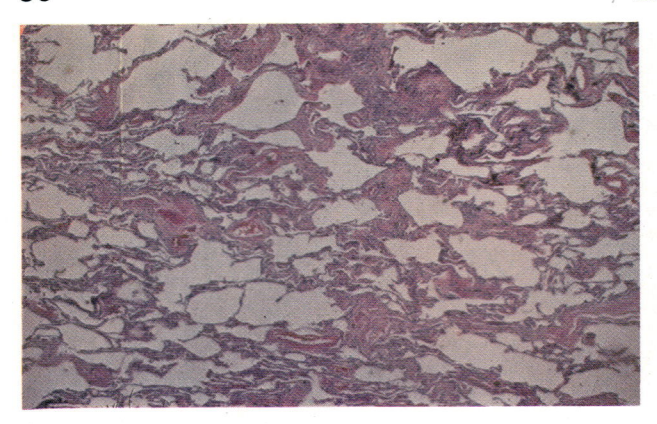

Figure 14.8 An area regarded as Grade 2 shows a prominent lymphoid infiltrate, sometimes encountered in asbestosis as is the rarer DIP component. H & E × 38.4.

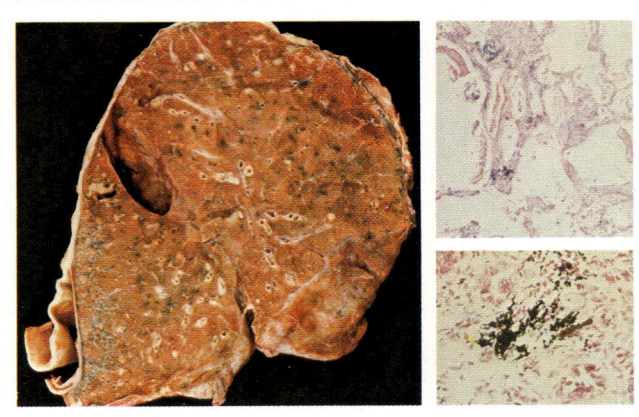

Figure 14.9 *Left:* Clearly recognizable fibrosis is affecting the lower lobe posteriorly. The pleura is also diffusely thickened. *Top right:* Grade II fibrosis. H & E × 38.4. *Bottom right:* Asbestos bodies found in relation to the fibrosis. H & E × 240.

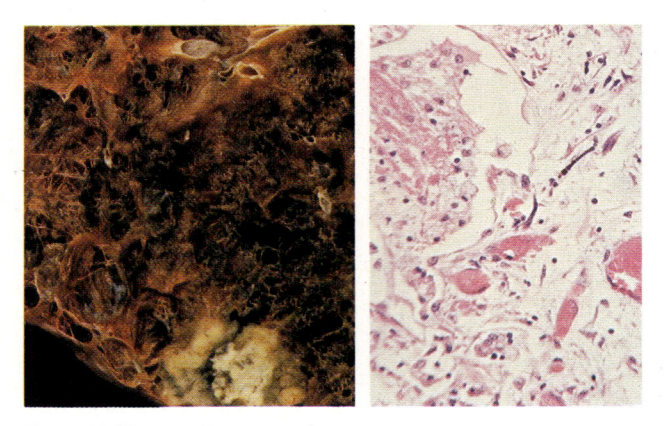

Figure 14.10 *Left:* 'Emphysematous' lung with a peripheral carcinoma. *Right:* Asbestos bodies seen in relationship to the adenocarcinoma. H & E × 240.

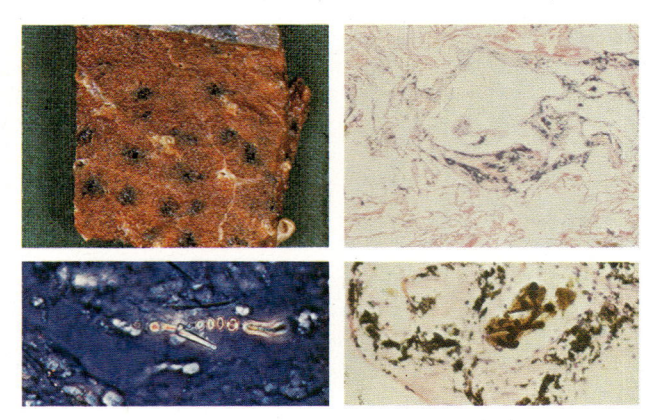

Figure 14.11 *Top left:* Cut surface of the lung with brownish parenchyma and dark central dust foci with questionable fine fibrosis. *Top right:* Grade 1 asbestosis. H & E × 38.4. *Bottom right:* Enlargement of the area shows clusters of asbestos bodies together with coal dust. H & E × 240. *Bottom left:* Phase contrast examination of lung juice.

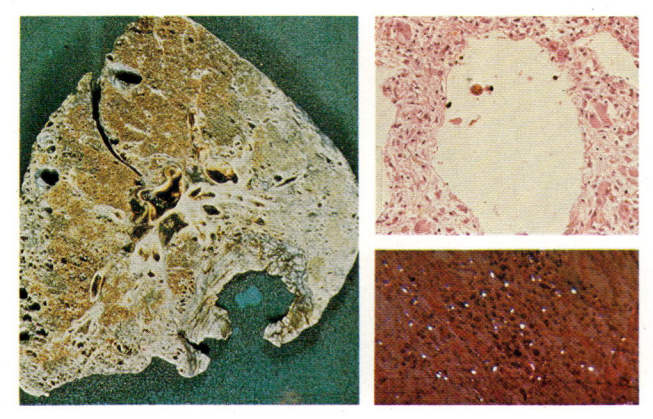

Figure 14.12 *Left:* The lung from a rubber worker showing interstitial fibrosis and honeycombing, most marked in the lower and posterior zones of the lung. *Top right:* Microscopy reveals interstitial pneumonitis and fibrosis with giant cells. H & E × 96. *Lower right:* Numerous clearly refractile needle shaped 'talc' crystals. H & E × 384.

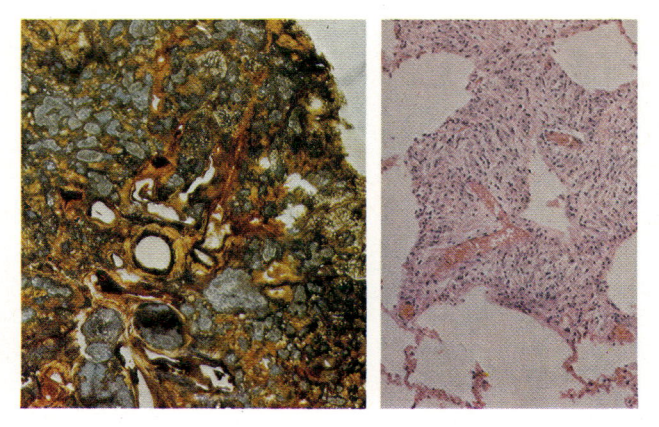

Figure 14.13 *Left:* Whole lung section from a china clay worker showing nodular grey lesions with coalescence in the parachyma and grey pigmentation of enlarged hilar nodes. *Right:* Part of central focus with grey slightly refractile material within macrophages. H & E × 384.

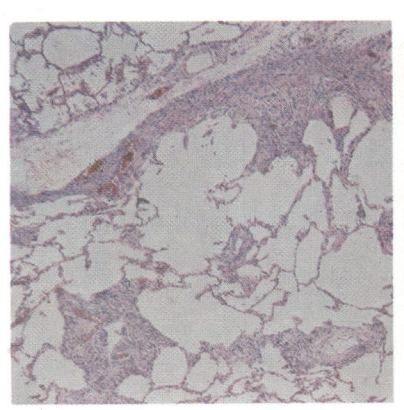

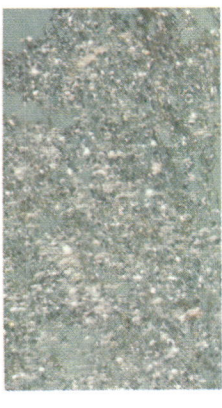

Figure 14.14 *Left:* Low power H&E with central dust focus as above but including interlobular septum also delineated by dust-laden macrophages. There is slight fibrosis. H&E × 24. *Right:* Polarization reveals innumerable doubly refractile non-fibrous material. H&E × 384.

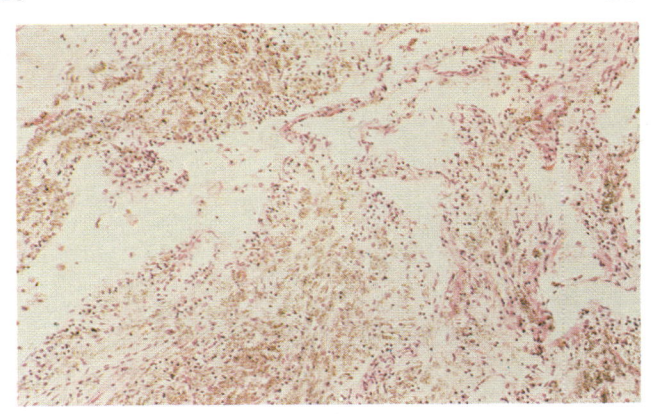

Figure 14.15 A biopsy from a fuller's-earth miner showing macrophages containing greenish brown material admixed with collagen. There also appears to be interstitial change. H&E × 38.4.

of random collagen fibres and large quantities of strongly birefringent dust, surrounded by numerous dust-laden macrophages (Figures 14.13 and 14.14).

Occasionally diffuse interstitial fibrosis, usually mild, may occur together with a prominent alveolar exudate containing dust-laden macrophages.

Fuller's Earth Pneumoconiosis

This is a clay consisting mainly of calcium montmorillonite, but may also have mica, glauconite and variable slight quartz content[11]. Pathological studies of pneumoconiosis due to fuller's earth have been few and its effects are debatable.

It appears that prolonged exposure to fuller's earth may produce a relatively benign pneumoconiosis[12], although exceptionally massive pneumoconiosis occurs.

The lungs contain black, irregular, soft nodules, mainly in the upper lobes, which comprise aggregations of macrophages containing translucent, brownish, doubly refractile particles[13] which are also extracellular, admixed with reticulin and a minimal amount of collagen (Figure 14.14). The lesions are situated around respiratory bronchioles.

References

1. Ashcroft, T. and Heppleston, A. G. (1973). The optical and electron microscopic determination of pulmonary asbestos fibre concentration, and its relation to the human pathological reaction. *J. Clin. Pathol.*, **26**, 224
2. Whitwell, F., Scott, J. and Grimshaw, M. (1977). Relationship between occupations and asbestos fibre content of the lungs in patients with pleural mesothelioma, lung cancer and other diseases. *Thorax*, **32**, 377
3. Pooley, F. D. (1973). Methods for assessing asbestos fibres and asbestos bodies in tissue by electron microscopy. In *Biological Effects of Asbestos*. IARC Scientific Publications, No. 8, p.50. (Lyon: International Agency for Research on Cancer)
4. Abraham, J. L. (1978). Recent advances in pneumoconiosis: the pathologist's role in etiologic diagnosis. In Thurlbeck, W. M. *The Lung Structure, Function and Disease*, I.A.P. Monograph No. 19. (Baltimore: Williams and Williams)
5. Churg, A. and Warnock, M. L. (1977). Analysis of the cores of ferruginous (asbestos) bodies from the general population. I. Patients with and without lung cancer. *Lab. Invest.*, **37**, 280
6. Gough, J. (1965). Differential diagnosis in the pathology of asbestosis. *Ann. N.Y. Acad. Sci.*, **132**, 368
7. Heard, B. E. (1958). A pathological study of emphysema of the lungs with chronic bronchitis. *Thorax*, **13**, 136
8. Wagner, J. C. (1965). The sequelae of exposure to asbestos dust. *Ann. N.Y. Acad. Sci.*, **132**, 691
9. Hinson, K. F. W., Otto, H., Webster, I., and Rossiter, C. E. (1973), Criteria for the diagnosis and grading of asbestosis. In *Biological Effects of Asbestos*. I.A.R.C. Scientific Publications No. 8, p.54. (Lyon: International Agency for Research in Cancer)
10. Hale, L. W., Gough, J., King, E. J. and Nagelschmidt, (1955). Pneumoconiosis of kaolin workers. *Brit. J. Ind. Med.*, **13**, 251
11. Parkes, W. R. (1974). *Occupational Lung Disorders*. p.344. (London: Butterworths)
12. Tonning, H. O. (1949). Pneumoconiosis from fuller's earth. *J. Ind. Hyg. Toxicol.*, **31**, 41
13. Sakula, A. (1961). Pneumoconiosis due to fuller's earth. *Thorax*, **16**, 176

Occupational Lung Disorders – III. Metals, Fumes and Organic Materials

15

Metals and Fumes

Aluminium Pneumoconiosis (including Shaver's Disease)

Both metallic aluminium dust[1] and fumes from the smelting of bauxite[2] (Al_2O_3) may cause pulmonary damage. The pathology is similar with both, but there is marked individual idiosyncrasy. The lungs are heavy, greyish black with thick pleural adhesions, and on cut section there are radiating bands of dense interstitial fibrosis, most prevalent in the upper lobes. Severe irregular emphysema is usually present (Figure 15.1).

Microscopically, the interstitium shows a mononuclear infiltrate, fibrosis and black dust (Figure 15.1). Macrophages are present within the alveoli.

Tungsten Carbide (Hard Metal) Pneumoconiosis

Respiratory disease attributable to the manufacture and grinding of tungsten carbide has been recognized on occasions. It is probable that cobalt is responsible for the pulmonary damage since tungsten carbide in the absence of cobalt appears to be inert. Reversible airways obstruction or an interstitial pneumonia may occur; the latter varies from chiefly collagenous (Figures 15.2 and 15.3), to predominantly desquamative[3], to giant cell type[4] (Figure 15.3). Granulomata may be present (Figure 15.3).

Berylliosis

Exposure to beryllium metal or its compounds may result in an acute or chronic form of disease according to the intensity of exposure[5].

The *acute* form, due to heavy exposure, results in a chemical pneumonia. The majority of cases recover in a few weeks but in those who have died, the pulmonary changes are those of diffuse alveolar damage.

The *chronic* form is characterized by multisystem granulomatous involvement, with pulmonary manifestations predominating. It may be due to repeated exposures or follow an acute episode. It sometimes presents 10–15 years following exposure. Chronic berylliosis is indistinguishable from sarcoidosis pathologically, apart from a greater degree of interstitial pneumonitis in the former (Figure 15.4). The chronic form of extrinsic allergic bronchioloalveolitis can be distinguished from chronic berylliosis by the persistence of granulomata in the presence of interstitial fibrosis in the latter.

The detection of beryllium in tissues and urine gives evidence of recent or past exposure, but does not, by itself, establish the diagnosis of beryllium disease.

Siderotic Lung Disease

This is due to inhalation of iron oxide either in a pure form or mixed with other dusts. Inhalation of pure iron, which is relatively inert, causes siderosis – seen in its purest form in silver polishers. In arc welders and oxyacetylene cutters the exposure is, in most cases, due to pure iron oxide but in some there are exposures to multiple agents, particularly asbestos. Many iron miners are exposed to silica as well as iron which may lead to silicosiderosis (haematite pneumoconiosis), but this seldom occurs without at least 10 years exposure.

Three gross forms of *haematite pneumoconiosis* occur: (a) diffuse (Figure 15.5), (b) nodular (Figure 15.5) and (c) massive fibrotic (Figures 15.5 and 15.6). Circumscribed secondary lesions, similar to those seen in silicosis, but reddish brown, may occur in haematite miners, either because of a high exposure (silicotic nodule) or rheumatoid diathesis (Caplan nodule).

Histologically, particles of haematite and silica are present in the alveoli and the bronchioles, and in relation to blood vessels. Fibrosis around bronchioles and arterioles occurs. The massive fibrotic lesions consist of dense collagen admixed with iron and silica. On polarized light the haematite appears as orange luminous dots, whereas the silica appears white (Figure 15.7).

Siderosis, as seen in arc welders, oxyacetylene cutters and silver polishers, is seldom associated with respiratory disability and there is usually little fibrosis. The iron lies free in alveoli and respiratory bronchioles and within macrophages. In silver polishers, silver as well as iron oxide particles are given off and the silver combines chemically with protein of the lung, resulting in the elastic tissue of vessels and alveoli being stained black.

Occasionally some arc welders and oxyacetylene cutters are exposed to other dusts and fumes in addition to iron oxide depending on the welding operation performed, the metal welded and the casting of the rods, which may result in pulmonary fibrosis, e.g. oxides of nitrogen, ozone, silica, asbestos, etc. (Figure 15.8). This may result in more complex pathology which often requires more sophisticated techniques for clarification.

Inert Dusts

Inhalation of these dusts may result in marked radiological changes but no clinical symptoms and no significant production of reticulin or collagen fibres. Amongst these dusts are tin (stannosis), barium (baritosis), titanium and antimony. The lungs reveal a fairly uniform distribution of macules, 2–5 mm in

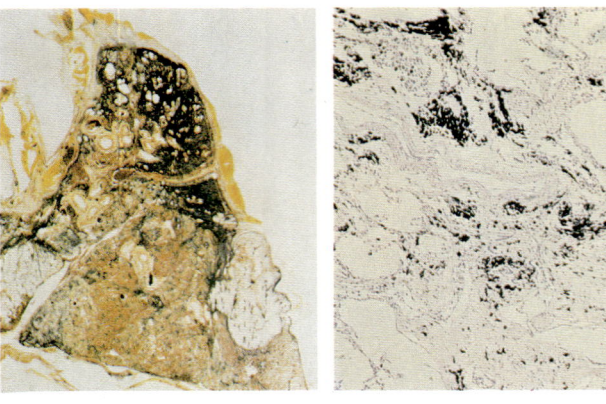

Figure 15.1 *Left:* The left lung of an aluminium worker showing dust impregnated interstitial fibrosis with confluence in and contraction of the upper lobe and apex of the lower. There are some areas of 'irregular' emphysema posteriorly in the lower lobe and also in the lingular anteriorly. *Right:* Microscopy shows the dust impregnated interstitial fibrosis. H & E × 38.4.

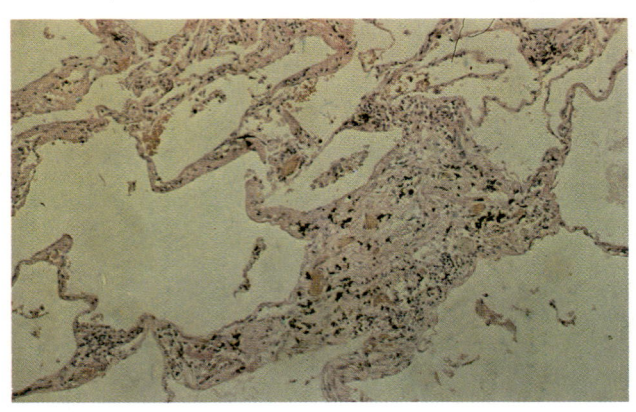

Figure 15.2 The lungs of a hard-metal worker showing collagenous thickening of interalveolar septa with a minimal inflammatory infiltrate. Suggesting an extrinsic inorganic aetiology is the focal dust-impregnated area of fibrosis with a mild mononuclear infiltrate. H & E × 96.

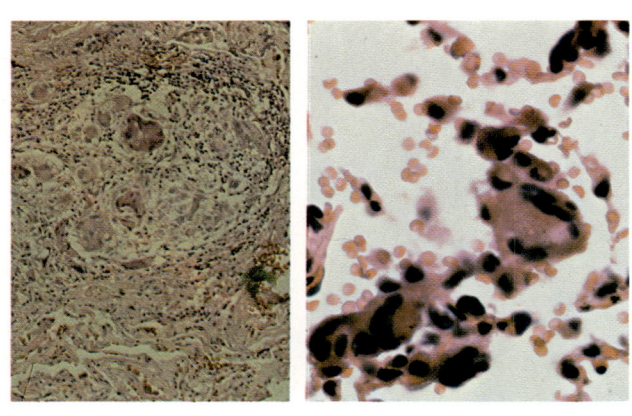

Figure 15.3 *Left:* Granuloma formation and fibrosis. This worker's exposure had been to silica and later to 'hard metals' and illustrates the problem of attributing pathology to a particular exposure. Recourse to sophisticated analytical EM procedures is necessary. H & E × 240. *Right:* This could easily be called by the pathologist GIP, since it fulfils all the necessary criteria. However, exposure to tungsten carbide was elicited and EDXA analysis demonstrated the inorganic material intracellularly. H & E × 480.

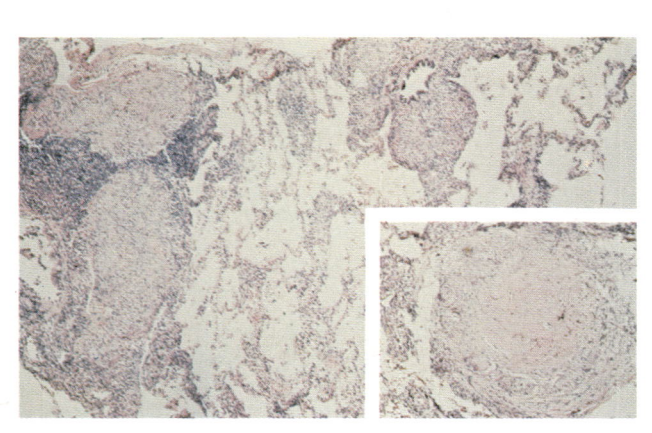

Figure 15.4 Beryllium worker illustrating several discrete giant cell granulomata, some around respiratory bronchioles, together with interstitial fibrosis and lymphocytic infiltrate. *Insert:* A granuloma exhibiting central hyalinization, not vitiating the diagnosis of berylliosis. H & E × 72.

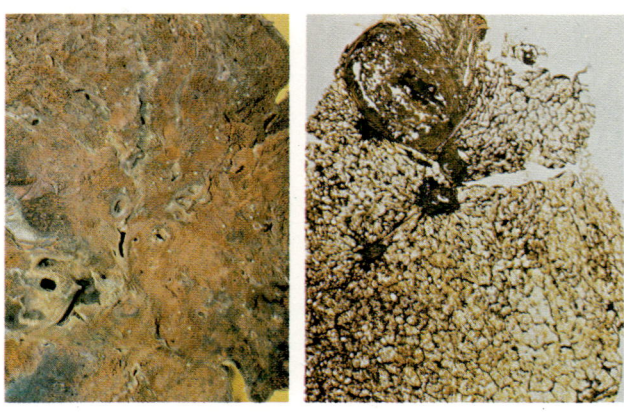

Figure 15.5 *Left:* A museum specimen of the lung of a haematite miner showing the diffuse brick red appearance. In this form there is often focal emphysema but minimal fibrosis. *Right:* Gough–Wentworth paper section showing delineation of interlobular septa, also soft central dust foci with no related emphysema but with stellate complicated secondary foci and a large apico-posterior massive lesion. Massive lesions usually correlate with the silica content of the lung..

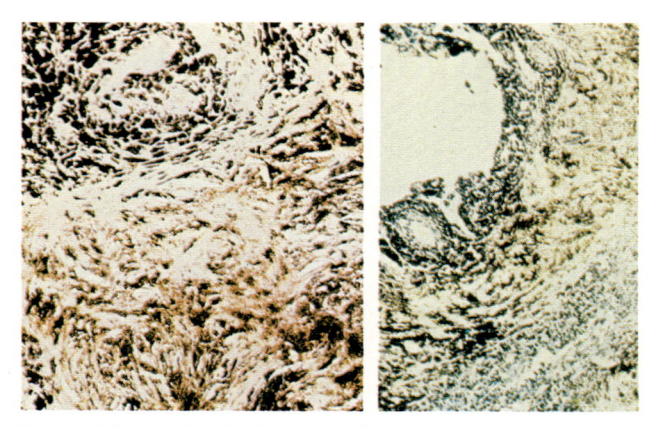

Figure 15.6 *Left:* Section from area of massive dust fibrosis showing collagenous tissue containing anthracotic and brown dust-laden macrophages. H & E × 40. *Right:* The haematite appears brown on Perls staining but there is also haemosiderin present, which is Prussian-blue positive. PERLS × 38.4.

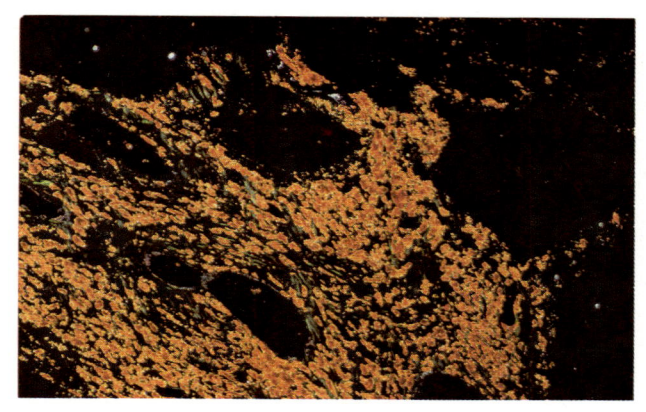

OCCUPATIONAL LUNG DISORDERS – III. METALS, FUMES AND ORGANIC MATERIALS

Figure 15.7 Haematite appears as orange luminous clots; there is also some white birefringent material present representing silica. H&E × 384.

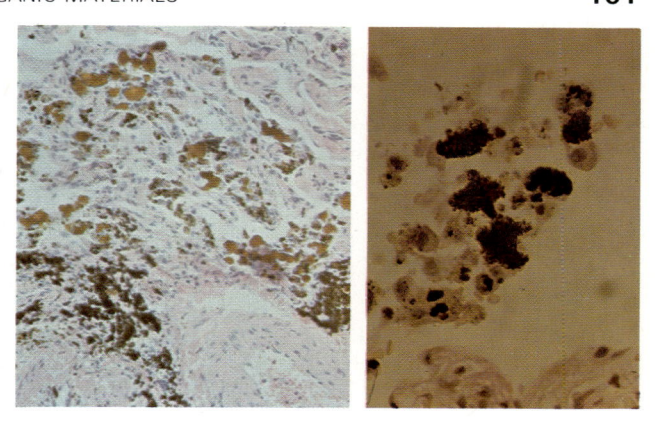

Figure 15.8 An arc welder in the ship-building industry who complained of progressive dyspnoea and a restrictive lung function profile. Lung biopsy revealed interstitial fibrosis and numerous ferruginous bodies. Modified asbestosis bodies were also found with ease. In such cases, clearly it is either the exposure to the fibrogenic asbestosis fibre or metal fumes, other than the iron, which are responsible for the fibrosis. *Left:* H&E × 96. *Right:* H&E × 384.

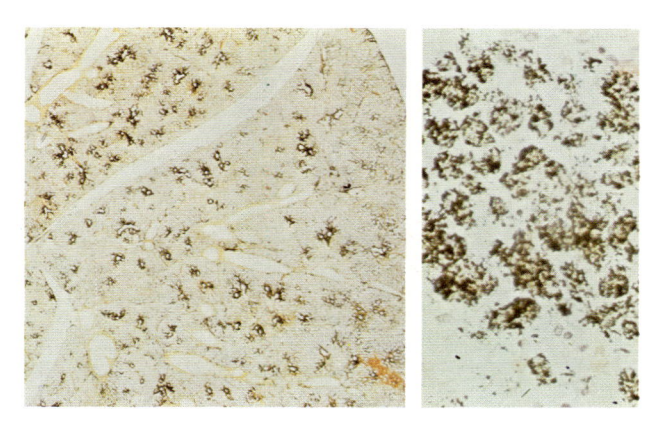

Figure 15.9 Gough–Wentworth paper section of a 35-year-old tin worker who died from trauma, who during life had extensive radiological nodular opacities. *Left:* Numerous, small central dust foci with no related emphysema. *Right:* Collection of heavily stannous-oxide laden macrophages. H&E × 96.

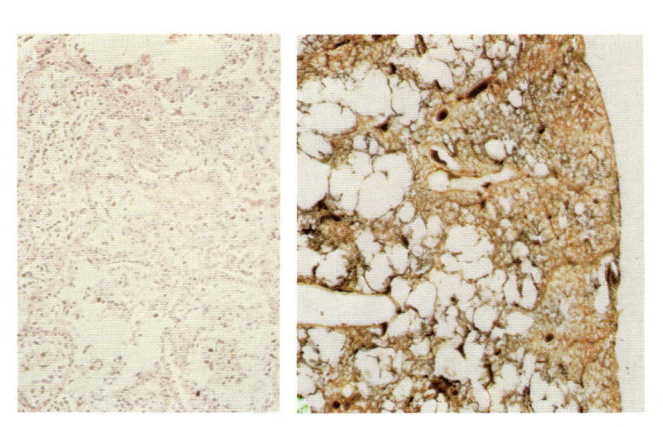

Figure 15.10 *Left:* A welder, working in an enclosed space, cutting cadmium steel bolts died approximately one week after exposure. The histology shows inflammatory thickening of interalveolar septa, intraalveolar mononuclear cells and inflammatory oedema resulting in a small focus of 'hyaline membrane' formation. H&E × 96 *Right:* Centrilobular emphysema with sparing of the subpleural area in a cadmium miner. Gough–Wentworth × 7.2.

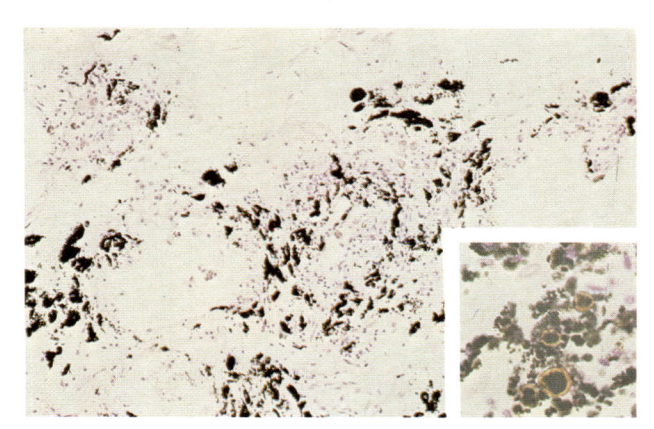

Figure 15.11 Lung from a cotton worker shows collections of dust-laden macrophages with some associated fibrosis. *Inset:* Numerous dust-laden macrophages and a typical 'byssinotic' body.

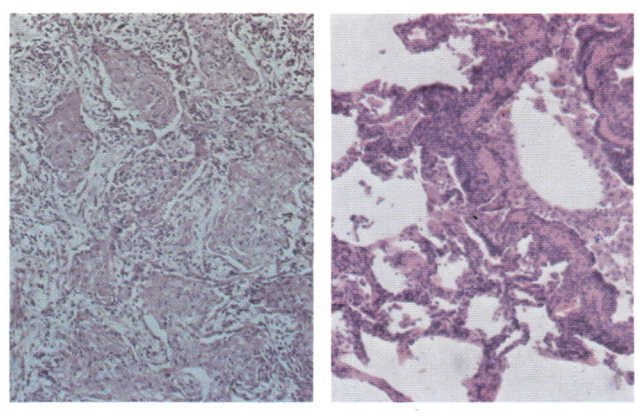

Figure 15.12 Open biopsy from a toluene diisocyanate worker. *Left:* Organizing intraalveolar fibrinous exudate and thickening of interalveolar septa. H&E × 96 *Right:* Centrilobular accentuation of disease with a mononuclear infiltrate and collagenous thickening of interalveolar septa. H&E × 78.

diameter, which consists of collections of dust-laden macrophages situated around respiratory bronchioles (Figure 15.9).

Cadmium

Inhaled cadmium metal or its compound can result in either acute or chronic disease. The former is due to inhalation of high concentrations of fumes and the features are those of diffuse alveolar damage (Figure 15.10). The disease is often fatal from a combination of respiratory and renal insufficiency, acute renal damage being also a feature of this exposure. The chronic form of the disease occurs as a result of repeated short exposures to low or moderate concentration of cadmium fumes and the picture is one of centrilobular emphysema[8]. An alleged pathognomonic feature, in this form of emphysema, is the 'sparing' of the subpleural area (Figure 15.10).

Mercury

Inhalation of high concentrations of mercury vapour may cause diffuse alveolar damage.

Silo Filler's Disease

Nitrogen dioxide is present in greatest amount 7-10 days after the silo is filled and exposure results in the pathological picture of diffuse alveolar damage. Some patients go on to develop bronchiolitis obliterans and pulmonary fibrosis.

Organic Materials

Organic substances resulting in extrinsic bronchioloalveolitis are discussed in Chapter 7.

Byssinosis

Cotton workers suffering from byssinosis complain of 'chest tightness' on returning to work after the weekend or holiday which gets better after a few hours and does not re-appear until after the following weekend. As the disease progresses, the symptoms may occur on Tuesday and Wednesday and in the most severe cases may extend over the whole week. Monday, however, remains the worst day. It is the result of exposure to the dust of raw or waste cotton, soft hemp or flax.

The pathological changes are usually non-specific and include mucous gland hyperplasia and muscular hypertrophy of lobar bronchi, and sometimes centrilobular emphysema. Byssinosis bodies are demonstrable in only a small percentage of cases[9]. These specific structures consist of spherical nodules (up to 10 um diameter) with a central black nidus surrounded by a clear yellow halo up to 2 um thick.

All cases show pigmentation by black dust with minimal associated fibrosis situated mainly around distal bronchi and vessels (Figure 15.11). A small number of cases have been described in whom established interstitial fibrosis has been attributed to their occupation[10].

Organic Isocyanates

These substances are used in the manufacture of foams, synthetic rubbers, adhesives and paints; toluene diisocyanate (TDI) is the most widely used.

It is well recognized that organic isocyanate vapour may cause airways obstruction but less well appreciated is that it may result in a 'hypersensitivity pneumonitis'. This is characterized by interstitial 'pneumonitis' and fibrosis, filling of alveoli by large mononuclear cells (DIP-like) and a fine fibrinous network within alveoli; the changes are most conspicuous in the centre of lobules. A prominent eosinophilic component is present within interalveolar septa and alveolar spaces[11] (Figure 15.12).

References

1. Mitchell, J., Manning, G. B., Molyneux, M. and Love, R. E. (1961). Pulmonary fibrosis in workers exposed to finely powdered aluminium. *Br. J. Ind. Med.*, **18,** 10
2. Shaver, C. G. and Riddell, A. R. (1947). Lung changes associated with manufacture of alumina abrasives. *J. Ind. Hyg. Toxicol.*, **29,** 145
3. Coats, E. O. and Watson, J. H. L. (1971). Diffuse interstitial lung disease in tungsten carbide workers. *Ann. Int. Med.*, **75,** 709
4. Abraham, J. L. and Hertzberg, M. A. (1981) Inorganic particles associated with desquamative interstitial pneumonia. *Chest*, **805,** 675-705
5. Hazard, J. B. (1959). Pathological changes of beryllium disease. *Arch. Ind. Med.*, **19,** 179
6. Jones Williams, W. (1958). A histological study of the lungs in 52 cases of chronic beryllium disease. *Br. J. Ind. Med.*, **15,** 85
7. Guidotti, R. L., Abraham, J. L., DeNee, P. B. and Smith, J. R. (1978). Arc welders' pneumoconiosis: application of advanced scanning electron microscopy. *Arch. Environ. Health*, **33,** 117
8. Gough, J. (1960). Emphysema in relation to occupation. *Ind. Med. Surg.*, **29,** 283
9. Edwards, C., Macartney, J., Rooke, G. and Ward, F. (1975). The pathology of the lung in byssinotics. *Thorax*, **30.** 612
10. Ruttner, J. R., Spycher, M. A. and Engeler, M. L. (1968). Pulmonary fibrosis induced by cotton fibre inhalation. *Pathol. Microbiol.*, **32,** 1
11. Charles, J., Bernstein, A., Jones, B., Jones, D. J., Edwards, J. H., Seal, R. M. E. and Seaton, A. (1976). Hypersensitivity pneumonitis after exposure to isocyanates. *Thorax*, **31,** 127

Lung Carcinomas

Major Categories of Carcinomas of the Lung

Lung carcinomas present as either central or peripheral tumours. Central tumours occlude partially or completely main, lobar, segmental or subsegmental bronchi. If partially obstructing a major airway, haemoptysis may be the sole manifestation. Where smaller airways are occluded the distal lung will either be collapsed with little inflammatory change, (Figure 16.1), or more usually there will be collapse consolidation (so-called obstructive pneumonitis) (Figure 16.2). This distal change may constitute a large proportion of the radiological opacity. Very rarely, slowly growing tumours may result in lobar obstructive emphysema due to a ball-valve action. Bronchiectasis may also be a consequence (Figure 16.3). Occasionally the distal lung is the seat of frank suppurative pneumonia as may be a localized abscess. Occasionally central growths occlude a pulmonary artery causing infarction of the distal lung. These features are represented in the right lung of plate 16.1.

Peripheral growths may be immediately subpleural with thickening of the overlying pleura and sometimes puckering, suggesting the presence of a pre-existing scar (Figure 16.4). Peripheral tumours may be located deeper within the parenchyma and even extend toward the hilum and involve hilar nodes, but by definition not occlude major bronchi. Peripheral tumours may cavitate (Figure 16.5) and mimic, radiologically, lung abscess or tuberculous cavities.

Bronchiolo-alveolar carcinomas may 'consolidate' lung parenchyma to simulate type 3 pneumococcal pneumonia (Figure 16.6). Less frequent are multiple nodular lesions. Bronchiolo-alveolar carcinomas often arise in previously damaged lungs. Secondary lung involvement by tumour, classically the pancreas, may mimic bronchiolo-alveolar carcinoma.

Diffuse lymphatic permeation, either from a primary lung cancer or a secondary from gastrointestinal tract or breast, produces the characteristic appearance of thickened interlobular septa and prominence of vessels and bronchi ('lymphangitis carcinomatosa') (Figure 16.7).

These latter macroscopic appearances of lung cancer are illustrated in the left lung of plate 16.1.

We base our histological typing of lung carcinomas on the WHO International Classification[1]. Although it has some imperfections, it is comprehensive – in our experience and others[2] fewer than 1% of lung tumours remain unclassified – and reproducible, provided that strict criteria are adhered to. Reproducibility is greater the more material available for study since a significant proportion of pulmonary tumours show diversity from one area to another. Where possible, at least three blocks from a tumour should be examined. Sometimes typing of a biopsy specimen may later be altered as a consequence of more tissue being available. This is most likely to happen when the initial diagnosis is large-cell carcinoma since further material may reveal small foci of squamous or glandular differentiation resulting in a diagnosis of poorly differentiated squamous or adenocarcinoma. However, it must be realized that radiotherapy treatment may modify the histology of the tumour. For every lung tumour we routinely use PAS and the combined haemalum–erythrosin–saffron and alcian green stains[1]. The latter demonstrates keratin and mucin.

Tumours are only classified as undifferentiated if no foci of squamous or glandular differentiation are evident. Tumours showing more than one type of differentiation are categorized as combined tumours of their respective types, e.g. adenosquamous carcinoma. However, by convention[3], small foci of glandular or squamous structures within a predominantly small cell carcinoma still retains the latter designation.

Rarely, a metastasis may reveal a different cell type to the primary lung tumour.

Squamous Cell Carcinoma (Epidermoid Carcinoma)

In most series of lung carcinomas in Britain and the USA squamous cell carcinoma appears to be the most frequent type. The majority are central, show a tendency to cavitation, and are less frequently inoperable than the other major categories.

To qualify as squamous cell carcinoma in the WHO classification, a tumour must show either keratin and/or intercellular bridges. Although these criteria are rather restrictive – stratification and whorl formation are ignored – it does result in more consistent typing of poorly differentiated and undifferentiated tumours.

Squamous cell carcinoma can be subdivided into well, moderate and poorly differentiated. Abundant keratin, epithelial pearls and numerous intercellular bridges are seen in the well differentiated tumours (Figure 16.2). By contrast, intercellular bridges and/or keratin are found with difficulty in the poorly differentiated tumours. Moderately differentiated tumours show intermediate features (Figure 16.3). Areas of sqamous metaplasia, dysplasia and *in-situ* carcinoma are frequently found in the bronchial epithelium which is in proximity to the invasive tumour.

It might be expected that the histopathologist might encounter a full range of epithelial change

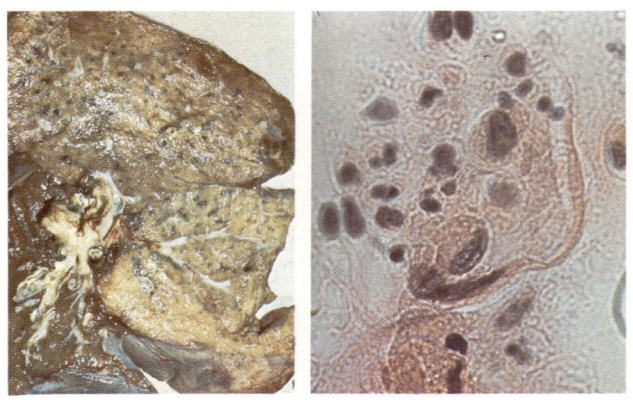

Figure 16.1 *Left:* Pneumonectomy specimen with central carcinoma in apical lower segmental bronchus occluding lower part of left main bronchus. The lower lobe is completely collapsed. *Right:* The cell type was established pre-operatively by sputum cytology as squamous carcinoma.

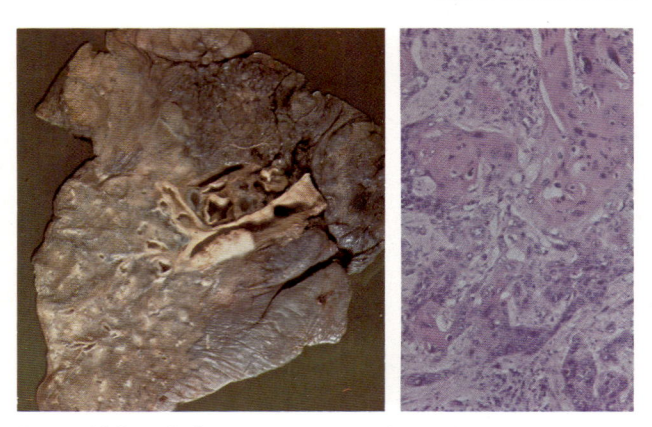

Figure 16.2 *Left:* Pneumonectomy specimen showing a carcinoma involving right lower lobe bronchus resulting in obstructive pneumonitis of basal segments. *Right:* Bronchoscopy showed a well differentiated squamous carcinoma H&E × 240.

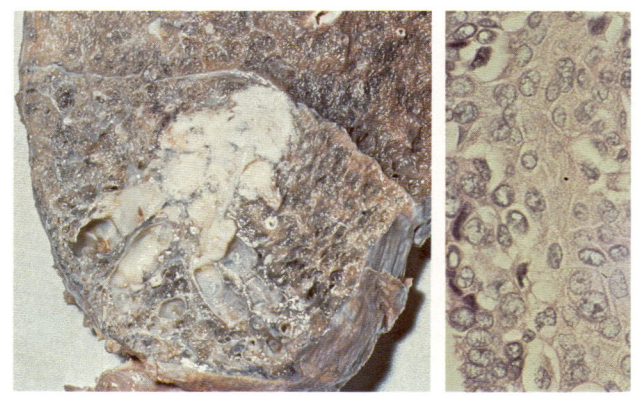

Figure 16.3 *Left:* Central carcinoma with distended bronchi containing mucopus. *Right:* Both criteria – keratin and intercellular bridges – were discernible in this moderately differentiated squamous carcinoma. H&E × 240.

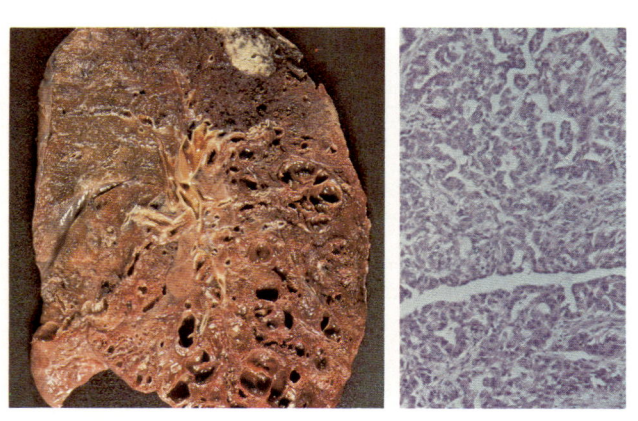

Figure 16.4 *Left:* Post-mortem lung specimen revealing a peripheral subpleural carcinoma with associated pleural thickening and puckering in the right upper lobe. There is saccular bronchiectasis of lower lobe. *Right:* The histology was that of a papillary adenocarcinoma. H&E × 38.4.

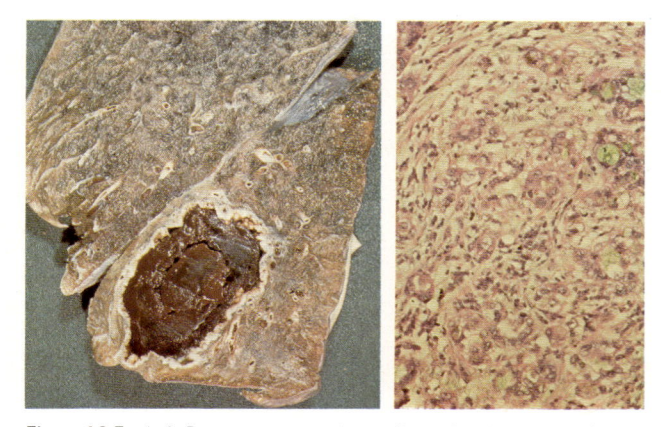

Figure 16.5 *Left:* Post-mortem specimen of lung showing cavitated carcinoma containing recent haemorrhage. This patient died suddenly of massive haemoptysis. *Right:* The tumour histology was that of a mucin secreting acinar adenocarcinoma. WHO × 96.

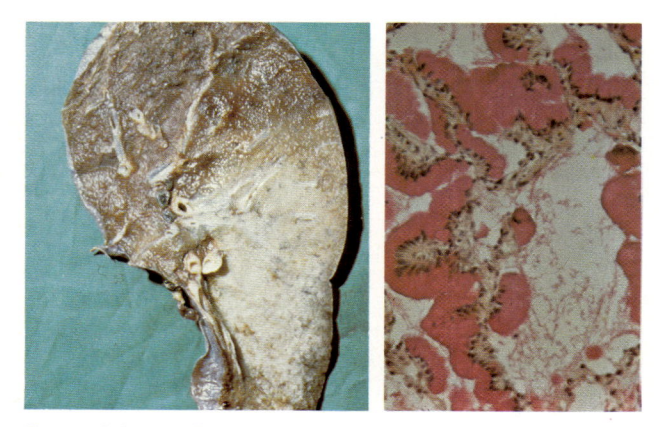

Figure 16.6 *Left:* Pneumonectomy specimen showing typical 'consolidated' appearance of alveolar cell carcinoma. The cut surface of the tumour was slimy to the touch. *Right:* There is intense mucin secretion within the tumour cell cytoplasm and alveolar space. Mucorrhea can be easily understood. PAS diastase × 192.

LUNG CARCINOMAS

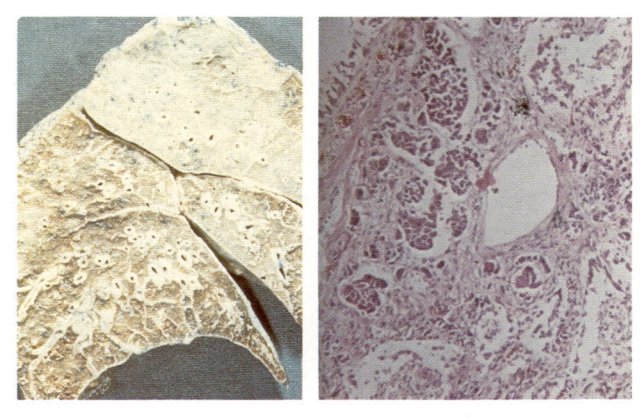

Figure 16.7 *Left:* Post-mortem specimen of right lung demonstrating carcinoma extensively involving the upper lobe and the typical apearance of 'lymphangitis carcinomatosa' in the middle and lower lobes. *Right:* There is tumour within bronchial submucosal lymphatics and a septum. The perilobular alveoli reveal atypical metaplastic change. H&E × 96.

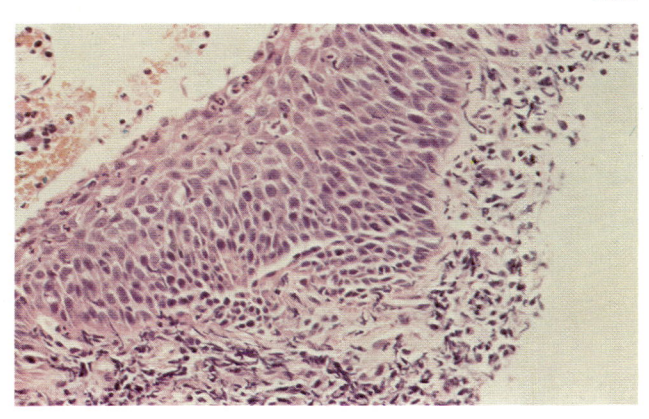

Figure 16.8 This biopsy showed dysplastic and *in-situ* neoplastic changes but no definite invasion. The resected specimen revealed an overt invasive central squamous carcinoma. H&E × 192.

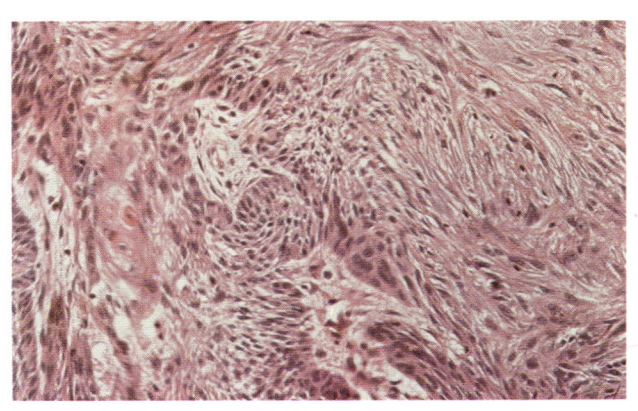

Figure 16.9 This shows a moderately differentiated squamous carcinoma with a prominent spindle celled component. H&E × 192.

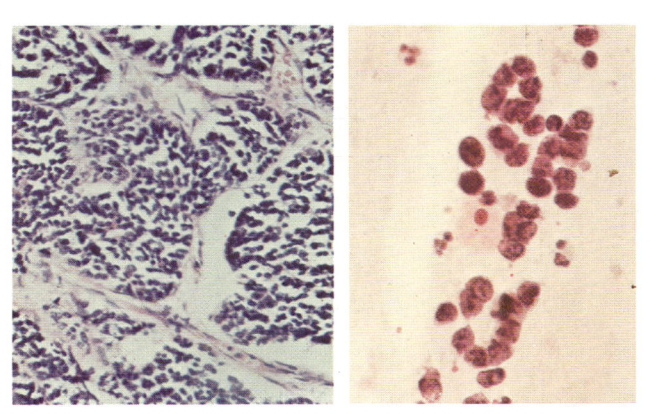

Figure 16.10 *Left:* Typical oat cell carcinoma. H&E × 96. *Right:* Another case in which oat cell carcinoma was diagnosed by sputum cytology.

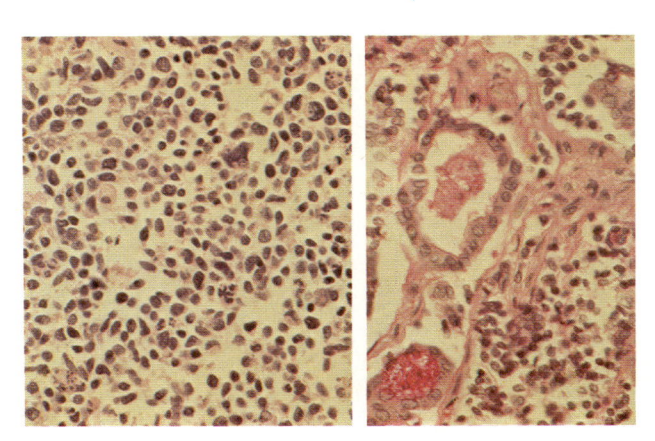

Figure 16.11 *Left:* Most of the cells are lymphocyte-like, but some have more cytoplasm than classical 'oat' cells and occasional tumour giant cells. By definition this would be classified as oat cell carcinoma rather than small cell intermediate. H&E × 240. *Right:* Oat cell carcinoma with tubules containing mucin. H&E × 240.

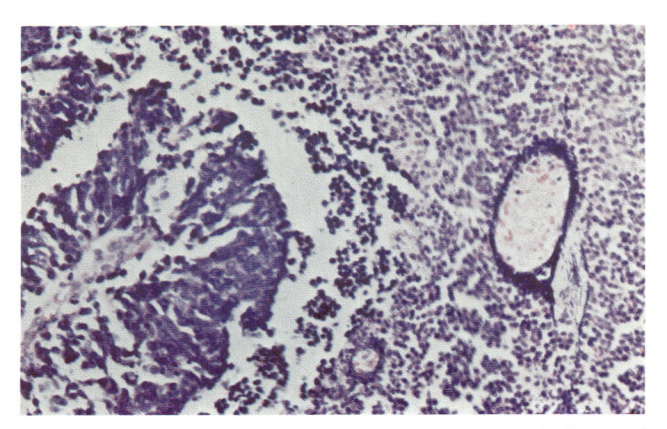

Figure 16.12 The viable tumour on the left is sufficiently fusiform and polygonal to be regarded as 'intermediate' rather than 'oat', but pyknotic nuclei around this tumour mimic 'oat'. Far right the tumour is more necrotic and the vessel wall impregnated with DNA. H&E × 74.4.

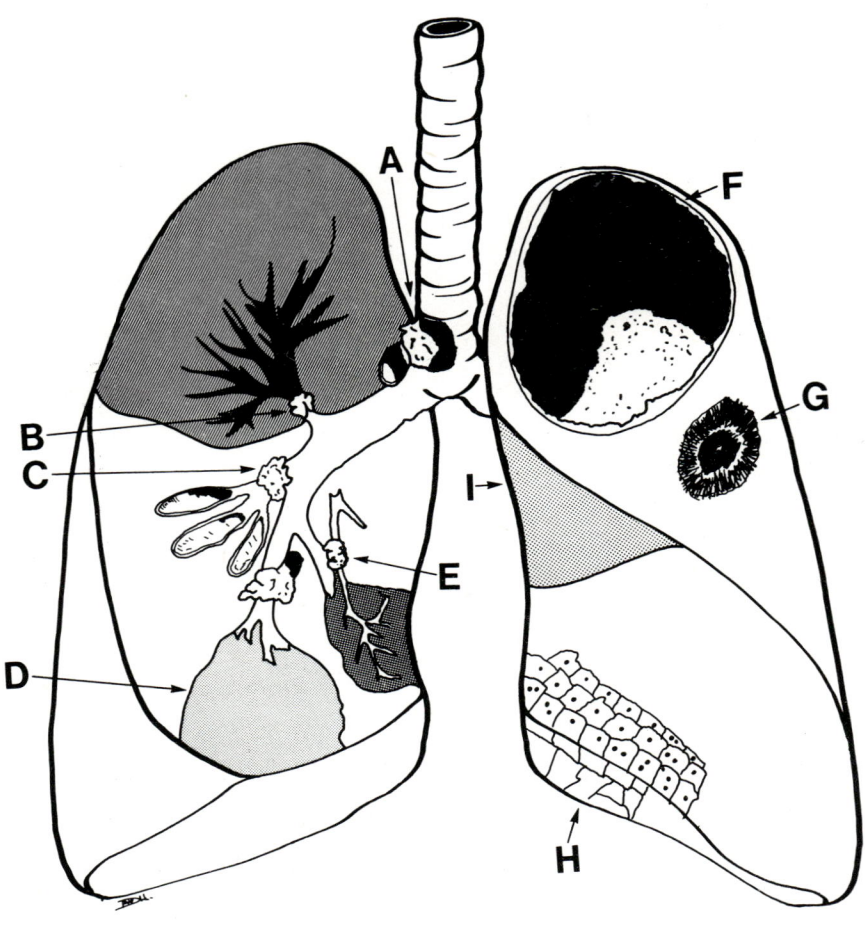

Plate 16.1 Macroscopic appearance and consequences of lung carcinoma A: Central growth with no distal obstructive consequences; B: Central growth occluding lobar bronchus with 'obstructive pneumonitis'; C: Central growth with distal bronchiectasis or mucoceles; D: Central growth with suppurative pneumonia or lung abscess; E: Central growth causing obstruction of pulmonary artery with distal infarct; F: Peripheral cavitating carcinoma; G: Solid peripheral 'scar' carcinoma; H: 'Lymphangitis carcinomatosa; I: Pneumonic appearance in alveolar cell carcinoma

ranging through squamous metaplasia, mild and severe dysplasia, *in-situ* carcinoma to invasive malignancy. Metaplasia is frequently observed in patients who are proven to have no neoplasm. However, severe dysplasia and *in-situ* carcinoma, when apparently encountered in small biopsy material, are almost invariably part of an invasive central squamous carcinoma (Figure 16.8).

Biopsy specimens, especially when small, are often evaluated more by cytological than morphological criteria, and this should be clearly stated in the histopathologist's report.

Since our routine employment of stains for mucin on every lung tumour, we have observed foci of mucin containing cells in about 10% of what appear to be typical squamous carcinomas. There was no other evidence of glandular differentiation and it did not appear to be due to entrapped mucous glands since we have observed it in metastases. The significance of this finding has still to be evaluated and we still categorize these tumours as squamous cell carcinomas.

An uncommon variant of squamous cell carcinoma is the spindle celled type. This demonstrates a definite sqamous component admixed with a spindle celled element, with transitions between the two (Figure 16.9). It is usually polypoid and situated within a bronchus. Great difficulty may be experienced in differentiating this from a carcinosarcoma (see Chapter 18).

Small Cell Carcinoma

This accounts for approximately one third of lung carcinomas. It is extremely malignant and extensive metastasis may be present even when the primary tumour is small. The majority are located within the larger central bronchi.

Although the behaviour of small cell carcinoma appears quite dissimilar to that of the bronchial carcinoid, there are grounds for considering small cell carcinoma as a highly malignant counterpart of bronchial carcinoid[5]. Both tumours contain neurosecretory granules within their cells at electron microscopy; both are associated with ectopic hormone production; and occasionally, carcinoid-like areas may be observed in what are otherwise typical small cell carcinomas. Bensch *et al.*[5] proposed that the derivation of both was from Kultschitsky cells.

The WHO classification subdivides small cell carcinomas into: (a) oat cell type; (b) intermediate cell type, and (c) combined oat-cell carcinoma.

Oat Cell Carcinoma

More than half of the small cell carcinomas are of the oat cell type. The tumours are composed of sheets, ribbons and rosettes of lymphocyte-like cells which have round or oval dense nuclei and sparse cytoplasm (Figure 16.10). The cells are slightly larger than lymphocytes. Occasional giant cells with large, irregular, dark nuclei may be present (Figure 16.11). Necrosis is frequently evident and, in relation to this, darkly staining haematoxophilic material (DNA) is frequently observed in vessel walls[3] – a feature not seen in other varieties of lung carcinoma (Figure 16.12). Tubules and ductules sometimes containing small amounts of mucin within their centres but not within the cells may be present[3] (Figure 16.11). Reticulin stains demonstrate argyrophilic membranes around individual cells[6]. Fisher et al.[6] found argyrophil granules in 15% of oat cell carcinomas. Vascular and perineural invasion is frequently evident.

Intermediate Cell Type

This tumour is similar to oat cell carcinoma but the cells have more cytoplasm and may be polygonal and/or fusiform in shape. Its behaviour is similar to that of the oat cell type (Figure 16.13).

Combined Oat-cell Carcinoma

These are very rare tumours exhibiting foci of squamous carcinoma and/or adenocarcinoma in addition to a definite oat cell component (Figure 16.14).

Biopsies of this group of tumours provide the histopathologist with a problem, when as frequently happens, there is considerable crushing of the tissue, particularly as the forceps become blunt with constant use (Figure 16.15). Recognizable neoplastic cells then have to be searched for. Under these circumstances the histopathologist should alert his clinical colleagues, who now treat these tumours with radiotherapy and cytotoxic drugs. Endoscopic biopsy is often the sole proof of diagnosis. Related to this problem is that squamous carcinoma may have areas resembling small cell intermediate tumours (Figure 16.16), which clinicians will regard as not suitable for surgery unless the report is very carefully worded.

Adenocarcinoma

The majority of adenocarcinomas arise in the periphery of the lung. They may show tubules, acini, papillae, solid areas and colloid areas (Figures 16.4 and 16.5). Great care must be taken to exclude secondary adenocarcinoma, since pulmonary metastases from primary intra-abdominal glandular malignancies may resemble very closely both adenocarcinoma and bronchiolo-alveolar carcinoma. In our experience any adenocarcinoma found on central bronchial biopsy, but particularly those with tall columnar epithelium, are more frequently secondary and therefore extrathoracic primary malignancies should be considered (Figure 16.17). It is well recognized that secondary deposits may present as visible tumours bronchoscopically, mimic primary tumours in their presentation, and also may involve hilar nodes.

The WHO subdivides adenocarcinoma into: (a) acinar type; (b) papillary type; (c) bronchiolo-alveolar type; and (d) solid carcinoma with mucus formation[1].

Acinar Adenocarcinoma

This shows a predominance of acini and tubules with or without a minor component of papillary structures or solid areas (Figure 16.5).

Papillary Adenocarcinoma

The predominant pattern consists of papillary structures with or without a lesser component of acinar or solid structures (Figure 16.4).

Both the acinar and papillary types may be graded into well, moderately, or poorly differentiated adenocarcinomas according to the amount of gland formation and cellular pleomorphism. Occasionally, equal quantities of acinar and papillary elements may be present; the tumour should be designated acinar and papillary adenocarcinoma.

Bronchiolo-alveolar Carcinoma

This comprises 1–8% of primary lung malignancies. It is characterized by tumour cells growing along the pre-existing alveolar walls, at times so well differentiated that distinction from atypical epithelial hyperplasia may be difficult[7] (Figure 16.18). Two main cell patterns occur, often within the same tumour[8]. One pattern is particularized by delicate alveolar septa lined by tall columnar cells, containing mucus in the cytoplasm and basal nuclei (Figure 16.6, right), forming single rows for the most part and occasional papillary infolding. The other consists of low columnar or cuboidal pleomorphic cells, containing little or no mucin, lining slightly thickened septa. These tumours generally have a low mitotic rate. Alveoli, some distance from the main tumour mass, may be packed with tumour cells.

At first, the tumour forms a solitary mass but it may become multinodular or diffuse and frequently bilateral – usually attributed to aerogenous spread because tumour cells still line intact alveolar walls. When the tumour is diffuse and mucin-secreting it may resemble a type 3 pneumococcal pneumonia macroscopically (Figure 16.6).

Bennett et al.[7] emphasized that ordinary adenocarcinoma (acinar or papillary) may contain foci typical of bronchiolo-alveolar carcinoma and the converse may also occur. They concluded that separation of bronchiolo-alveolar carcinoma from ordinary adenocarcinoma was rather arbitrary. Both are peripherally located, both are frequently associated with localized scar or diffuse fibrosis, and both may exhibit papillary foci containing psammoma bodies. We retain the separation but appreciate the difficulties that may sometimes occur in doing so.

Solid Carcinoma with Mucus Formation

Previously included under the category of large cell carcinoma, the revised WHO classification now regards this as a subcategory of adenocarcinoma. It consists of sheets of large cells with abundant cytoplasm, some containing mucin (Figure 16.19). It lacks acini, tubules and papillae. Histochemical stains for mucin are essential for diagnosis.

Large Cell Carcinoma

This category should be reserved for tumours which exhibit no evidence of small cell, squamous or glandular differentiation and are composed of large cells, with large nuclei, prominent nucleoli, well defined cytoplasmic borders, conspicuous cytoplasm and which lack mucin[1] (Figure 16.20).

In practice this has proven the most problematic group with regard to consistency of diagnosis. The greater the amount of material examined the more likely one is to find a small focus of differentiation which necessitates reallocation to another category. If the criteria are strictly adhered to this accounts for a relatively small percentage of lung tumours. This may be of academic importance only since Churg[9] concluded, based on ultrastructural studies, that the majority of large cell carcinomas were very poorly differentiated adenocarcinomas or squamous carcinomas.

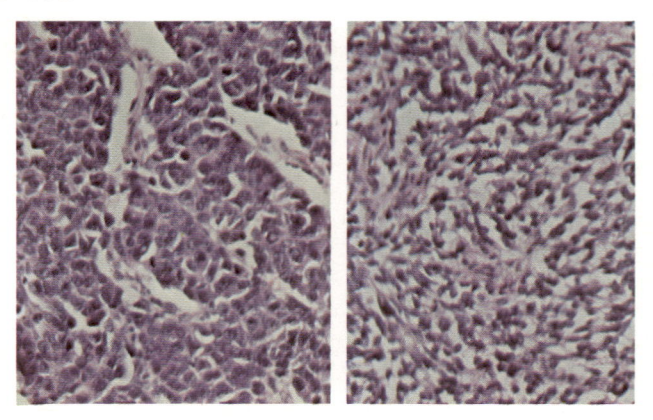

Figure 16.13 *Left:* An intermediate (polygonal) small cell carcinoma. H & E × 192. *Right:* An intermediate (fusiform) small cell carcinoma. H & E × 192.

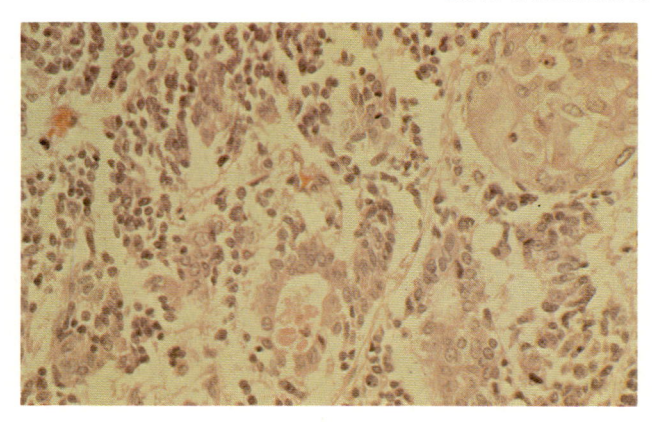

Figure 16.14 Small cell carcinoma showing tubules and squamous areas. H & E × 240.

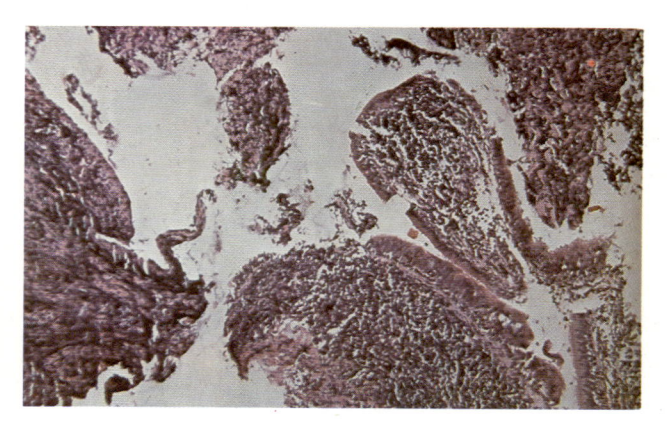

Figure 16.15 Most of the biopsy was crushed as in the top right and bottom left of the picture. However, the central areas reveal recognizable densely packed malignant lymphocyte-like cells in the submucosa. (This biopsy presented a further problem in that there was a history of previous therapy for diffuse lymphocytic lymphoma. Cytological differentiation is difficult.) H & E × 96.

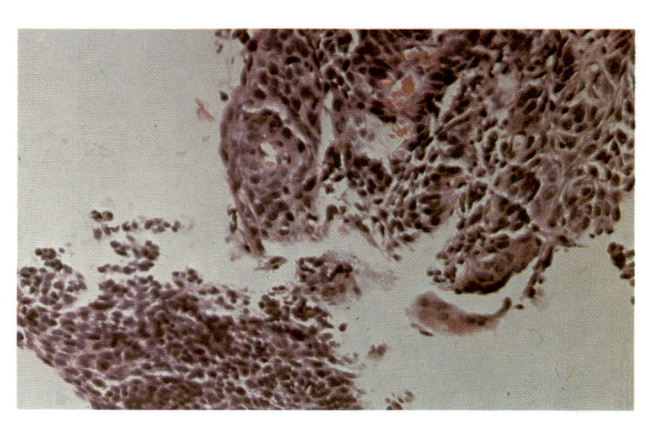

Figure 16.16 Endoscopy specimen showing, at bottom left a poorly differentiated carcinoma where intercellular bridges were observed, but in the top right an area which could be mistaken for oat cell carcinoma. However, the amount of cytoplasm and fusiform appearance should alert the histopathologist to the possibility of a poorly differentiated squamous carcinoma. H & E × 96.

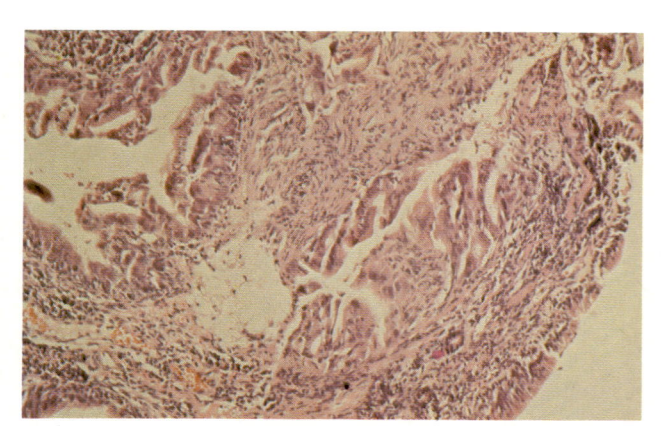

Figure 16.17 A bronchoscopy biopsy showing secondary adenocarcinoma from ovary. H & E × 96.

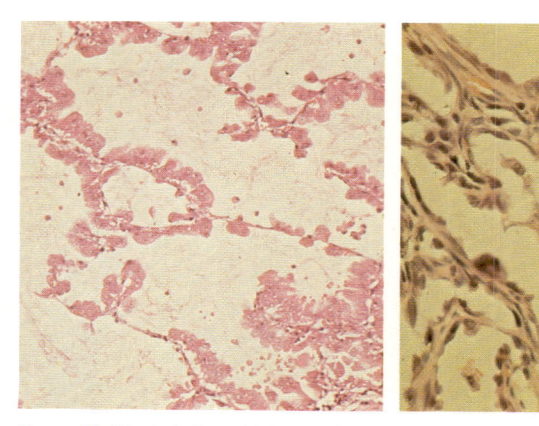

Figure 16.18 *Left:* Bronchiolo-alveolar cell carcinoma with rows of cells lined up along the alveolar framework. H & E × 96. *Right:* The same case but a focus of atypical? neoplastic epithelial proliferation occurring in a separate lobe from the main tumour mass. H & E × 240.

LUNG CARCINOMAS

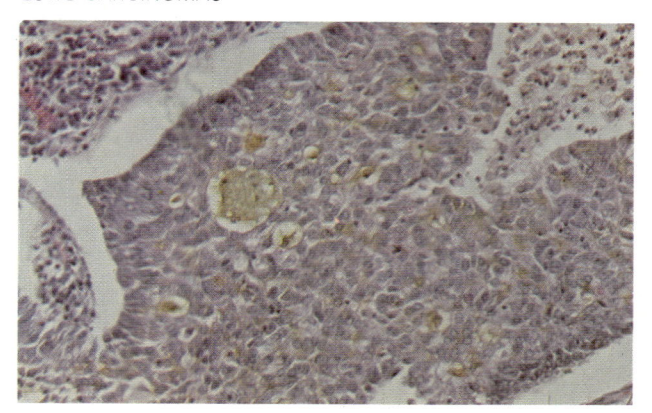

Figure 16.19 An undifferentiated large cell tumour containing much mucin. WHO × 192.

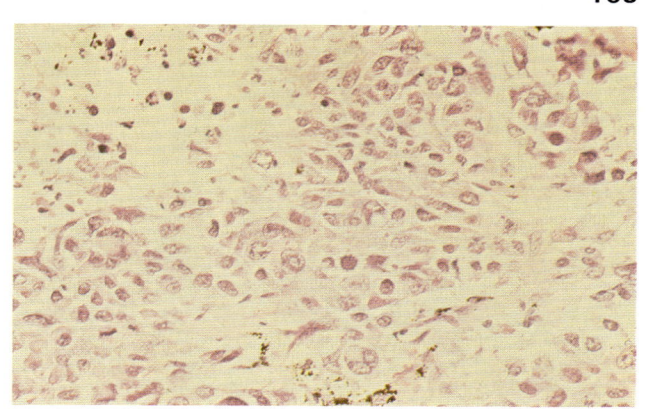

Figure 16.20 Sheets of large pleomorphic cells with moderate to copious amounts of cytoplasm. Giant cells are seen but these are not as bizarre or prolific as in giant cell carcinoma. H&E × 240.

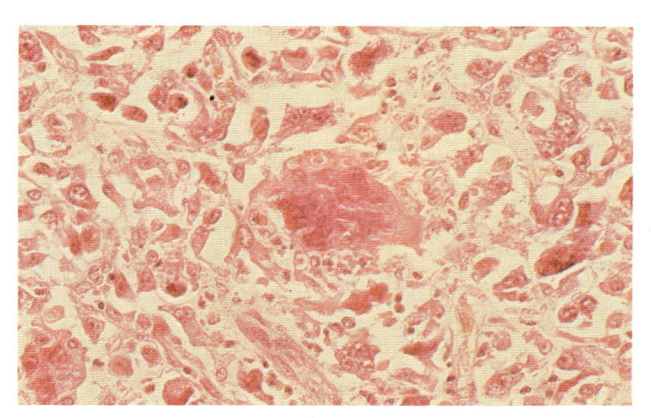

Figure 16.21 Giant cell carcinoma exhibiting bizarre tumour cells. The giant cell in the centre of the picture contains ingested red blood cells. H&E × 100.

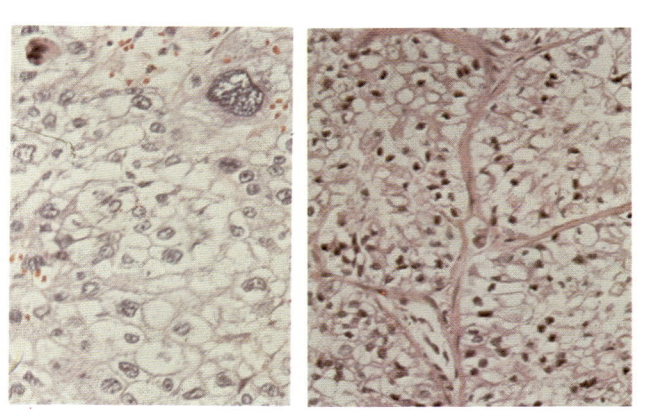

Figure 16.22 Clear cell carcinoma showing a sheet-like arrangement on the left and an alveolar pattern on the right. H&E × 240.

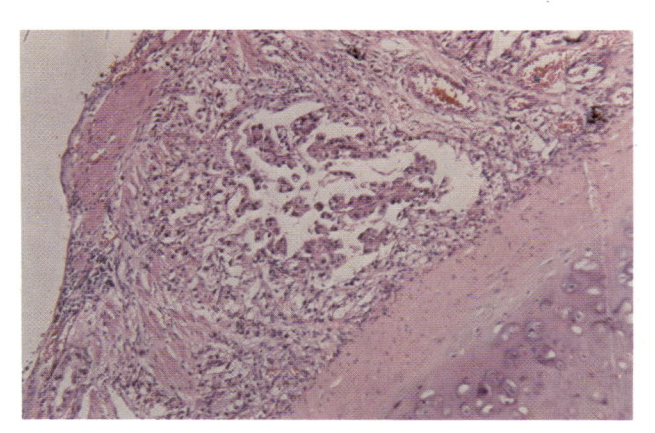

Figure 16.23 A bronchus showing a secondary deposit of renal cell carcinoma in the submucosa. H&E × 74.4.

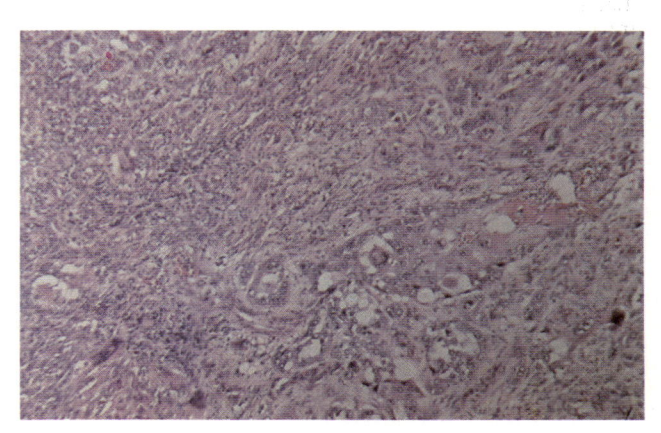

Figure 16.24 A carcinoma showing an intermingling of squamous and glandular elements – adenosquamous carcinoma. H&E × 192.

Giant Cell Carcinoma

Regarded by the WHO[1] as a variant of large cell carcinoma this is characterised by large, bizarre cells, often multinucleated, with strongly eosinophilic cytoplasm (Figure 16.21). The large cells often contain neutrophils and small tumour cells within their cytoplasm. The tumour is typically peripheral, highly malignant and has often invaded the chest wall by the time of presentation[10].

Criteria for the diagnosis of giant cell carcinoma have varied between different authors; some accept the diagnosis only if the tumour appears pure and exhibits no evidence of squamous or glandular differentiation whereas other include under giant cell carcinoma tumours which show glandular or squamous structures in addition to the typical giant cell areas. To avoid confusion we classify the latter as giant cell carcinoma plus adenocarcinoma or squamous carcinoma. However, the behaviour appears to be determined by the giant cell component.

Giant cell carcinoma of the lung has to be distinguished from irradiated squamous cell carcinomas, in which giant cells may occur, and rhabdomyosarcoma[11]. For the latter diagnosis we require the demonstration of cross-striations.

Clear Cell Carcinoma

The WHO[1] defines this as a tumour composed of cells with clear or foamy cytoplasm, which may contain glycogen but not mucin, and which does not show squamous or glandular structures (Figure 16.22). However, the earliest report of clear cell carcinoma[12] described mucin within the clear cells, and concluded that it was a form of adenocarcinoma. If the WHO's criteria are strictly adhered to clear cell carcinoma is a very rare tumour – less than 1% of lung carcinomas[13]. However, if tumours composed of greater that 50% of clear cells but containing foci of adenocarcinoma or glandular carcinoma are included then the incidence is 4–5% of lung carcinomas[13]. Moreover, a tumour composed of clear cells on initial biopsy may lose this appearance later. Katzenstein *et al.* concluded that clear cell carcinoma could be a variant of squamous carcinoma, adenocarcinoma or large cell carcinoma and found no effect on prognosis[13].

Tumours composed purely of clear cells have to be differentiated from secondary renal cell carcinoma and this may necessitate intravenous pyelography. It has been reported that, in most thoracic units, tumours of clear cell type seldom prove to be of renal origin. However, we have experienced several examples of renal carcinomas, presenting with polypoid intrabronchial lesions[14] (Figure 16.23).

Adenosquamous Carcinoma

This is a tumour showing malignant glandular and squamous elements. The latter requires the demonstration of intercellular bridges and/or keratin. It is said to behave similarly to adenocarcinoma (Figure 16.24).

Scar Carcinoma

Lung cancers may develop in relation to focal scars (e.g. infarcts, tubercle) and diffuse interstitial fibrosis (e.g. asbestosis, systemic sclerosis). In scarred lungs all gradations from hyperplasia, atypical hyperplasia to malignancy of bronchiolar epithelium may be seen.

The majority are adenocarcinomas but squamous, large cell and adenosquamous carcinomas may arise within scars. Scar cancers may invade lymphatic and blood vessels at a very early stage and give rise to distant metastases even when small[11].

References

1. World Health Organization (1977). International Histological Classification of Tumours. Histological Typing of Lung Tumours (Revision) (Geneva: World Health Organization)
2. Larsson, S. and Zettergren, L. (1976). Histological typing of lung cancer. Application of the World Health Organization classification of 479 cases. *Acta Pathol. Microbiol. Scand.*, **A84**, 529
3. Azzopardi, J. G. (1959). Oat cell carcinoma of the bronchus. *J. Pathol. Bacteriol.*, **78**, 513
4. Lichtiger, B., Mackay, B. and Tessmer, C. F. (1970). Spindle cell variant of squamous carcinoma. A light and electron microscopic study of 13 cases. *Cancer*, **26**, 1311
5. Bensch, K. G., Corrin, B., Pariente, R. and Spencer, H. (1968). Oat cell carcinoma of the lung. Its origin and relationship to bronchial carcinoid. *Cancer*, **22**, 1163
6. Fisher, E. R., Palekar, A. and Paulson, J. D. (1977). Comparative histopathologic, histochemical, electron microscopic and tissue culture studies of bronchial carcinoids and oat cell carcinomas of lung. *Am. J. Clin. Pathol.*, **69**, 165
7. Bennett, D. E. and Sasser, W. F. (1969). Bronchiolar carcinoma: a valid clinicopathological entity? A study of 30 cases. *Cancer*, **24**, 876
8. Greenberg, S. D., Smith, M. N. and Spjut, H. J. (1975). Bronchiolo-alveolar carcinoma – cell of origin. *Am. J. Clin. Pathol.*, **63**, 153
9. Churg, A. (1978). The fine structure of large cell undifferentiated carcinoma of the lung. Evidence for its relation to squamous cell carcinomas and adenocarcinomas. *Hum. Pathol.*, **9**, 143
10. Wang, N., Seemayer, T. A., Ahmed, M. N. and Knaask, J. (1976). Giant cell carcinoma of the lung. A light and electron microscopic study. *Hum. Pathol.*, **7**, 3
11. Spencer, H. (1977). *Pathology of the Lung*. 3rd Ed. (Oxford: Pergamon Press)
12. Morgan, A and Mackenzie, D. (1964). Clear-cell carcinoma of the lung. *J. Pathol. Bacteriol.*, **87**, 25
13. Katzenstein, A.-L., Prioleau, P. G. and Askin, F. B. (1980). The histological spectrum and significance of clear-cell change in lung carcinoma. *Cancer*, **45**, 943
14. Jariwalla, A. G., Seaton, A., McCormack, R. M. J., Gibbs, A. R., Campbell, I. and Davies, B. (1981). Intrabronchial matastases from renal carcinoma with recurrent tumour expectoration. *Thorax*, **36, 179**

Carcinoid and Salivary-Gland Type Tumours 17

This group, which includes carcinoids, adenoid cystic and mucoepidermoid tumours amongst others, comprises approximately 1% of lung tumours. Although historically termed adenomas, the majority of tumours within this group tend to recur and in a small proportion metastasize. Adenoma is therefore an inappropriate term and the tumours should be named carcinoid, etc.

Based on ultrastructural characteristics, Hage has described three types of endocrine cell in the human fetal lung[1], and one type of endocrine cell in the normal adult lung. She has demonstrated the three corresponding types of cell in small-cell undifferentiated carcinoma and two of the three types in pulmonary carcinoids. This supports the earlier concept proposed by Bensch et al.[2] that carcinoid tumours and oat-cell carcinomas are, respectively, the locally malignant and highly malignant form of tumour arising from the endocrine cells of the lung. However, it must be stressed that their behaviour is vastly dissimilar – the 5 year overall survival of pulmonary carcinoid tumours being approximately 80% and that of small-cell undifferentiated carcinomas less than 5%.

Several varieties of tumour discussed in this section have direct histological counterparts in the salivary glands, including adenoid cystic, mucoepidermoid, pleomorphic (mixed) adenoma, oncocytoma and the acinic cell tumour and are thought to arise from different components of the bronchial mucous glands.

Carcinoid Tumours

Approximately 70% of pulmonary carcinoids are central and 30% peripheral in distribution[3]. The central carcinoids are usually polypoid and show invasion of the underlying cartilage. The central carcinoids tend to be larger than their peripheral counterparts[1], sometimes reaching as large a size as 10 × 5 cm (Figure 17.1).

The typical carcinoid is composed of ribbons, solid nests, rosettes or tubules of fairly uniform round cells with hyperchromatic or vesicular nuclei (Figures 17.2 and 17.3). The nuclear–cytoplasmic ratio is low, mitoses rare and necrosis absent or minimal[4]. The overlying bronchial epithelium is frequently intact over central carcinoids. Ossification occurs in about 16% of pulmonary carcinoids[5] (Figure 17.3). Sometimes carcinoids mimic oncocytomas (Figure 17.4).

Argyrophilic techniques are positive in approximately 70% and argentaffin techniques positive in small numbers of cells in 30% of pulmonary carcinoids[6]. About 60% of the tumours contain PAS positive, diastase-resistant material[4].

Peripheral carcinoids tend to show more cellular variability than the central variety, and the former may evince pronounced spindling of the tumour cells (Figures 17.5 and 17.6).

Arrigoni et al.[7] have drawn attention to a group of tumours that they have termed atypical carcinoid tumours of the lung (Figure 17.5). They listed four histological features, any one, or a combination of which, would qualify a tumour for this designation:

(1) increased mitotic activity;
(2) pleomorphism of nuclei with increased nuclear–cytoplasmic ratio;
(3) areas of increased cellularity with disorganization of architecture;
(4) areas of tumour necrosis.

They found that metastasis was much more likely in this group.

Carcinoid Tumourlet (Pulmonary Tumourlet)

There is now reliable evidence that these tumours are a variety of peripheral carcinoid[8]. They are minute tumours, usually less than 3 mm in diameter, situated within the periphery of the lung, and are discovered incidentally on microscopic examination. They may be multiple and are often seen in association with previously damaged lungs (Figures 17.7 and 17.8). They may metastasize to lymph nodes but clinically significant metastases have not been reported.

Adenoid Cystic Carcinoma (Cylindroma)

These uncommon tumours occur within the trachea and major bronchi (Figure 17.9), frequently invade the bronchial or tracheal cartilage and show a marked tendency to neural involvement. A large proportion of them recur locally after resection and a significant proportion metastasizes[9].

Mucoepidermoid Carcinoma

Analogous to the salivary gland tumours, both low- and high-grade variants have been reported in the trachea and major bronchi, explaining the wide discrepancy between reported survival rates of tumours[9,10].

The low-grade variant (Figure 17.10) is usually polypoid, and covered by intact mucosa. Invasion of the bronchial wall often occurs but metastases are rare and the prognosis excellent[11].

The high-grade variant (Figure 17.10) is usually circumscribed and invades parenchyma without a conspicuous intrabronchial component. The 5 year survival rate was as low as 5% in Turnbull et al.'s series[10]. Histologically, the high grade tumours

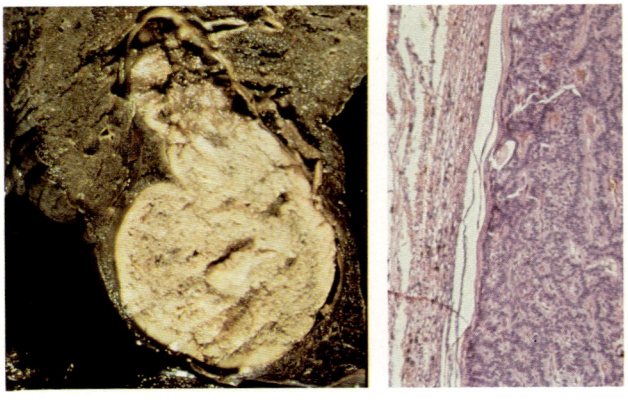

Figure 17.1 *Left:* Occasionally central carcinoids grow slowly to produce a large tumour mass, which on first appearance mimics a peripheral lesion. Closer examination reveals that the whole of the neoplasm has slowly expanded the bronchus outwards and peripherally toward the basal pleura. *Right:* Histology of the tumour reveals a mixed mosaic and tubular pattern with a single layer of respiratory epithelium and compressed lung at its periphery. H & E × 96.

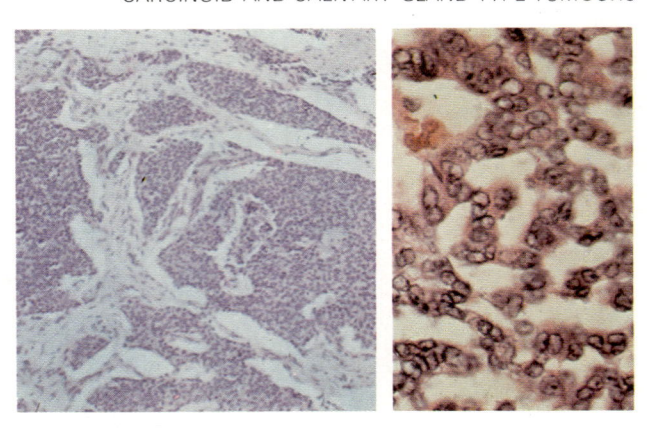

Figure 17.2 *Left:* This carcinoid reveals a purely mosaic pattern. H & E × 74.4. *Right:* This carcinoid shows a purely trabecular pattern. H & E × 480.

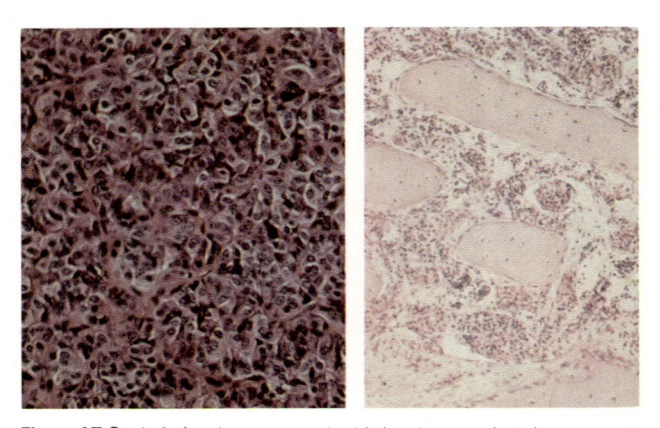

Figure 17.3 *Left:* A pulmonary carcinoid showing a packeted appearance and composed of some cells with a granular eosinophilic cytoplasm and some scattered cells with clear cytoplasm. H & E × 38.4. *Right:* Typical ossifying carcinoid. The ossification is usually attributed to stromal metaplasia. H & E × 300.

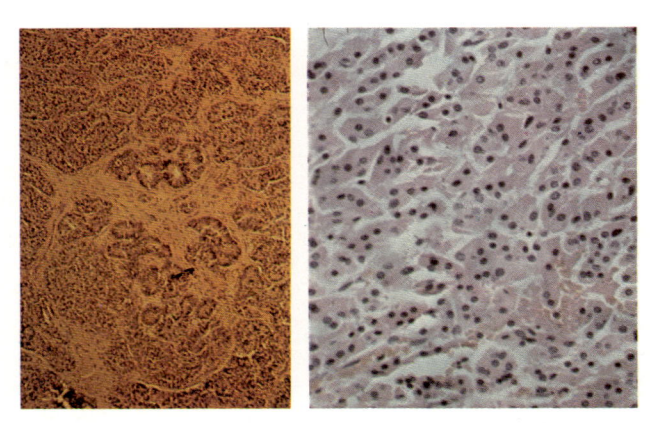

Figure 17.4 *Left:* Bronchial carcinoid showing an 'acinar' pattern. H & E × 74.4 *Right:* A carcinoid tumour composed purely of eosinophilic granular cells resembling the oncocytes of bronchial-gland and salivary-gland epithelium. H & E × 300.

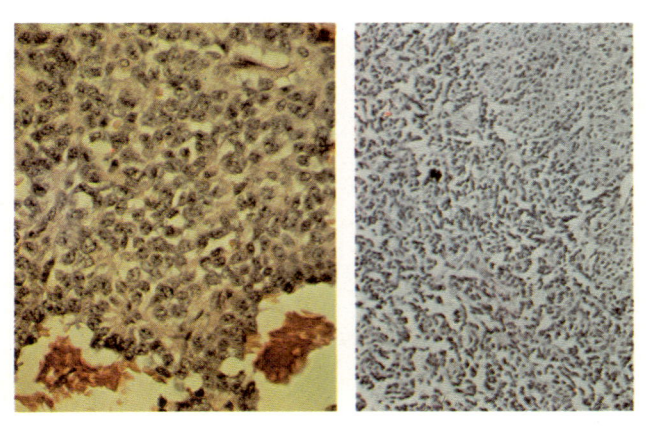

Figure 17.5 *Left:* A vascular tumour showing disconcerting hyperchromatism and pleomorphism warranting the diagnosis 'atypical' carcinoid. (Neurosecretory granules demonstrated on electron microscopy). Metastasis is said to occur in 70% of atypical carcinoids as opposed to 5.6% of typical carcinoids. H & E × 384. *Right:* Carcinoid tumour with spindle celled areas. This causes considerable diagnostic difficulty, particularly with haemangiopericytoma and smooth-muscle tumours. Electron microscopy is often of benefit. The appearance does not connote increased aggressiveness. H & E × 96.

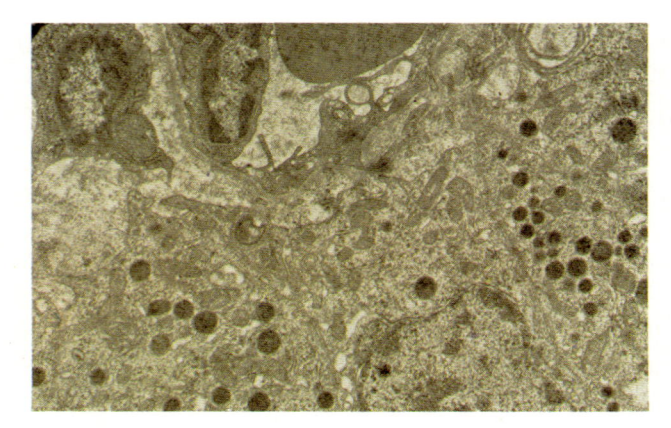

Figure 17.6 Electron micrograph of spindle celled tumour (Figure 17.5) showing neurosecretory granules, confirming that it is a bronchial carcinoid.

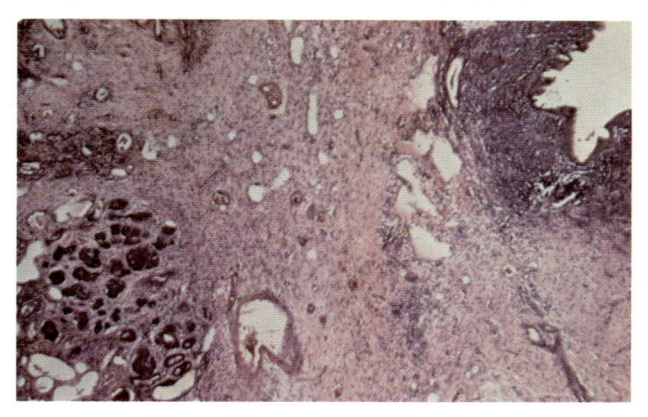

CARCINOID AND SALIVARY-GLAND TYPE TUMOURS

Figure 17.7 Follicular bronchiectasis (top right) with clusters of 'tumourlet' (bottom left).

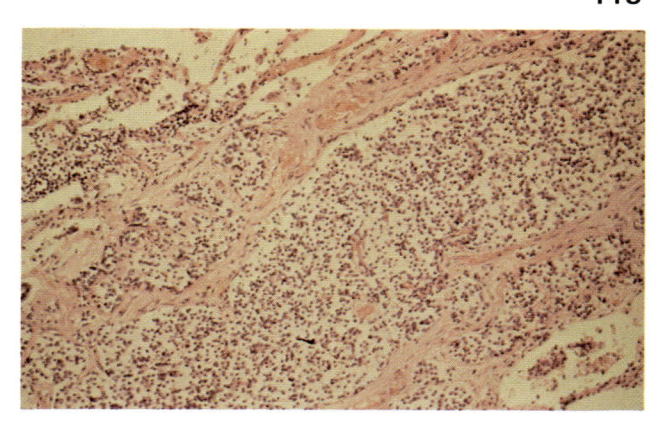

Figure 17.8 'Tumourlet' found incidentally at postmortem of a patient with cardiac failure. No other pulmonary pathology was observed. Tumourlets consist of multiple nests, often separated by fibrous tissue, of spindled or round dark cells. They must be distinguished from minute chemodectomas which are interstitial, related to veins and have a capillary barrier between the tumour cells and lumens of air spaces. Tumourlets are related to arteries and are not confined to the interstitium. H & E × 96.

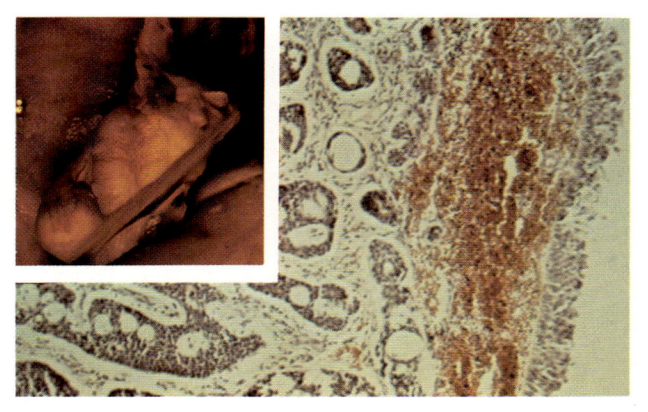

Figure 17.9 *Inset:* A nodular grey tumour present at the junction of the trachea and right main bronchus. *Main slide:* Histology reveals it to be a typical adenoid cystic carcinoma, identical to its salivary gland counterpart. The bronchial epithelium overlying them is frequently intact. H & E × 96.

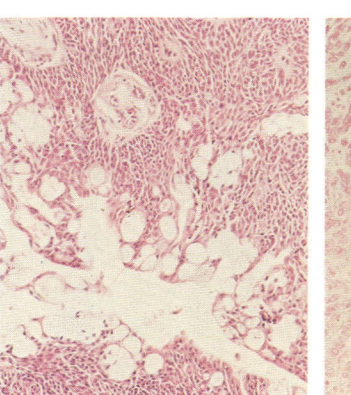

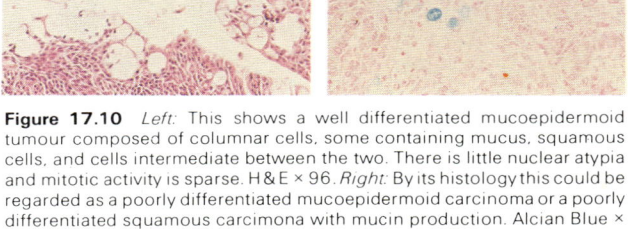

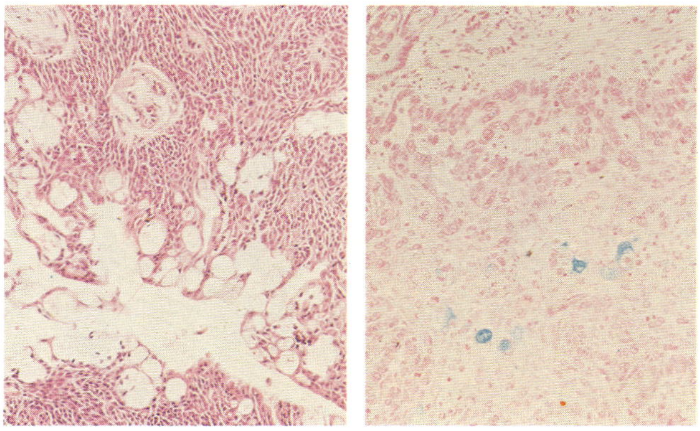

Figure 17.10 *Left:* This shows a well differentiated mucoepidermoid tumour composed of columnar cells, some containing mucus, squamous cells, and cells intermediate between the two. There is little nuclear atypia and mitotic activity is sparse. H & E × 96. *Right:* By its histology this could be regarded as a poorly differentiated mucoepidermoid carcinoma or a poorly differentiated squamous carcinoma with mucin production. Alcian Blue × 96.

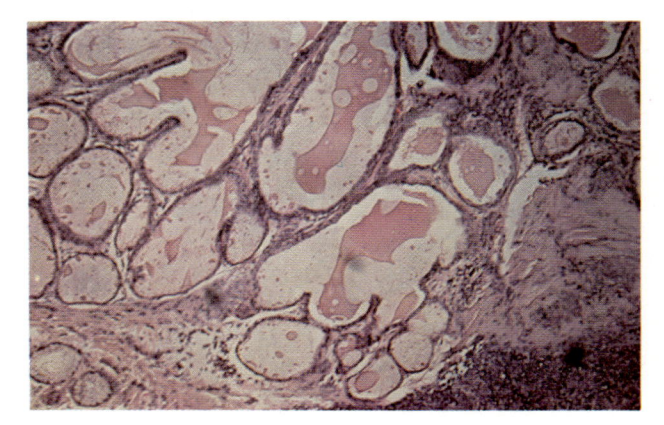

Figure 17.11 A typical mucous gland adenoma which had obstructed the bronchus and resulted in obstructive pneumonitis. H & E × 24.

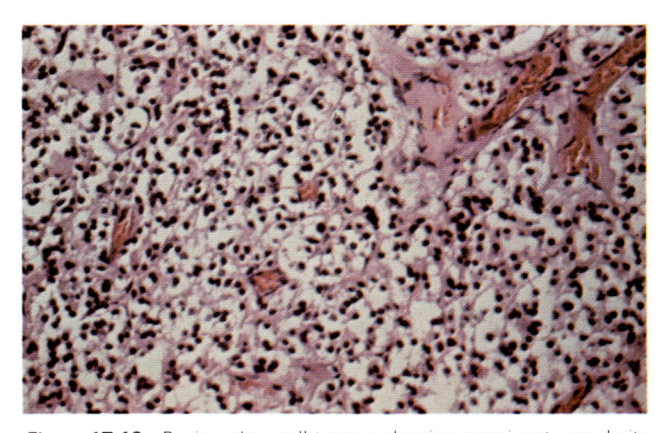

Figure 17.12 Benign clear cell tumour showing prominent vascularity and relatively uniform clear cells. It is readily distinguished from clear cell carcinoma of the lung by lack of pleomorphism, foci of necrosis and mitotic activity. The major difficulty is differentiating it from a secondary renal carcinoma, which may necessitate intravenous pyelogram. Lipid stains may be of value, since if positive, would indicate renal cell carcinoma. Electron microscopy is also of value since it should reveal large, membrane-bound cytoplasmic vesicles in the benign clear-cell tumour of lung.

show marked cellular and nuclear pleomorphism, a high mitotic rate and foci of necrosis. There may be difficulty in distinguishing this tumour from adenosquamous carcinoma. Although probably only of academic importance, features which favour the diagnosis of mucoepidermoid carcinoma are circumscription, intact, non-malignant bronchial epithelium over the tumour, and areas within the tumour which resemble the low grade variant of mucoepidermoid carcinoma. Large areas of keratinization, including individual cell keratinization, are suggestive of adenosquamous carcinoma[12].

Mucous Gland Adenoma

These are rare, benign tumours situated in the major bronchi. They are composed of dilated, mucin-filled spaces, lined by well differentiated mucus cells[13] (Figure 17.11).

Benign Clear Cell ('Sugar') Tumour

These are rare, benign peripheral tumours composed of large, polygonal or columnar, clear glycogen-containing cells[14] (Figure 17.12). Ultrastructural studies of this tumour have been conflicting: Becker and Soifer[15] found dense-core granules in some of the cells and proposed that it was derived from Kultschitzky cells, whilst Hoch et al.[16] considered it to be of pericytic origin.

Pleomorphic Adenoma (Benign Mixed Tumour)

This is similar to the tumour found in major salivary glands and is discussed in Chapter 18.

Acinic Cell Tumour

Fechner et al.[17] first described an acinic cell tumour in the right lower lobe of a 64-year-old male, histologically and ultrastructurally similar to those occurring in the salivary glands. The tumour was composed predominantly of light cells containing small vesicular nuclei and coarsely vacuolated cytoplasm. About 10% of the cells (dark) had dark granular cytoplasm and smaller denser nuclei. Both types of cells contained PAS positive diastase resistant granules, a feature helpful in distinguishing this tumour from the benign clear cell tumour which contains glycogen.

Oncocytoma

Up to 1977 two genuine examples of pulmonary oncocytoma had been described[18-19]. Microscopically, the tumours consisted of sheets, cords or alveolar collections of large ovoid or polygonal cells which had one or two spherical nuclei and finely granular, eosinophilic cytoplasm. Electron microscopy demonstrated that the cells were packed with mitochondria. This feature distinguishes the pulmonary oncocytoma form the oncocytic pulmonary carcinoid where the strongly eosinophilic cytoplasm is due to numerous large neurosecretory granules.

References

1. Hage, E. (1980) Light and electron microscopic charateristics of the various lung endocrine cell types. *Invest. Cell. Pathol.*, **3**, 345
2. Bensch, K. G., Corrin, B., Pariente, R. and Spencer, H. (1968). Oat cell carcinoma of the lung – its origin and relationship to bronchial carcinoid. *Cancer*, **22**, 1163
3. Goldstraw, P., Lamb, D., McCormack, R. J. M. and Walbaum, P. R. (1976). The malignancy of bronchial adenoma. *J. Thor. Card. Surg.*, **72**, 309
4. Fisher, E. R., Palekar, A. and Paulson, J. B. D. (1978) Comparative histopathologic, histochemical, electron microscopic and tissue culture studies of bronchial carcinoids, and oat cell carcinomas of lung. *Am. J. Clin. Pathol.*, **69**, 165
5. Kinney, F. J. and Kvorarik, J. L. (1965). Bone formation in bronchial adenoma. *Am. J. Clin. Pathol.*, **44**, 52
6. Williams, E. D. and Azzopardi, J. G. (1960). Tumours of the lung and the carcinoid syndrome. *Thorax*, **15**, 30
7. Arrigoni, M. G., Woolner, L. B. and Bernatz, P. E. (1972). Atypical carcinoid tumours of the lung. *J. Thor. Card. Surg.*, **64**, 413
8. Churg, A. and Warnock, M. L. (1976). Pulmonary tumourlet – A form of peripheral carcinoid. *Cancer*, **37**, 1469
9. Payne, W. S., Ellis, F. H., Woolner, L. B. and Moessch, H. J. (1959). The surgical treatment of cylindroma (adenoid cystic carcinoma) and mucoepidermoid tumours of the bronchus. *J. Thor. Card. Surg.*, **38**, 709
10. Turnbull, A. D., Huvos, A. G., Goodner, J. T. and Foote, F. W., Jr.(1971). Mucoepidermoid tumours of bronchial glands. *Cancer*, **28**, 539
11. Reichle, F. A. and Rosemund, G. P. (1966) Mucoepidermoid tumours of the bronchus. *J. Thor. Card. Surg.*, **51**, 443
12. Klacsmann, P. G., Olson, J. L. and Eggleston, J. C. (1979). Mucoepidermoid carcinoma of the bronchus. An electron microscopic study of low grade and high grade variants. *Cancer*, **43**, 1720
13. Kroe, D. J. and Pitcock, J. A. (1967). Benign mucous gland adenoma of bronchus. *Arch. Pathol.*, **84**, 539
14. Liebow, A. A. and Castleman, B. (1963). Benign clear cell ('sugar tumours') of the lung. *Am. J. Pathol.*, **43**, 13a abstr
15. Becker, N. H. and Soifer, I. (1971). Benign clear cell tumour ('sugar tumours') of the lung. *Cancer*, **27**, 712
16. Hoch, W. S., Patchefsky, A. S., Tokeda, M. and Gordon, G. (1974). Benign clear cell tumour of the lung. *Cancer*, **33**, 1328
17. Fechner, R. E., Bentinck, B. R. and Askew, J. B. (1972). Acinic cell tumour of the lung. *Cancer*, **29**, 501
18. Fechner, R. E. and Bentinck, B. R. (1973). Ultrastructure of bronchial oncocytoma. *Cancer*, **31**, 1451
19. Santos-Briz, A., Terron, J., Sastre, R., Romero, L. and Valle, A. (1977). Oncocytoma of the lung. *Cancer*, **40**, 1330

Mixed Tumours 18

This group of tumours has given rise to controversy with regard to both diagnosis and histogenesis. A detailed account of this group, summarizing the arguments for and against the various theories of histogenesis, is given in another publication by the authors[1].

Pleomorphic Adenoma (Mixed Salivary Tumour)

Rarely, this arises from bronchial or tracheal mucous glands and it is the counterpart of that tumour which commonly develops from the major salivary glands. It is usually polypoid, arises in a major bronchus and is locally infiltrative (Figure 18.1). The tumour has a slow rate of growth, tends to be locally recurrent, but does not metastasize. Payne et al.[2] reported four cases and found that they comprised 1% of tumours arising from bronchial mucous glands.

As in the pleomorphic adenoma of the salivary glands, it is possible for malignancy to develop in these tumours; carcinomatous transformation of one such tumour has been reported[3].

Hamartoma

A hamartoma is, by definition, a tumour composed of an abnormal mixture of tissues normally present within a particular organ and does not include foreign tissue. In the lung these tumours contain admixtures of mature tissue, including glandular spaces lined by columnar or ciliated epithelium resembling bronchial epithelium, fibrous tissue, smooth muscle, cartilage, fat and nerve.

Three types of pulmonary hamartoma are usually recognized, depending on the predominant component(s), viz. chondromatous hamartoma, leiomyomatous hamartoma and adenomatoid hamartoma. Some surgeons refer to arteriovenous aneurysms and other vascular abnormalities as vascular hamartomas when the only abnormality is of vascular tissue. We have considered these under congenital anomalies. Also dubiously coming under this heading are connective tissue malformations associated with generalized disease such as neurofibromatosis and tuberous sclerosis.

Chondromatous Hamartoma is the most common type of pulmonary hamartoma, the incidence at autopsy being estimated at approximately 0.25%. The majority are subpleural, but about 5% are endobronchial. They may be seen at any age but the majority are incidental findings within the fourth and fifth decades[5].

Grossly, they are characteristic, bluish-white, bosselated tumours varying from a few millimetres to three or four centimetres in diameter; rarely, they may be considerably larger. They are characteristically easily shelled out by the surgeon.

As their name implies, they show nodules of cartilage which may undergo calcification or ossification, separated by connective tissue containing varying amounts of epithelial lined clefts, fat, smooth muscle and nerve.

The occurrence of *malignancy in chondromatous hamartoma* is debatable. However, the case reported by Hayward et al.[6], in which adenocarcinoma occurred in a chondromatous hamartoma, would appear genuine. Theoretically it is possible that malignant transformation of a chondromatous hamartoma could result in adenocarcinoma, sarcoma of cartilage or smooth muscle, or malignant mixed tumour.

Fibroleiomyomatous Hamartomas are usually subpleural, often multiple and show a predominance of smooth muscle admixed with cysts and tubes lined by cuboidal or columnar epithelium. They may occur in association with chondromatous hamartoma[1,5].

Adenomatoid Hamartoma is called by Spencer[5] a non-cartilagenous local hamartoma; he likens it to a benign form of pulmonary blastoma. This should not be confused with the diffuse congential adenomatoid malformation of infancy. It is much less common that the other types and is often multiple and subpleural. It consists of epithelial lined tubules or spaces embedded in an undifferentiated mesenchymal type stroma, both components appearing benign.

Pulmonary Lymphangiomyomatosis lesions identical to those of tuberous sclerosis occur (rarely) in premenopausal women, who do not manifest neurological abnormalities. Characteristically, progression of these lesions over several years leads to death from respiratory failure.

The lungs reveal extensive honeycombing with emphysema and bullae, most severe in the upper and middle lobes. It is characterized by focal muscle proliferation of alveolar walls, septa, pleura, pulmonary vessels and lymphatics (Figure 18.5), siderosis and fibrosis[7].

Teratoma

This tumour, at its most differentiated, shows a mixture of adult tissues, derived from all three germ layers, some of which are foreign to the lung. At its least differentiated, only one primitive element may be present. Approximately 20 cases have been reported[8]. The age at presentation has varied between 16 and 60 years of age[9], apart from a malignant teratoma in an infant and an unreported case of

MIXED TUMOURS

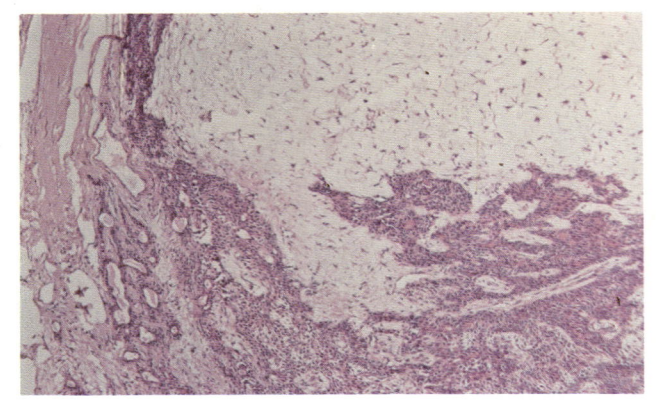

Figure 18.1 Polypoid bronchial tumour removed by lobectomy revealed the typical morphology of a pleomorphic adenoma (mixed salivary tumour). H&E × 96.

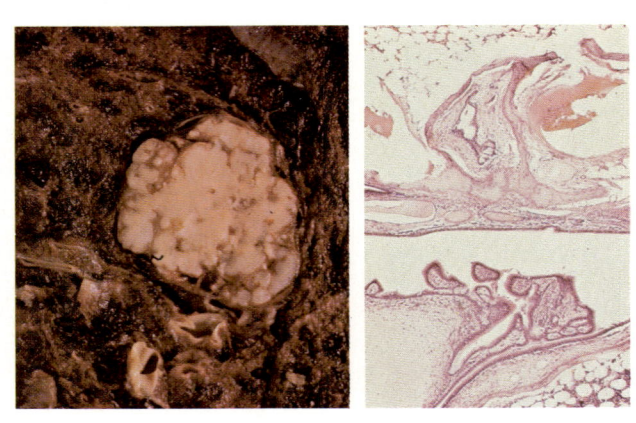

Figure 18.2 Chondromatous hamartoma. *Left:* The typical circumscribed, bosselated, greyish-blue, lobulated peripheral lesion. The background lung shows moderate simple pneumoconiosis. *Right:* Histology of the tumour reveals adult cartilage, bone, marrow, respiratory epithelium and smooth muscle. H&E × 38.4.

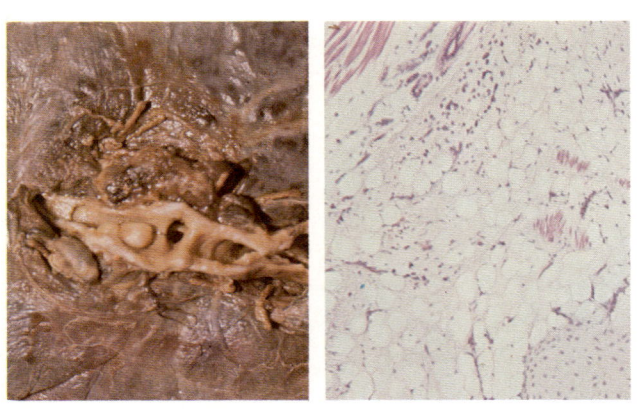

Figure 18.3 *Left:* A central chondromatous hamartoma ('chondroma') obstructing a segmental bronchus. *Right:* Histology of the tumour reveals mainly cartilage, fat and smooth muscle. Central tumours are more variable in structure than the peripheral variety, sometimes being so cartilagenous that they have been termed chondromas, others being so diverse that a teratomatous nature has had to be excluded. H&E × 74.4.

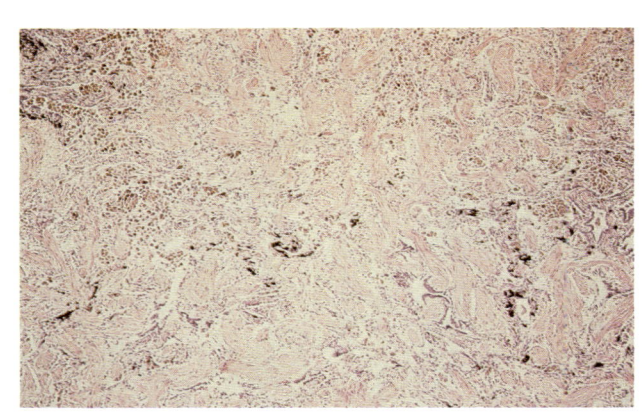

Figure 18.4. A peripheral leiomyomatous hamartoma found incidentally in the lobectomy specimen for a large central chondromatous hamartoma. These tumours have to be differentiated from smooth-muscle hyperplasia occurring in damaged lungs and in women from metastatic spread of uterine smooth-muscle tumours. The latter, however, do not contain an epithelial element. H&E × 38.4.

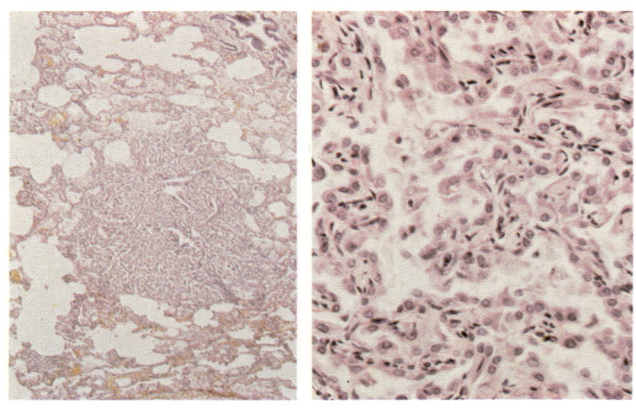

Figure 18.5 *Left:* One of numerous small nodules found in the lung of a subject with tuberous sclerosis. H&E × 24. *Right:* A lesion from the same case showing fibroleiomyomatous proliferation covered by cuboidal epithelium. H&E × 240.

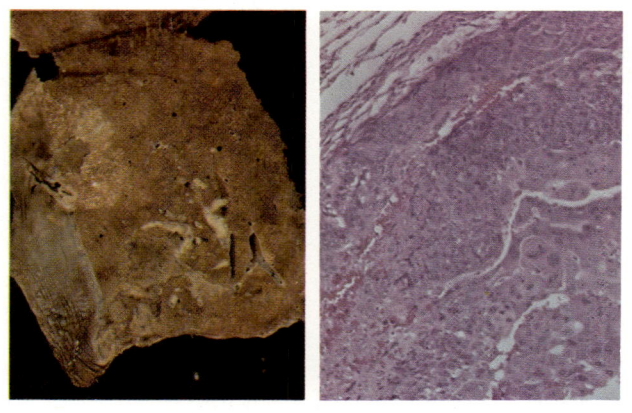

Figure 18.6 Primary choriocarcinoma of lung. *Left:* Cut surface of right lower lobectomy specimen with two ill-defined lesions in medial basal segment and occlusion of vessels in other segments by pale friable tissue. *Right:* Histology of the lesions reveal typical appearance of choriocarcinoma. H&E × 240.

MIXED TUMOURS

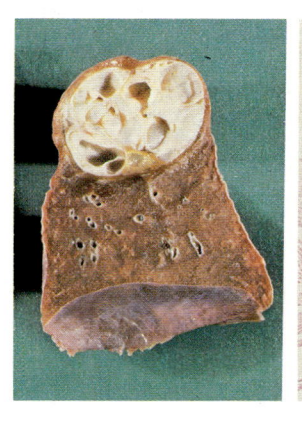

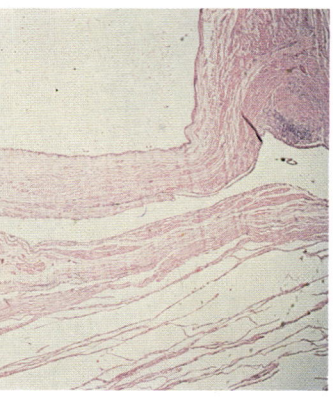

Figure 18.7 Secondary teratoma removed from a young male. This was, at first, considered to be a developmental lesion or a well differentiated teratoma, but the patient's history revealed that a teratoma from the testis had been removed some years earlier followed by treatment with chemotherapeutic agents. Solitary metastases to the lung from nephroblastoma and mixed mesodermal genital-tract tumours may also cause diagnostic errors.
Left: Multicystic lesion occupying much of apical segment of lower lobe.
Right: Microscopy reveals benign epithelial lined multilocular cyst with smooth muscle and collagenous wall. H&E × 24.

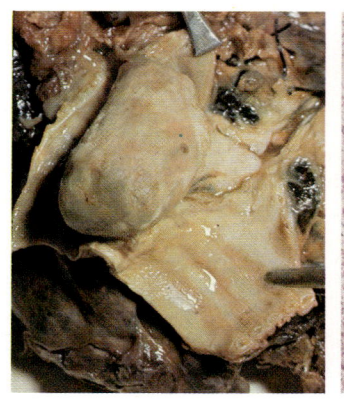

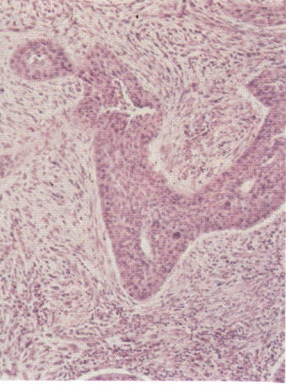

Figure 18.8 *Left:* Polypoid tumour protruding from a lobar bronchus. These often produce bronchial obstruction with consequent damage to the distal lung; changes of bronchiectasis or pneumonia may be seen. *Right:* Typical mixture of malignant squamous and spindle celled elements of a carcinosarcoma. H&E × 96.

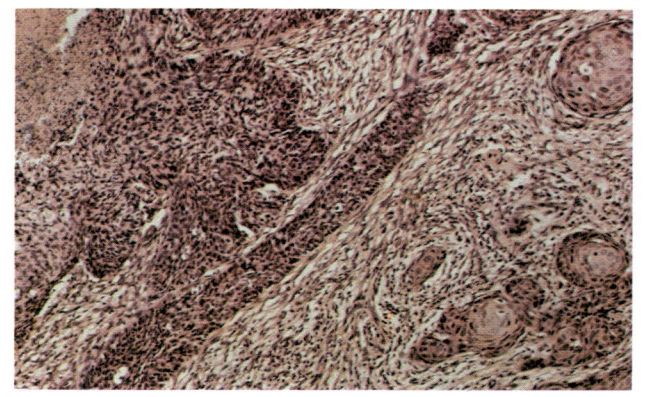

Figure 18.9 A central tumour showing islands of squamous and small-cell undifferentiated carcinoma within a sarcomatous stroma. H&E × 120.

Care has to be exercised in differentiating squamous carcinoma with spindle cell metaplasia (also a central tumour) from carcinosarcoma – a sarcomatous pattern on reticulin staining may be seen in the spindle celled foci in carcinosarcoma. Electron microscopic examination, even of formalin fixed material, may be of help, since squamous cell features may be revealed within the spindle-celled component. Carcinosarcoma could also be confused with malignancy occurring in a hamartoma; for the latter to be confidently diagnosed, at least one benign hamartomatous element should be identified.

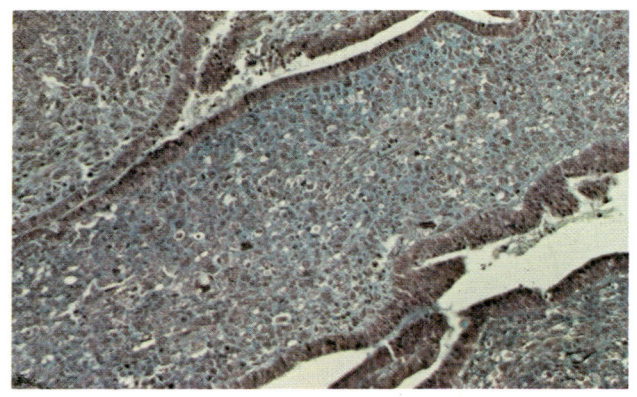

Figure 18.10 Pulmonary blastoma. Multilayered tubular structures composed of pleomorphic, hyperchromatic cells set in a 'myxoid' stroma in which there are spindle and plump cells with occasional mitoses. Trichrome × 74.4.

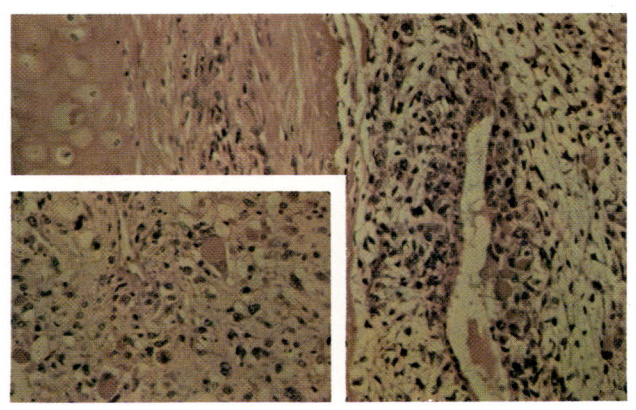

Figure 18.11 A central tumour showing a squamous component (not illustrated), cartilage (top left), tubular elements with spindle and plump stromal cells (right half) with occasional large plump cells reminiscent of rhabdomyoblasts (inset). This was regarded as a 'transitional tumour'. H&E × 240.

a benign teratoma in a three-month-old male infant. They have been most common in the left upper lobe.

Approximately two thirds of the cases have been well differentiated without producing metastases and have shown admixtures of mature tissues including squamous epithelium, sebaceous glands, apocrine and eccrine sweat glands, hair follicles, pancreatic acini and islets, muscle, fat and thymic tissue. Some have presented with the coughing up of hair. Amongst the malignant cases two cases of choriocarcinoma have been described[10].

We have also seen a case of choriocarcinoma which had apparently arisen within the lung of a young woman (Figure 18.6). However, the well known ability of gonadal teratomas to involute and at the same time be associated with distant metastases questions the nature of true primary pulmonary teratoma (Figure 18.7).

Carcinosarcoma and Blastoma

These are rare tumours of the lung, approximately 40 examples of each having been reported[1]. They are unpredictable in behaviour and are both equally capable of disseminating widely. Most of these tumours show distinct differences and are easily separable (Table 18.1). However, we have encountered a few cases which have shown histological features of both carcinosarcoma and blastoma. We have also met exceptions to the rule that carcinosarcomas are central lung tumours and blastomas are peripheral. This, to our minds, casts doubts upon Spencer's theory that pulmonary blastoma is mesodermal in origin. Although we think it semantically desirable to separate the two types of tumour, we regard pulmonary blastoma as a distinct variety of carcinosarcoma. An electron microscopical study of pulmonary blastoma by McCann et al.[11] gives further support to this conclusion.

Carcinosarcoma connotes simultaneous malignancy in both epithelial and stromal components of the tumour. These tumours are usually endobronchial polypoid lesions (Figure 18.8) but accompanying invasion of the surrounding extrabronchial tissues often occurs. Occasionally they may be solely extrabronchial.

The most common malignant epithelial element is squamous (Figure 18.8), but glandular or undifferentiated carcinomas may occur either solely or in combination[1,12] (Figure 18.9). The malignant stromal constituent is usually fibrosarcomatous, but differentiation to chondrosarcoma, osteogenic sarcoma, or rhabdomyosarcoma may occur. There is usually blending of the epithelial and sarcomatous elements.

Pulmonary Blastomas show a similarity to fetal lung, being composed of epithelial lined tubules, quite unlike acini of ordinary adenocarcinoma, embedded within a primitive mesenchymal stroma[5]. (Figure 18.10). There may be cytological evidence of malignancy of one or usually both components of the tumour. The histology is not helpful in predicting the behaviour of the tumour, however.

The tubules are lined by a single layer of cuboidal or columnar epithelium, or there may be pseudostratification of the epithelium. There may also be solid nests of epithelial cells. The tubules may contain mucin.

The stroma consists of plump oval or spindle cells set in a loose matrix. There may, in addition, be differentiation towards smooth muscle, cartilage or bone. In our experience, there has been little evidence of merging between the epithelial and stromal components.

Grossly, the tumour is well circumscribed, peripheral, without a bronchial connection, and has a fleshy, mucoid cut surface. The tumour may become large and occupy most of a lobe.

Transitional Tumours are malignant tumours which show features of pulmonary blastoma viz. tubules in a mesenchymal stroma, in what are otherwise typical carcinosarcomas[13]. We have encountered three such examples, which were all central in location (Figure 18.11). We have also seen areas of squamous differentiation in a peripheral pulmonary blastoma[1].

References

1. Seal, R. M. E. and Gibbs, A. R. (1982). Mixed tumours of the lung. In Shimosato, Y., Melamed, M. and Nettesheim, Y. (eds.) *Morphogenesis of Lung Cancer.* (Boca Raton C.R.C. Press) (In press)
2. Payne, W. S., Schier, J. and Woolner, L. B. (1965). Mixed tumours of the bronchus (salivary gland type). *J. Thor. Card. Surg.,* **49,** 663
3. Vadillo-Briceno, F., Feder, W. and Albores-Saavedra, J. (1970). Malignant mixed tumour of the lung. *Chest.* **58,** 84
4. McDonald, J. R., Harrington, S. W. and Clagett, O. T. (1945). Hamartoma (often called chondroma) of the lung. *J. Thor. Card. Surg.,* **14,** 128
5. Spencer, W. S. (1977). In *Pathology of the Lung,* 3rd ed., Chap. 23. (Oxford: Pergamon Press)
6. Hayward, R. H. and Carabasi, R. J. (1967). Malignant hamartoma of the lung: fact or fiction?. *J. Thor. Surg.,* **53,** 457
7. Corrin, B., Liebow, A. A. and Friedman, P. T. (1975). Pulmonary lymphangiomyomatosis. *Am. J. Pathol.,* **79,** 348
8. Day, D. W. and Taylor, S. A. (1975). An intrapulmonary teratoma associated with thymic tissue. *Thorax,* **30,** 582
9. Gautam, H. P. (1969). Intrapulmonary malignant teratoma. *Am. Rev. Resp. Dis.,* **100,** 863
10. Hakawa, K., Takahaski, M., Sasaki, K., Kawoioi, A., Okano, R., Osada, H., Otsuka, R. and Murota, Y. (1977). Primary choriocarcinoma of the lung – Case report of two male subjects. *Acta. Pathol. Jpn.,* **27,** 123
11. McCann, M. P., Fu, V. and Kay, S. (1976). Pulmonary blastoma – A light and electron microscopical study. *Cancer,* **38,** 789
12. Stackhouse, E. M., Harrison, E. G. and Ellis, F. H. (1969). Primary mixed malignancies of lung: carcinosarcoma and blastoma. *J. Thor. Card. Surg.,* **57,** 385
13. Davis, P. W., Briggs, J. C., Seal, R. M. E. and Storring, F. K. (1972). Benign and malignant mixed tumours of the lung. *Thorax,* **27,** 657

Table 18.1 **Major differences between carcinosarcoma and pulmonary blastoma**

	Carcinosarcoma	*Pulmonary Blastoma*
Age	35–81 years	All ages
Location	Usually central	Usually peripheral
Epithelial component	Most frequently squamous but adenocarcinoma and undifferentited carcinoma occur	Epithelial tubules, clefts and nests resembling fetal lung
Connective tissue component	Fibrosarcoma, sometimes chondrosarcoma, osteogenic sarcoma and rhabdomyosarcoma	Myxoid, spindle celled (fetal-like) stroma. Occasional differentiation to cartilage, bone or striated muscle

Primary Lymphoproliferative Conditions

19

This group of conditions is ill understood and their nomenclature is confusing. Some of the diseases have been described relatively recently, and it is probable that earlier reports did not utilize strict diagnostic criteria and have been inaccurate. Their natural histories are therefore not completely understood. In this chapter we attempt to elucidate these conditions and emphasize useful diagnostic features. However, it must be realized that there is overlap between the different diseases and that sometimes an individual case will not conform exactly to one particular entity.

Pre-malignant Lymphoma (Pseudolymphoma) and Malignant Lymphoma

Malignant lymphomas involving the lung are more likely to be secondary than primary (Figure 19.1). For a tumour to qualify as primary pulmonary lymphoma it should comply with Salzstein's definition[2], namely, the lesion must be confined to the lung and its regional lymph nodes without evincing any evidence of spread beyond these confines within three months of the initial diagnosis. Primary lymphoma of the lung is more likely to be of non-Hodgkin's type, primary Hodgkin's disease being exceedingly rare.

Table 19.1 shows clinico-pathological features which assist in distinguishing between malignant lymphoma and pre-malignant lymphoma (pseudo-

Table 19.1 A comparison of pulmonary pre-malignant lymphoma and malignant lymphoma

	Pre-Malignant Lymphoma	Malignant Lymphoma
(1)	Mixed cell infiltrate of mature cells	Uniform infiltrate (especially immature cells)
(2)	Germinal centres usually present	Germinal centres absent
(3)	Vascular invasion infrequent	Vascular invasion usually present
(4)	Pleural invasion infrequent	Pleural invasion often present
(5)	Lymph nodes not involved	Lymph node involvement often present

lymphoma)[1] (Figures 19.2–19.4). Salzstein believed that the latter represented a benign inflammatory disorder with, consequently, a good prognosis in contrast to that of a malignant neoplastic process.

However, there are certain conflicting facts. Various authors, including Greenberg et al.[2], have reported 'pseudolymphomas' developing into true malignant lymphomas, after varying intervals of time. Also, histologically-proven malignant lymphomas of the lung may exhibit long survival time (Figure 19.3). In our opinion the term pre-malignant lymphoma is more apt than pseudolymphoma since it is a pre-malignant condition, although it is of prognostic benefit to separate the two. Both diseases appear similar on gross examination – either appear as single or multiple rounded lesions, or may diffusely involve contiguous portions of more than one lobe. In contrast to Salzstein[1], Greenberg et al.[2] found that both conditions could infiltrate the pleura. Presence or absence of regional lymph node involvement appears the best indicator of behaviour. Loose epithelioid granulomata can occur at the periphery of either lesion which may cause considerable diagnostic confusion on biopsy.

Lymphoid Interstitial Pneumonia (LIP)

This is characterized by diffuse, interstitial collections of mature lymphocytes, plasma cells and large lymphoid cells with germinal centre formation[3] (Figures 19.5 and 19.6). Histologically, it is identical to pre-malignant lymphoma in individual microscopic fields but it is the extent of the changes that distinguishes LIP. If biopsy material only is available correlation with the radiographic features is essential; in LIP there is diffuse often bilateral shadowing; pre-malignant lymphoma reveals a discrete mass. Loose, poorly defined, sarcoid-like granulomata may be present in LIP. In one case we have seen, the centres of 'follicles' were composed of epithelioid cells instead of large lymphocytes (Figure 19.5).

In nearly all cases of LIP there are serum immunoglobulin abnormalities and an association with Sjögren's syndrome in 30%[3] (cf. lymphomatoid granulomatosis). LIP may culminate in interstitial fibrosis, resolve with steroid therapy or develop after varying periods of time into frank lymphoma (Figure 19.6)[4]. The latter is indicated by a predominance of immature cells in the infiltrate or the development of discrete masses. Amyloid-like material may be present in the lesions of both LIP and pre-malignant lymphoma.

Benign Lymphoid Hyperplasia

An occasional incidental finding, usually seen at autopsy, is the presence of numerous subpleural nodules, varying from a few millimetres to 1 or 2 cm in diameter, which have a normal lymph-node structure (Figure 19.7).

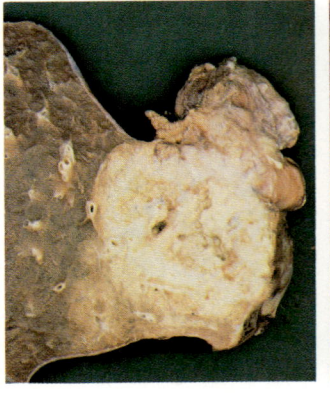

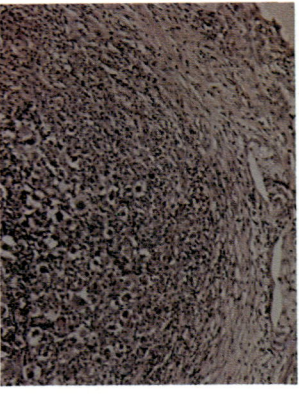

Figure 19.1 *Left:* Lobectomy specimen showing a circumscribed grey tumour medially. *Right:* Histology of the tumour showed the pleomorphic picture of mixed cellularity Hodgkin's lymphoma.

Hodgkin's disease and non-Hodgkin's lymphoma involve the lung in approximately 40% of cases. Grossly, deposits may appear as solitary nodules, miliary lesions or as large confluent masses of tumour.

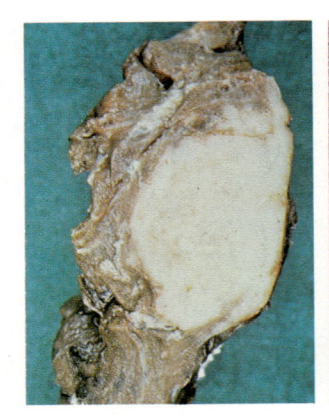

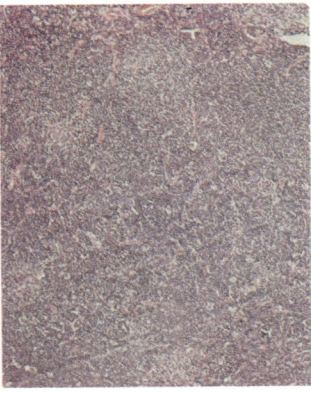

Figure 19.2 *Left:* Wedge resection of an ill-defined tumour nodule (2 cm diameter) removed from a patient with systemic lupus erythematosus. *Right:* Histology reveals the appearance of diffuse lymphocytic (non-Hodgkin's) lymphoma.

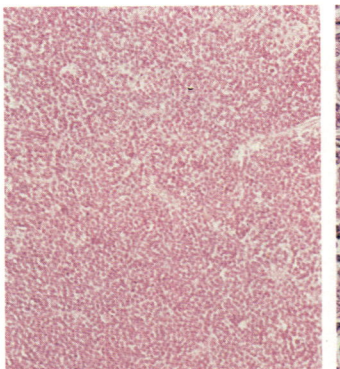

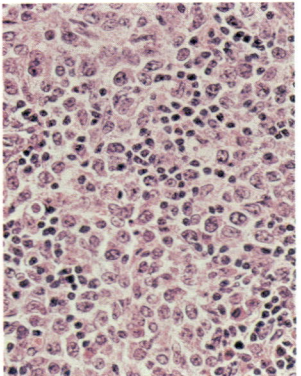

Figure 19.3 *Left:* Low power view of a non-Hodgkin's lymphoma removed from an 18-year-old female, who was still alive without recurrence 20 years later. H & E × 38.4. *Right:* High power view of the same case showing follicular centre cell lymphoma. H & E × 384.

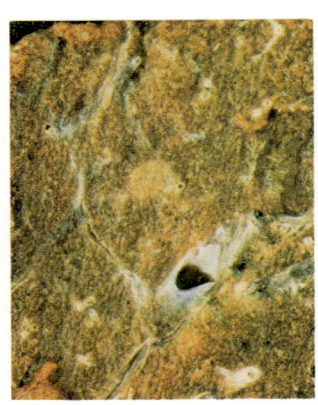

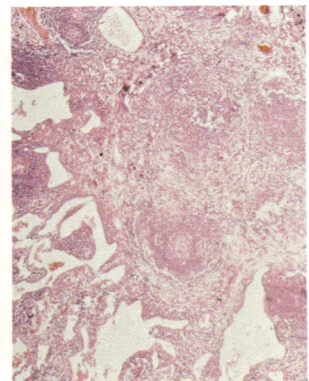

Figure 19.4 *Left:* A 1 cm diameter ill-defined grey tumour which was one of four in a resected lower lobe. *Right:* Histology reveals lymphoid collections with germinal centres and a lymphoid infiltrate extending into the neighbouring parenchymal interstitium. The dividing line between pre-malignant lymphoma and LIP is not sharp and borderline cases will be observed. This case was classified as multiple pre-malignant lymphomas, in spite of the fact that microscopy revealed several more lesions in addition to the four macroscopical lesions. H & E × 24.

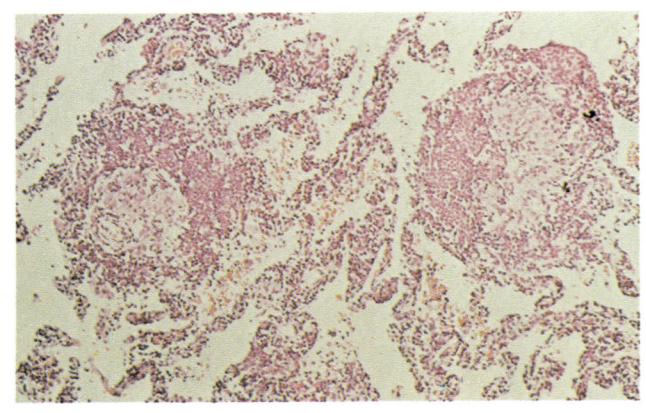

Figure 19.5 A diffuse lymphocyte infiltrate in interalveolar septa with lymphoid aggregates containing centres composed of epithelioid-like cells. This was interpreted as lymphocytic interstitial pneumonia. H & E × 96.

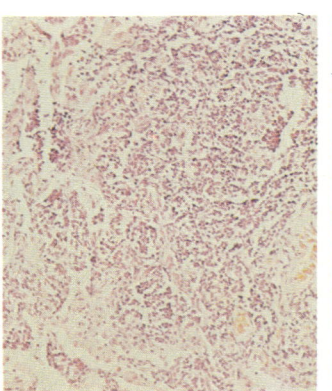

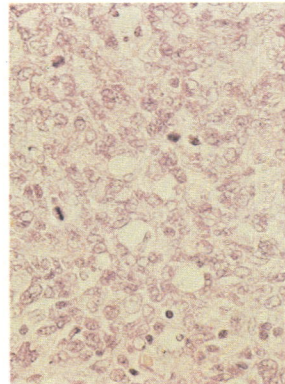

Figure 19.6 Limited thoracotomy specimen from a patient with interstitial disease of 4-years standing, recently complicated by larger ill-defined granules. *Left:* 'Normal lung' revealing appearances of LIP with some mural fibrosis. H & E × 38.4. *Right:* A tumour nodule composed of poorly differentiated, diffuse lymphosarcoma (centroblastic) from another area. H & E × 384. This was regarded as malignant lymphoma developing within a milieu of lymphocytic interstitial pneumonia.

PRIMARY LYMPHOPROLIFERATIVE CONDITIONS

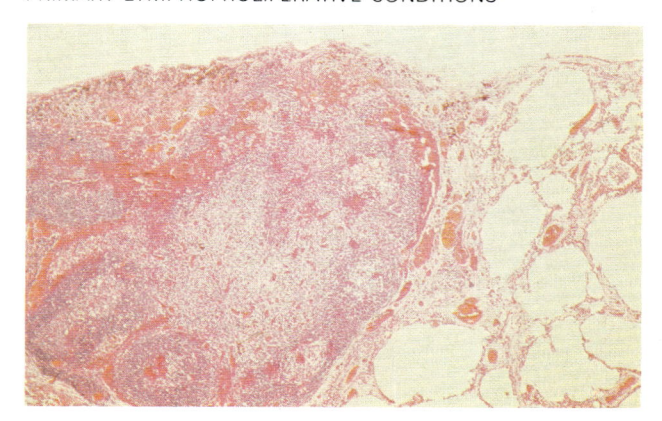

Figure 19.7 Typical subpleural lymph node – one of several found incidentally at postmortem. H&E × 24.

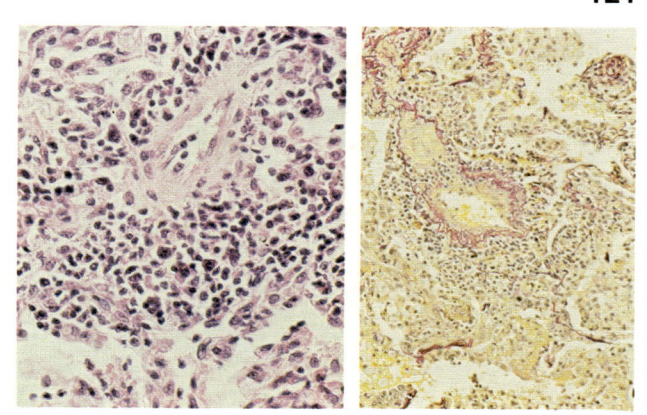

Figure 19.8 *Left:* Lymphomatoid granulomatosis – typical pleomorphic lymphoid infiltrate situated interstitially and around vessels. H&E × 240 *Right:* Elastic stain showing non-necrotizing vascular involvement. EVG × 38.4. LYG may be confused with LIP. Absence of germinal centres, atypical cells within the infiltrate, conspicuous involvement of vessels and areas of necrosis strongly favour LYG. Serum immunoglobulin abnormalities frequently present in LIP are unusual in LYG.

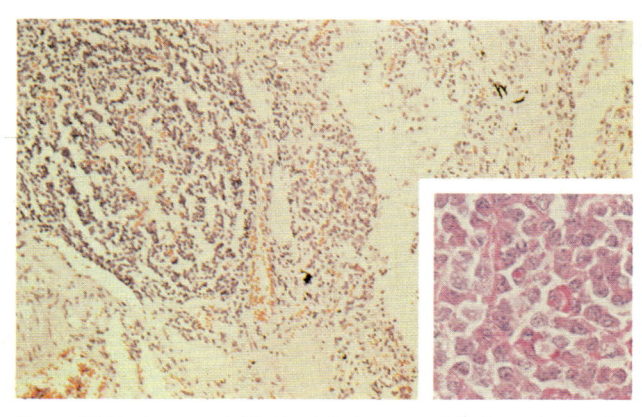

Figure 19.9 A case of Waldenström's macroglobulinaemia showing pulmonary infiltrates with similarities to lymphoid interstitial pneumonia. The infiltrate consists of mature and immature lymphocytes, histiocytes, plasma cells and plasmacytoid cells which may contain PAS positive inclusions. There is often accompanying fibrosis. H&E × 38.4 *Inset:* Intranuclear and cytoplasmic PAS-positive (Dutcher–Fahey) bodies sometimes seen in Waldenström's macroglobulinaemia. H&E × 384.

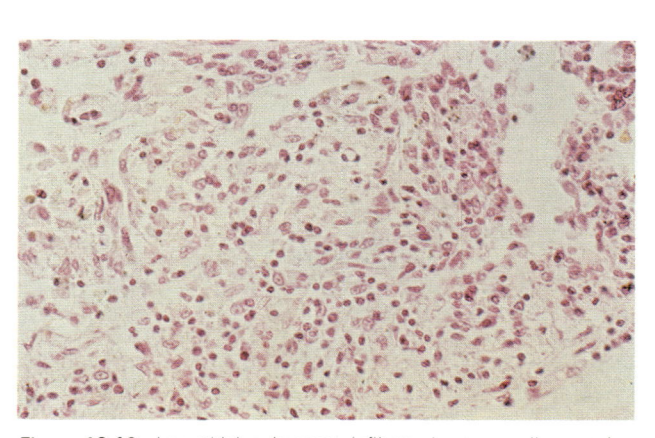

Figure 19.10 Interstitial pulmonary infiltrate in a case diagnosed as angioimmunoblastic lymphadenopathy, based on typical lymph node morphology and clinical features. The presence of numerous immunoblasts is the histological clue to diagnosis. Immunoblasts are typified by large, oval, open nuclei containing a single large or two or three prominent nucleoli, and cytoplasm that is intensely pyroninophilic on methyl green pyronin stain.

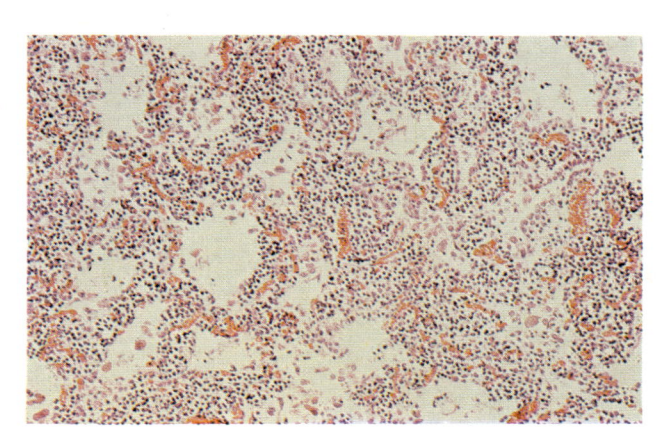

Figure 19.11 An interstitial leukaemic infiltrate in a patient with chronic lymphatic leukaemia. This mimics LIP but the lymphoid cells are more primitive, relatively uniform and germinal centres are absent. Also examination of blood vessels will reveal large numbers of cells which appear similar. Intrapulmonary haemorrhages are also frequently present. H&E × 240.

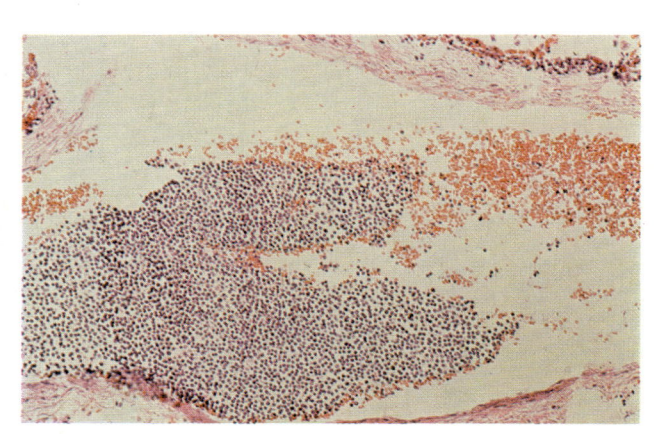

Figure 19.12 The same case as Figure 19.11 showing the leukaemic cells in a pulmonary artery. H&E × 240.

Lymphomatoid Granulomatosis (LYG)

In 1972, Liebow et al.[5] proffered the term lymphomatoid granulomatosis for a rare condition primarily involving the lung and showing similarities to both Wegener's granulomatosis and malignant lymphoma. Other organs, particularly skin, central and peripheral nervous system, were frequently involved by the disease, sometimes a considerable period of time prior to pulmonary manifestations. In contradistinction to malignant lymphoma, involvement of spleen and lymph nodes and bone marrow was not usually seen early on in the disease. The mortality in Liebow's series was high, the majority of cases succumbing to respiratory failure. A few patients apparently responded to therapy or spontaneously improved. Histology did not appear to be of value in predicting outcome. Thirteen per cent of the cases developed overt malignant lymphoma.

Recently, McDonald et al.[6] pointed out the histological similarities between LYG and lesions of lethal midline granuloma (polymorphic reticulosis) of the upper respiratory tract. They argued that they were one and the same disease. It is similar to Wegener's granulomatosis in that there is vasculitis, varying amounts of necrosis and an accompanying cellular response, composed of varying proportions of lymphocytes, plasma cells, histiocytes, primitive lymphoid cells and large atypical cells, resembling the 'reticulum cell' element of Hodgkin's disease. This lymphoma-like infiltrate invades the walls of both arteries and veins, resulting in varying degrees of occlusion, destruction and obliteration of the vessels (Figure 19.8). By contrast, in Wegener's granulomatosis the infiltrate involving vessels is predominantly polymorphonuclear, and also the tuberculoid lesions conspicuous in the latter are rare in LYG. Lesions similar to those seen in the lung in LYG may be seen in the kidney but glomerulonephritis does not occur.

Benign Lymphocytic Angiitis

Saldana et al.[7] coined the term 'benign lymphocytic angiitis' for a condition that they regard as the benign counterpart of LYG. Characterized by dense benign infiltrates of lymphocytes, plasma cells and histiocytes with angiitis of mild or moderate degree and minimal or no necrosis it would appear to us to have similarities to LIP. The validity of this term therefore remains to be established.

Three other conditions – Waldenström's macroglobulinaemia, angioimmunoblastic lymphadenopathy and leukaemia – may involve the lungs and cause confusion with LIP and LYG. This is particularly important to the pathologist on biopsy material as, in leukaemias and lymphomas under treatment when an interstitial pulmonary infiltrate develops he will be asked, given minimal material, to distinguish between neoplasia, opportunistic infection and drug induced pneumonitis.

Waldenström's Macroglobulinaemia

This typically affects the elderly and is particularized by anaemia, raised erythrocyte sedimentation rate, lymphocytic infiltration of the bone marrow and a monoclonal IgM paraproteinaemia, an infiltrate which may be exclusively interstitial and mimic LIP very closely[3] (Figure 19.9). The alveoli may contain homogenous eosinophilic PAS positive material, presumably macroglobulin[8]. Regional lymph nodes, usually normal in LIP, show infiltration by cells intermediate between plasma cells and lymphocytes, some containing PAS-positive globules.

Angioimmunoblastic Lymphadenopathy

Infiltration of the lung by cells similar to those seen in the lymph nodes may occur in angioimmunoblastic lymphadenopathy[9] (Figure 19.10). The lymph nodes in this condition show blood-vessel proliferation, amorphous material within the stroma and proliferation of immunoblasts. Also present are plasma cells, lymphocytes and occasional multinucleated cells similar to but distinguishable from Reed–Sternberg cells.

Leukaemic infiltration of the lung occurs in about 25% of those dying from the condition, but rarely does it cause disturbance in lung function. Microscopically, this could cause diagnostic difficulties with LIP and LYG (Figures 19.11 and 19.12).

References

1. Salzstein, S. L. (1963). Pulmonary malignant lymphomas and pseudolymphomas: classification, therapy and prognosis. *Cancer*, **16**, 928
2. Greenberg, S. D., Heisler, J. G., Gyorkey, F. and Jenkins, D. E. (1972). Pulmonary lymphoma versus pseudolymphoma: a perplexing problem. *South. Med. J.*, **65**, 775
3. Liebow, A. A. and Carrington, C. B. (1973). Diffuse pulmonary lymphoreticular infiltrations associated with dysproteinaemia. *Med. Clin. N. Am.*, **57**, 809
4. Gibbs, A. R. and Seal, R. M. E. (1978). Primary lymphoproliferative conditions of lung. *Thorax*, **33**, 140
5. Liebow, A. A., Carrington, C. B. and Friedman, P. J. (1972). Lymphomatoid granulomatosis. *Human Pathol.*, **3**, 457
6. McDonald, T. J., DeRemee, R. A., Harrison, E. G., Facer, G. W. and Devine (1976). The protean clinical features of polymorphic reticulosis (lethal midline granuloma). *Laryngoscope*, **86**, 936
7. Saldana, M. J., Patchefsky, A. S., Israel, H. L. and Atkinson Jr., G. W. (1977). Pulmonary angiitis and granulomatosis. The relationship between histological features, organ involvement and response to treatment. *Human Pathol.*, **8**, 391
8. Winterbauer, R. H., Riggins, R. C. K., Griesman, F. A., Bauermeister, D. E. (1974). Pleuropulmonary manifestations of Waldenström's Macroglobulinaemia. *Chest*, **66**, 368
9. Iseman, M. D., Schwarz, M. I. and Stanford, R. E. (1976). Interstitial pneumonia in angioimmunoblastic lymphadenopathy with dysproteinaemia. *Ann. Int. Med.*, **85**, 752

Miscellaneous Rare Pulmonary Tumours

20

Sclerosing Angioma of the Lung (Sclerosing Haemangioma, Xanthoma, Histiocytoma, Xanthofibroma, Fibroxanthomatous Pseudotumour)

This rare benign tumour occurs predominantly in young and middle-aged females and manifests usually by haemoptysis or as an incidental 'coin' lesion radiologically.

The tumour is usually solitary, circumscribed, often encapsulated, and situated in the parenchyma, more commonly of the lower lobes. Grey-pink or yellow on cut surface, mottled with red areas, it may be solid or exhibit cystic spaces.

The great variety of terms given to this tumour reflects the varied histology of the tumour. Several authors have confused plasma cell granuloma and fibrous histiocytoma with sclerosing angioma, either not distinguishing each entity separately or putting individual examples under the incorrect category.

The characteristic feature is the presence of blood-filled channels, which may be large and thin walled or small with thick hyaline walls[1] (Figure 20.1). Between the channels a hyaline stroma or sheets of cells, similar to those lining the channels, may be present. Papillary projections are also present (Figure 20.1). The cells appear similar whether forming solid groups or lining papillae or channels. They vary from lightly stained with round nuclei and a delicate chromatin structure to darkly stained with small round nuclei having coarse chromatin (Figure 20.2).

Varying amounts of fibrosis are seen within the tumours. Foci of foamy macrophages, lymphocytes, plasma cells and mast cells are present. Haemosiderin deposition may be marked.

The few electron microscopical studies of this tumour have been conflicting; two reports[2,3] demonstrated epithelial cells lining the blood-containing channels, whereas others concluded that the tumour was derived from endothelial cells[4,5]. One of the authors (A.R.G.) has examined five of these tumours ultrastructurally and found the channels lined by epithelial cells.

Plasma Cell Granuloma (Pseudotumour, Post-inflammatory Pseudotumour, Histiocytoma, Xanthoma and Fibroxanthoma)

This is an uncommon tumour, usually asymptomatic and situated in the periphery of the lung (Figure 20.3). It is occasionally intrabronchial. It has not infrequently been misdiagnosed as sclerosing angioma or pseudolymphoma.

Grossly, it is usually circumscribed but not encapsulated, firm, yellow-white, grey or brown in colour and may show foci of haemorrhage, necrosis or calcification (Figure 20.3). It may form a sessile mass if located within a bronchus[6].

It is characterized by a proliferation of plasma cells (Figure 20.3) which are usually mature but may be multinucleated admixed with large lymphoid cells, lymphocytes and occasional neutrophils and eosinophils[6]. Russell bodies may be present and collections of lymphoid cells may form germinal centres. The stroma consists of bundles and whorls of fibroblasts, collagen and hyalinized homogenous eosinophilic material resembling, but not staining, for amyloid (Figure 20.4). Foci of calcification and even ossification may be present. Fat-laden histiocytes, often occurring in clumps, may be present and if prominent may make distinction from histiocytoma difficult (Figure 20.5). Germinal centres, if conspicuous, may mimic pseudolymphoma.

Fibrous Histiocytoma

The majority of reports of pulmonary fibrous histiocytomas have been, in fact, sclerosing angiomas or plasma cell granulomas. However, true fibrous histiocytomas arising in the lung do occur. Nair et al.[7] described a 1.2 cm yellow nodule in the right upper lobe of a 23-year-old female, which was composed of plump spindle cells, arranged in a storiform pattern, and showing foci of foamy cells resembling histiocytes.

Two examples of primary malignant fibrous histiocytoma of the lung have recently been documented[8,9], and we have also encountered a case (Figure 20.6).

Intravascular Bronchiolo-Alveolar Tumour (IVSBAT)

Fewer than 30 cases of this tumour have been reported. Typically, it is multifocal, occurs in young females, although the age has varied from 14 to 71 years[10], and progresses to fatal respiratory failure which may take several years.

Characteristically, numerous nodules (as many as 100) are present in the lungs, each measuring from a few millimetres to 2 cm in diameter. The nodules are composed of short cords or groups of epithelial-like cells embedded in a hyaline fibrous stroma. The tumour tends to fill arteries, veins and bronchioles even at a distance from the main mass (Figures 20.7 and 20.8). At the edges, the tumour appears to spread through the interalveolar pores. In early stages, the stroma is positive with PAS and alcian blue staining. The central parts may be necrotic or calcified[11].

Corrin et al.[11] based upon ultrastructural examination of three cases, proposed that the tumour originated from a vasoformative reserve cell.

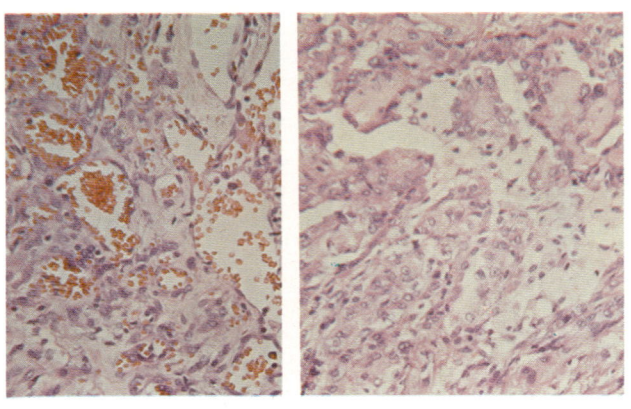

Figure 20.1 *Left:* Blood-containing channels lined by flattened or cuboidal cells. H & E × 240 *Right:* A papillary area, some showing sclerosis and lined by cuboidal cells. Some foamy cells are present within a space. H & E × 240.

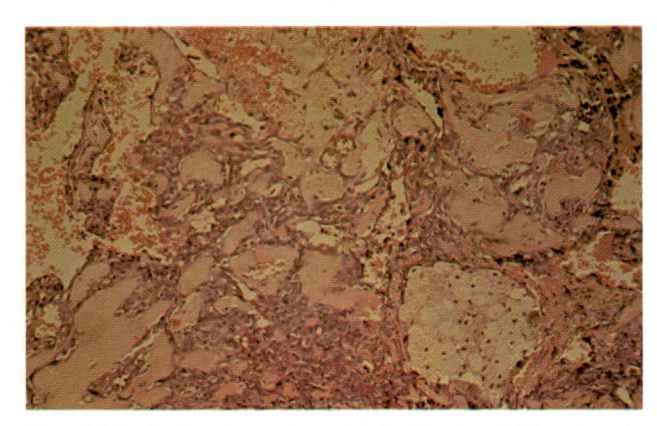

Figure 20.2 A sclerosing angioma showing blood-containing channels, sclerotic areas, solid areas and a focus of foamy cells. H & E × 96.

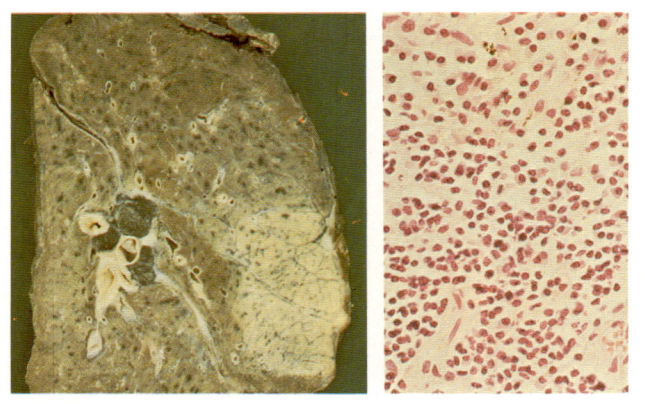

Figure 20.3 *Left:* Right pneumonectomy specimen showing involvement of most of middle lobe and part of the upper lobe by a greyish, firm, fairly-well demarcated lesion. *Right:* Microscopy revealed plasma cells to be a prominent component of the lesion. H & E × 384.

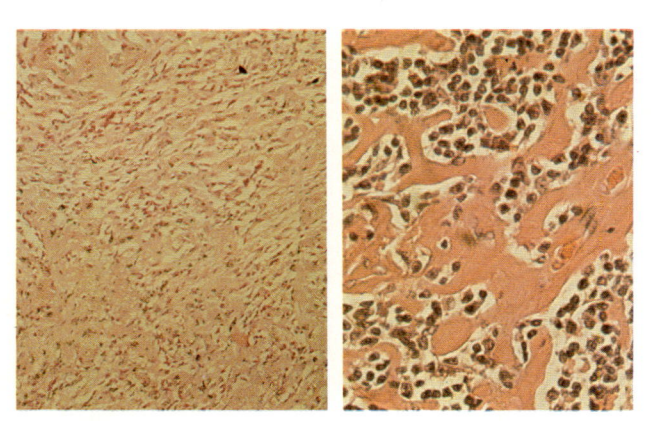

Figure 20.4 (Same specimen as Figure 20.3.) *Left:* Areas of the lesion were composed of a fibrous stroma in which numerous plasma cell, lymphocytes and histiocytes were present. H & E × 38.4 *Right:* An area where plasma cells and amyloid-like material were prominent. H & E × 384.

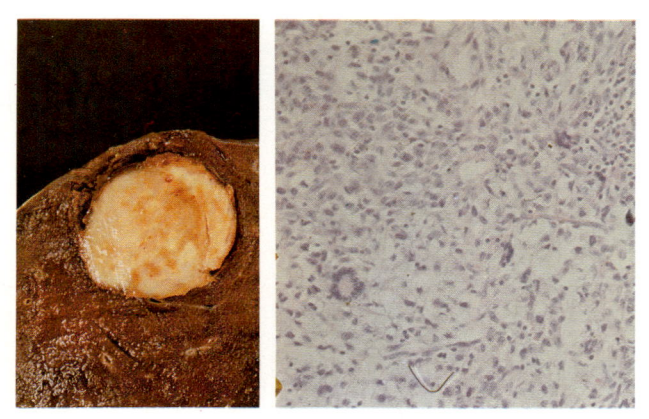

Figure 20.5 *Left:* A right lower lobectomy specimen showing a yellow circumscribed 3 cm diameter tumour in the subpleural area. *Right:* Microscopy revealed areas rich in plasma cells, foamy histiocytic cells and giant cells including Touton types. This tumour manifested features of both histiocytoma and plasma cell granuloma and was difficult to assign solely to either entity. H & E × 240.

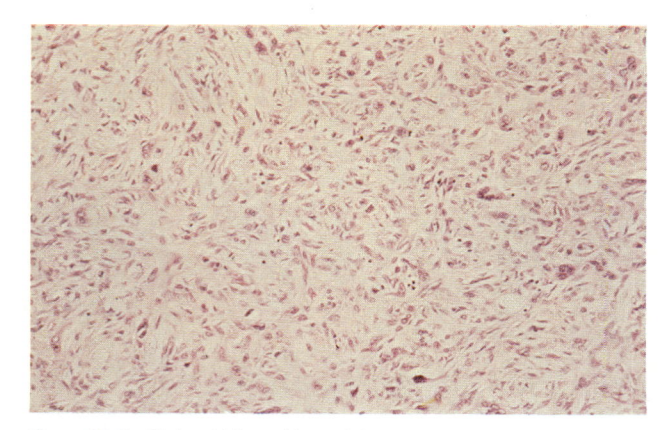

Figure 20.6 Right middle and lower lobectomy specimen was received in which a tumour appeared to occupy the whole of medial basal segment and indented the adjacent lung. Microscopy revealed cells interpreted as histiocytic, fibroblasts and giant cells. It showed a storiform pattern in areas. Mitoses and pleomorphism were marked in some foci. It was interpreted as a fibrous histiocytoma of borderline malignancy. H & E × 240.

MISCELLANEOUS RARE PULMONARY TUMOURS

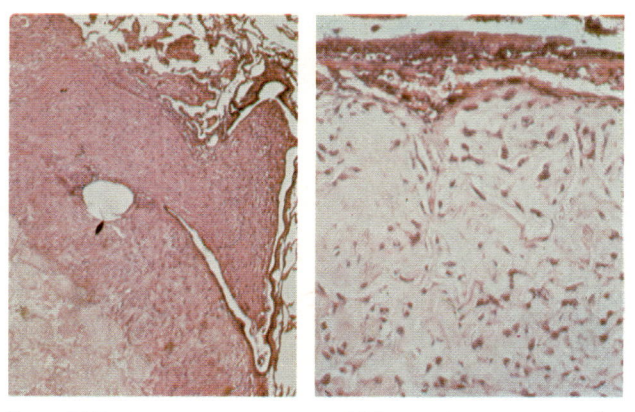

Figure 20.7 *Left:* Low power view of IVSBAT, showing tumour spreading into a bronchiole. H & E × 38.4. *Right:* The tumour shows marked hyalinization in which are scattered irregularly shaped, eosinophilic tumour cells with regular nuclei. H & E × 180.

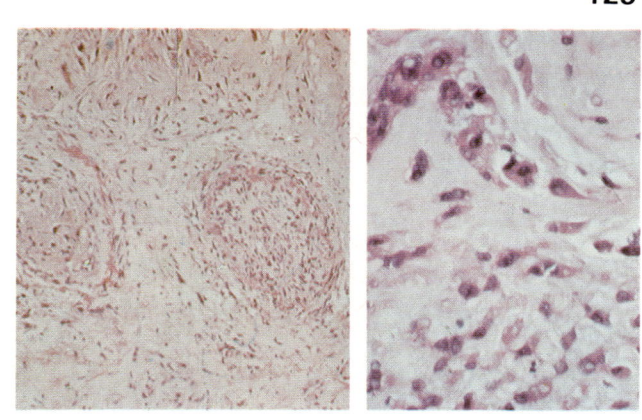

Figure 20.8 *Left:* Vessels occluded by cellular and hyalinized tumour. Similar tumour surrounds the vessels. H & E × 96. *Right:* High power view of tumour cells which appear similar both within the stroma and lining nodules. H & E × 384.

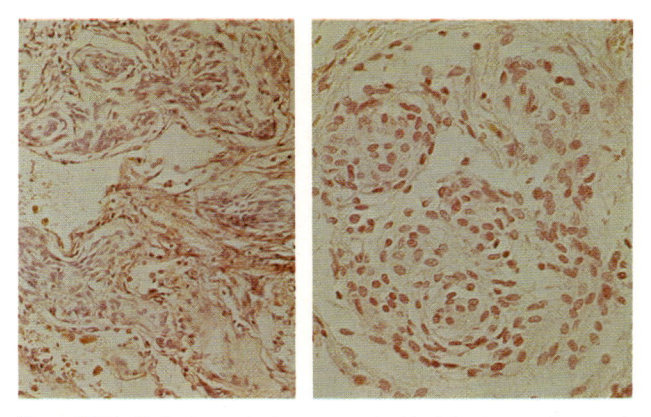

Figure 20.9 Both chemodectomas were incidental autopsy microscopic findings. *Left:* The relationship of the tumour to a vein. H & E × 38.4 *Right:* The characteristic 'cell balls'. H & E × 240.

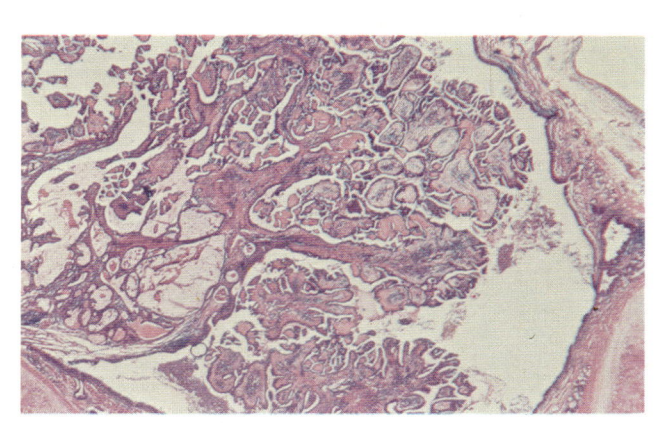

Figure 20.10 The wall of a large bronchus bearing a benign papillary tumour. It presented with an obstructive pneumonitis. H & E × 9.6.

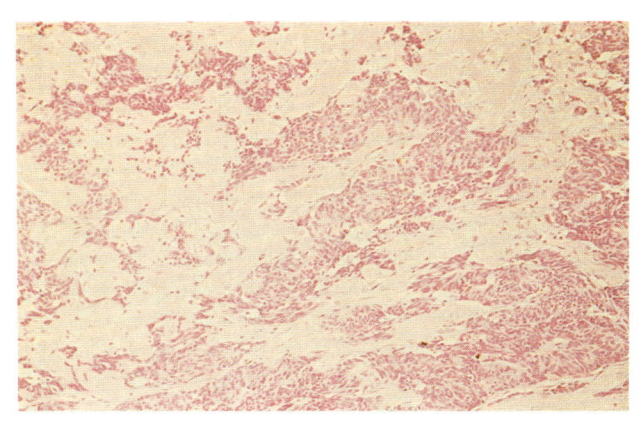

Figure 20.11 This tumour was an incidental autopsy finding in the lung; no thyroid tumour was found. Microscopy reveals pink amorphous material, which stained for amyloid, and tumour cells resembling those seen in medullary carcinoma of thyroid. H & E × 96.

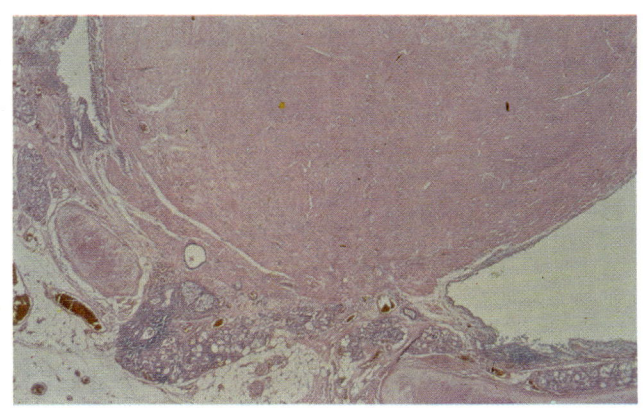

Figure 20.12 A benign leiomyoma arising from the wall of a large bronchus. H & E × 96

Minute Pulmonary Chemodectoma

First described by Korn et al.[12], these tumours are often multiple, small and usually detected incidentally in greater than 0.3% of autopsies. Reports have usually shown a female preponderance, and an association with cardiac failure, thromboemboli and obstructive airways disease[13].

The majority of the tumours are situated deep within the pulmonary parenchyma and measure up to 2 mm in diameter. If observed macroscopically they appear as a grey speck. They are located interstitially in relation to small veins. They consist of nests of elongated cells, arranged concentrically, with indistinct cytoplasmic borders, eosinophilic cytoplasm and delicate oval nuclei (Figure 20.9). Alveolar capillaries appear stretched over the nests. The nests are separated by a small quantity of reticulin or sometimes wider bands of collagen. Argentaffin and argyrophil stains are negative[13]. These tumours have to be distinguished from the carcinoid tumourlet (see page 111).

Ultrastructural examination of these tumours by Churg and Warnock[13] revealed a meningioma-like structure and did not demonstrate any characteristics of paraganglioma.

Surface Papillary Tumours

Rarely, solitary or multiple, non-invasive, papillary tumours occur in the trachea and bronchi. Multiple tumours are frequently associated with laryngeal papillomatosis[14].

The tumours have a connective-tissue core lined by a variety of epithelial types – squamous, transitional, squamous epithelium containing goblet cells, columnar epithelium, ciliated epithelium – either alone or in combination (Figure 20.10). The epithelium may be benign or show foci of dyplasia and in-situ carcinoma. Invasive carcinoma may supervene[15]. This risk is greater in those cases commencing in adulthood; disease beginning in childhood is usually self-limiting[14].

Granular Cell Tumours (Granular Cell Myoblastoma)

Benign tumours composed of closely packed cells with regular oval or round nuclei and eosinophilic cytoplasmic granules, identical histologically to the granular cell tumour situated within the tongue, may arise in the bronchial tree. Up to 1974, 43 cases had been reported[16]. Local excision results in cure.

Medullary Carcinoma of the Lung with Amyloid Stroma

A rare amyloid-containing tumour which appears to be the histological counterpart of medullary carcinoma of the thyroid has been described, arising primarily within the lung[17]. We, the authors, have observed a similar case (Figure 20.11).

Primary Sarcoma of the Lung

Several types of malignant connective-tissue tumours have been described in the lung, including fibrosarcoma, leiomyosarcoma, rhabdomyosarcoma, neurogenic sarcoma, chondrosarcoma, osteosarcoma and haemangiopericytoma. Great care must be taken to exclude a primary focus in another organ. Cameron[18] encountered nine primary lung sarcomas in 6 000 cases of bronchogenic carcinoma. Fibrosarcoma and leiomyosarcoma appear to be the most frequent types seen. An endobronchial location is associated with a better prognosis than an intraparenchymal position. Mitotic rate and size are also helpful prognostic indicators[19].

Other Rare Tumours

Other rare pulmonary tumours that have been described include neurofibroma, neurilemmoma, lipoma, fibroma, leiomyoma (Figure 20.12) and malignant melanoma.

References

1. Liebow, A. A. and Hubbell, D. S. (1956). Sclerosing haemangioma (histiocytoma, xanthoma) of the lung. *Cancer*, **9**, 53
2. Mikuz, G., Szinicz, G. and Fischer, H. (1979). Sclerosing angioma of the lung. Case report and electron microscope investigation. *Virchows Arch. A. Anat. Hist.*, **385**, 93
3. Hill, G. S. and Eggleston, J. C. (1972). Electron microscopic study of so-called 'pulmonary sclerosing haemangioma'. *Cancer*, **30**, 1092
4. Kay, S., Still, W. J. S. and Borochovitz, D. (1977). Sclerosing haemangioma of the lung: An endothelial or epithelial neoplasm? *Human Pathol.*, **8**, 468
5. Haas, J. E., Yunis, E. J. and Totten, R. S. (1972). Ultrastructure of a sclerosing haemangioma of the lung. *Cancer*, **30**, 512
6. Bahadori, M. and Liebow, A. A. (1973). Plasma cell granulomas of the lung. *Cancer*, **31**, 191
7. Nair, S., Nair, K. and Weisbrot, I. M. (1974). Fibrous histiocytoma of the lung (sclerosing haemangioma variant?). *Chest*, **65**, 465
8. Bedrossian, C. W. M., Verani, R., Unger, K. M. and Salman, Joanne (1979). Pulmonary malignant fibrous histiocytoma. *Chest*, **75**, 186
9. Kern, W. H., Hughes, R. K., Meyer, B. W. and Harley, D. P. (1979). Malignant fibrous histiocytoma of the lung. *Cancer*, **44**, 1793
10. Dail, D. A. and Liebow, A. A. (1975). Intravascular bronchioloalveolar tumour. *Am. J. Pathol.*, **78**, 6a
11. Corrin, B., Manners, B., Millard, M. and Weaver, L. (1979). Histogenesis of the so-called 'intravascular bronchioloalveolar tumour'. *J. Pathol.*, **128**, 163
12. Korn, D., Bensch, K., Liebow, A. A. and Castleman, B. (1960). Multiple minute pulmonary tumours resembling chemodectomas. *Am. J. Pathol.*, **37**, 641
13. Churg, A. M. and Warnock, M. L. (1976). So-called 'Minute Pulmonary Chemodectoma' – A tumour not related to paragangliomas. *Cancer*, **37**, 1759
14. Al-Saleem, T., Peal, A. R. and Norris, C. M. (1968). Multiple papillomatosis of the lower respiratory tract. Clinical and pathological study of eleven cases. *Cancer*, **22**, 1173
15. Spencer, H., Dail, D. H. and Arneaud, J. (1980). Non-invasive bronchial epithelial papillary tumours. *Cancer*, **45**, 1486
16. Korompai, F. L., Awe, R. J., Beall, A. C. and Creerley, S. D. (1974). Granular cell myoblastoma of the bronchus: A new case, 12 year follow-up report, and review of the literature. *Chest*, **66**, 578
17. Gordon, H., W., Miller, R. and Mittman, C. (1973). Medullary carcinoma of the lung with amyloid stroma: A counterpart of medullary carcinoma of the thyroid. *Hum. Pathol.*, **4**, 431
18. Cameron, E. W. J. (1975). Primary sarcoma of the lung. *Thorax*, **30**, 516
19. Guccion, J. G. and Rosen, S. H. (1972). Bronchopulmonary leiomyosarcoma and firbrosarcoma – A study of 32 cases and review of the literature. *Cancer*, **30**, 836

Pleural Tumours

Localized Pleural Fibroma (Localized Fibrous Mesothelioma)
This is a slowly-growing neoplasm which shows a peak age incidence in the sixth decade. A considerable proportion of subjects manifest joint symptoms and changes similar to rheumatoid arthritis. The symptoms tend to disappear on removal of the tumour. Complete surgical resection of the tumour results in cure.

Macroscopically, the tumours are circumscribed, encapsulated, protrude into the pleural cavity and have a pedicle attached to the visceral pleura. They may reach a considerable size but do not invade the parietal pleura or lung parenchyma. On cut section they are pink-grey, whorled or lobulated and firm. Foci of haemorrhage may be evident[1], as may small smooth-walled cystic areas containing protein-rich straw-coloured fluid (Figure 21.1).

Microscopically, the tumours are composed of fascicles of spindle cells forming bundles and whorls, interspersed with reticulin and collagen fibres (Figure 21.1). Slight pleomorphism and occasional mitoses may be observed without connoting malignancy. Sparsely cellular areas composed of hyalinized collagen and foci of loose myxomatous tissue are frequently present. Vessels are usually conspicuous and there is perivascular hyalinization. The tumours are often covered by a single layer of mesothelial cells with an underlying thin eosinophilic, PAS positive zone[1]. In some tumours mesothelial lined clefts may be observed[2].

Malignant Mesothelioma
A malignant neoplasm arising from pleura or peritoneum, this was first associated with asbestos-dust exposure by Wagner et al.[3] in 1960. Nowadays, in urban populations, over 85% of malignant mesotheliomas can be linked to asbestos-dust exposure. In certain rural areas where mesothelioma is conspicuous the tumour results from exposure to naturally occurring fibrous minerals (Turkey). In areas where mesothelioma is excessively rare, there may well be examples of apparently naturally occurring malignant mesotheliomas. In these cases asbestosis may or may not be present, but variable numbers of asbestos bodies, from a few to numerous, are present within the lung parenchyma. Exposure to the crocidolite type of asbestos constitutes the greatest risk of developing malignant mesothelioma, but chrysotile and amosite also predispose. There is probably a dose–response relationship between exposure to asbestos and the likelihood of developing malignant mesothelioma, particularly with the chrysotile and amosite forms, but it must be remembered that exposure may be brief with a long latent interval to the development of the tumour – approximately 40 years – particularly with the crocidolite form.

The ability of the mesothelial cell to differentiate along diverse pathways results in marked histological variability both from field to field within the same tumour and between one mesothelioma and another. It is essential, therefore, to examine several blocks from the same tumour. In spite of this histological variability, the gross characteristics of the tumour are surprisingly constant[4].

Malignant mesotheliomas exhibit a striking tendency to grow along serosal membranes, which, in the case of the pleura, results in envelopment and compression of the lung by dense grey-white tumour tissue. Pleural mesotheliomas also tend to grow along fissures. Invasion of the lung frequently occurs both by direct spread and lymphatic permeation (Figures 21.2 and 21.3). A considerable proportion eventually metastasize widely.

Mesothelioma cells most commonly differentiate into lining cells, resembling epithelial cells, and stromal cells, which range from innocent looking spindle cells to sarcoma-like cells. Cells intermediate between the two types are evident[5].

Whitwell et al.[6] divided malignant mesotheliomas into four histological subgroups: (a) tubulopapillary; (b) sarcomatous; (c) undifferentiated polygonal and (d) mixed.

Tubulopapillary Type
This comprises tubules, papillae and cords composed of fairly regular columnar, low cuboidal or flattened cells with delicate vesicular nuclei (Figures 21.2–21.4). Branching papillary fronds, composed of fine connective tissue and lined by cells similar to the above, project into distended acini. Psammoma bodies occur in papillary areas in about 2% of cases. Vacuolation of cells may occur with signet ring forms, or cystic spaces may be found giving an adenomatoid appearance (Figure 21.4). These vacuoles and spaces contain hyaluronic acid. The cells are usually relatively uniform with a low mitotic rate. Occasionally, pleomorphism may be considerable, the mitotic rate high and bizarre tumour giant cells found. The pleomorphic tumours may be difficult and sometimes impossible to distinguish from undifferentiated carcinomas, as may pure tubulopapillary tumours from some examples of peripheral pulmonary and metastatic adenocarcinoma (particularly from ovary and kidney). Mesothelial tumour cells may contain dust or carbon particles within the cytoplasm – a helpful diagnostic feature[6].

Sarcomatous Type
In this type, appearances vary from large areas of dense hyaline collagen, to loose delicate collagen fibres, to bizarre pleomorphic spindle cells resembling fibrosarcoma (Figure 21.5). The stromal cells may be oval to spindle shaped with delicate vesicular

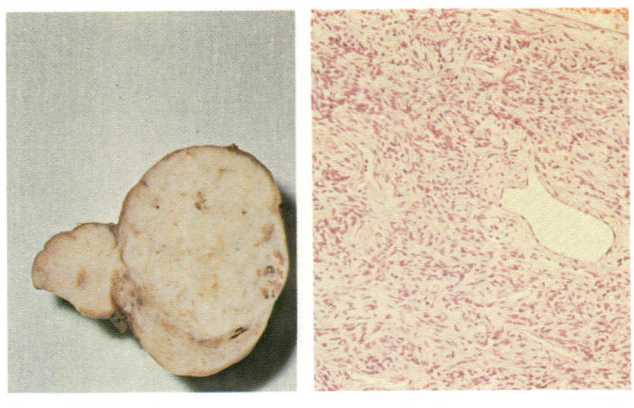

Figure 21.1 *Left:* A pedunculated, circumscribed, bossed tumour easily removed from the parietal pleura of a 52-year-old male. The cut surface appeared white and fibrous with small cystic spaces at one pole. *Right:* Histology reveals a cellular spindled tumour containing a few small clefts lined by flattened cells. H & E × 96.

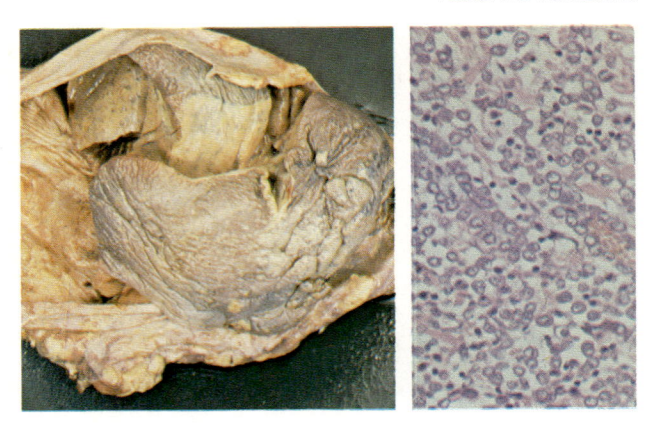

Figure 21.2 *Left:* Pleuropneumonectomy specimen of early mesothelioma presenting as an effusion. The most extensive visceral involvement is in fissures. There are also confluent nodules in upper lobe and involvement of the diaphragm. *Right:* Histology revealed tubulopapillary areas invading the diaphragm, but much of the tumour exhibited only a suggestion of papillary structures, the nuclei having a delicate open structure H & E × 384.

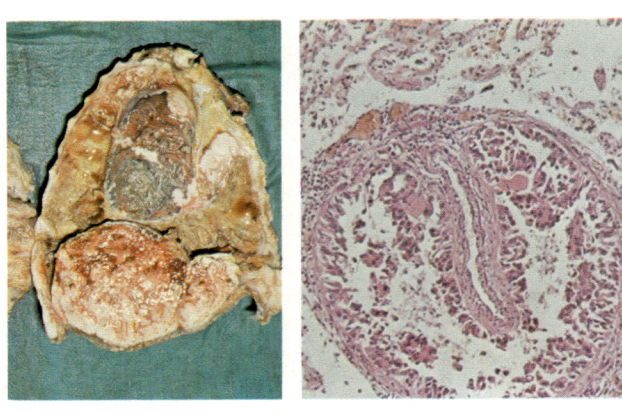

Figure 21.3 *Left:* Post-mortem specimen showing extensive encepahloid tumour between lung and diaphragm, involvement of fissure and direct invasion of lung. *Right:* Lymphatics invaded by tubulopapillary mesothelioma. H & E × 96.

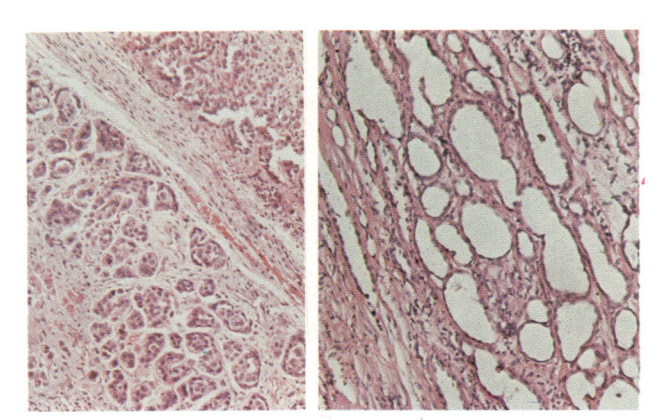

Figure 21.4 *Left:* A mesothelioma showing a variable tubulopapillary pattern. H & E × 96. *Right:* A mesothelioma showing capillary-like (adenomatoid) areas in a dense collagenous stroma. H & E × 96.

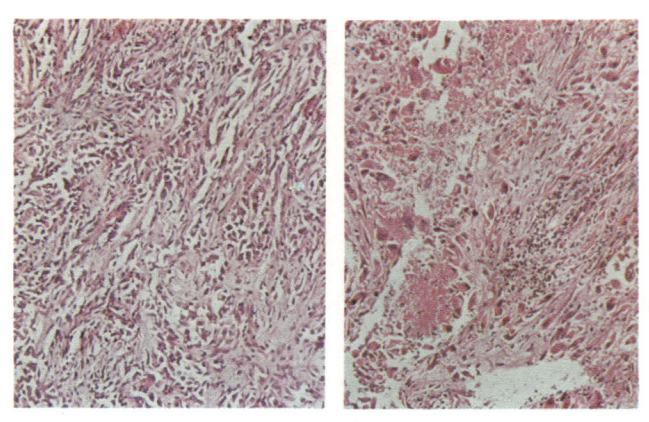

Figure 21.5 *Left:* Mainly cellular spindle celled sarcoma-like appearance where a tubular component is barely discernible. H & E × 96. *Right:* A spindle celled mesothelioma with scattered bizarre giant cells, some of which resemble rhabdomyoblasts. H & E × 192.

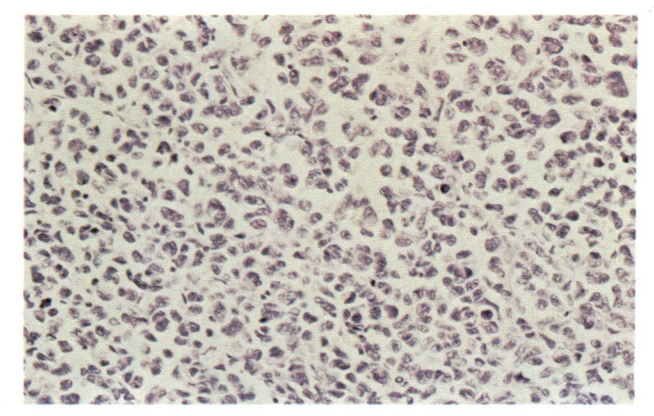

Figure 21.6 Sheets of epithelial cells in a mesothelioma which in other areas exhibited tubulopapillary differentiation. H & E × 480.

PLEURAL TUMOURS 129

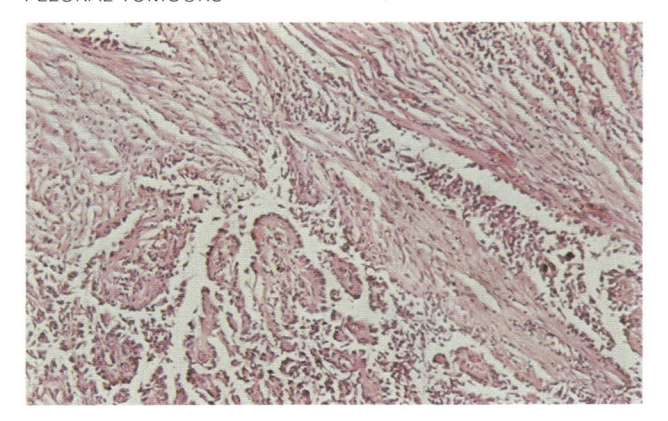

Figure 21.7 An admixture of papillary and ill-defined tubular (bottom right) with spindle celled area (left). H&E × 150.

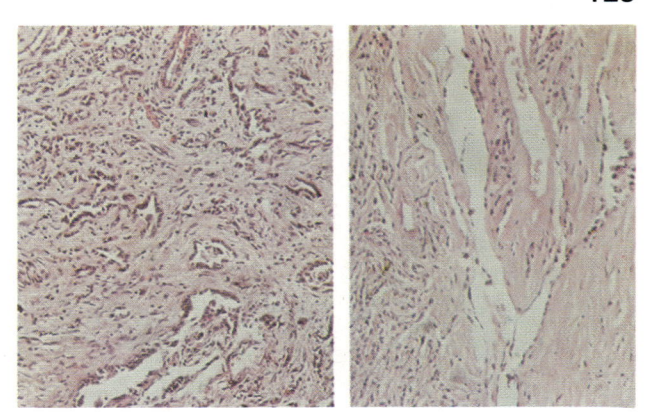

Figure 21.8 Photomicrographs taken from different parts of the same malignant mesothelioma. They illustrate the variability and the fact that many areas likely to be encountered on small biopsies will be non-diagnostic of neoplasia, let alone mesothelioma. Left: H&E × 96. Right: H&E × 240.

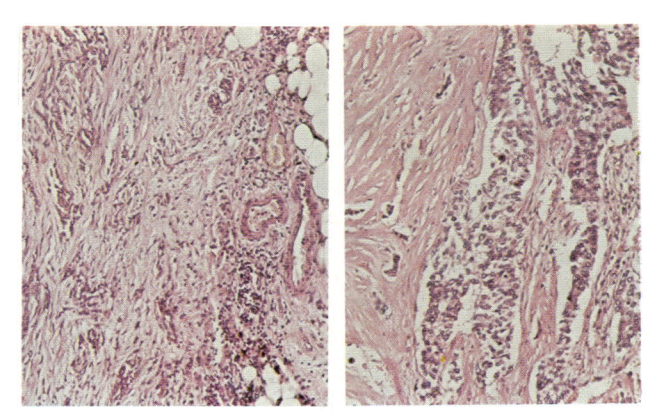

Figure 21.9 As Figure 21.8 Left: H&E × 96. Right: H&E × 192.

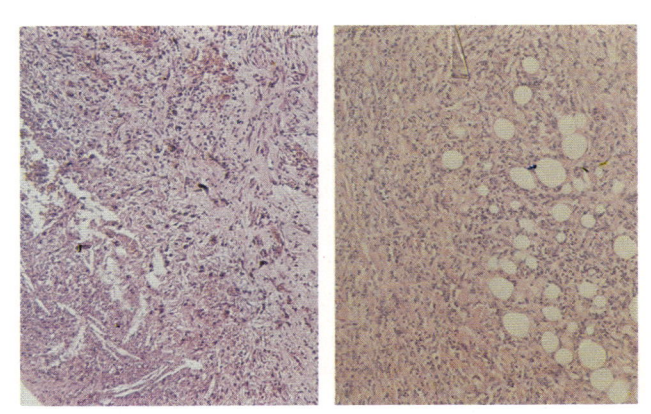

Figure 21.10 Left: Inflammatory pleural thickening (rheumatoid arthritis) with spindle celled areas. H&E × 96. Right: Edge of proven mesothelioma infiltrating fat. H&E × 96. In biopsies of inflammatory pleuritis it is difficult to exclude mesothelioma and in small biopsies of mesothelioma it is difficult to substantiate malignancy.

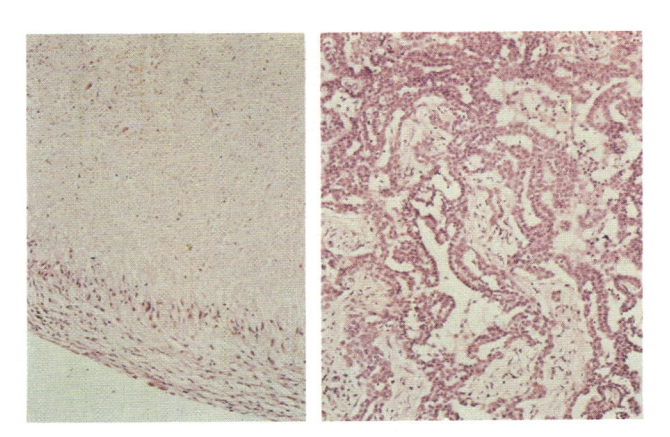

Figure 21.11 Multiple biopsies revealed (left) rheumatoid, nodules (H&E × 38.4) in the pleura and (right) proliferated mesothelium (H&E × 38.4) which has shown no progression over 10 years.

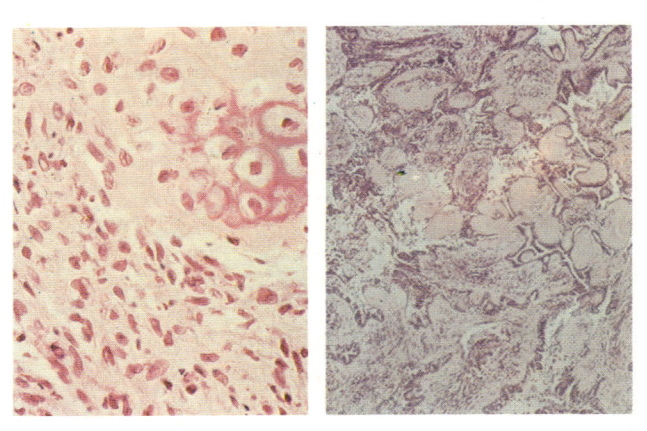

Figure 21.12 Left: An otherwise typical mesothelioma exhibiting chondroid differentiation. H&E × 384. Right: A mesothelioma showing an unusual pattern of sclerosis of papillae. H&E × 96.

nuclei[5], and/or markedly pleomorphic, bizzare, large and sometimes multinucleated. Atypical mitoses may be evident. Strap-like cells, simulating rhabdomyoblasts, may be present, but we have never demonstrated cross-striations within them (Figure 21.5). Areas with parallel orientation of fibres and a storiform pattern may occur which resemble histiocytic neoplasms. Tumours sometimes reveal prominent areas of myxoid change.

Undifferentiated Polygonal Cell Type
Occasionally occurring in a pure form, this pattern is more frequently observed in conjunction with the other types (Figure 21.6). It consists of sheets of regular benign-looking epithelial cells with abundant eosinophilic cytoplasm which produce a pavement-like effect. Occasionally the cellular sheets demonstrate considerable anaplasia, pleomorphism and mitotic activity with tumour giant cell formation. This is probably the most difficult form to distinguish from carcinoma.

Mixed Type
This exhibits a variety of combinations of the above types (Figure 21.7). This, and the tubulopapillary form, account for over 80% of malignant mesotheliomas. All stages of transition are observed between the various elements. It is a very characteristic tumour and is the most easily identified. The frequency of this type is likely to increase with the greater number of blocks examined from each tumour. Not infrequently, only one element may be evident in metastases from the mixed type.

It used to be argued that widespread metastasis made the diagnosis of malignant mesothelioma unlikely, but it is now realized that extensive blood-borne and lymphogenous spread is by no means uncommon. The sarcomatoid type appears to show the greatest tendency to blood-borne metastasis[6]. Extensive lymphogenous spread within the lungs may result in the picture of 'lymphangitis carcinomatosa'.

A number of problems occur in relation to the differential diagnosis of malignant mesothelioma, particularly with regard to biopsy material. At times a confident answer may only be given when the full clinico-pathological information is available, which may require autopsy. The two major problems regularly encountered are: (1) is a neoplasm present or not and (2) is this mesothelioma or some other type of tumour?

With regard to the first problem, inflammatory conditions of the pleura may produce vascular spindle celled areas difficult to distinguish from spindle celled mesothelioma. Indeed, even when examining a known malignant mesothelioma it may be difficult to decide exactly which are reactive stromal cells and which are neoplastic cells (Figures 21.8–21.10). Hourihane[7] found that the degree of inflammatory infiltrate and the cytology of the cells were the points of greatest value in distinguishing inflammation from neoplasia. He found only slight inflammatory cell infiltrate in malignant mesothelioma unless necrosis was conspicuous. He also found that cells with vesicular nuclei and prominent eosinophilic nucleoli argued in favour of malignant mesothelioma, since he did not observe them in inflammatory reactions. Occasional mitoses may be present in reactive and neoplastic mesothelium. In certain circumstances, e.g. pulmonary infarction, rheumatoid disease, etc. the mesothelium may proliferate to produce papillary structures and inflammatory tissue apparently containing entrapped innocent reactive mesothelium, which in biopsy material may be falsely interpreted as invasion. Indeed, it must be admitted that diagnosis is sometimes impossible; a case we would have confidently diagnosed as malignant mesothelioma has shown no progression over 10 years (Figure 21.11).

The most common neoplasm to simulate malignant mesothelioma, both macroscopically and histologically is a peripheral adenocarcinoma of the lung. Mesothelioma is favoured by regularity and orderliness of tumour cells which have delicate vesicular nuclei. Help may be obtained from histo-chemical stains, since if tumour cells or glandular lumina contain periodic acid–Schiff diastase-resistant material (neutral mucin) this would strongly support a diagnosis of adenocarcinoma[8]. Further, demonstration of hyaluronic acid within the tumour would favour mesothelioma. However, fixatives such as formal–alcohol–acetic, alcohol or Bouin's are more suitable for the preservation of hyaluronic acid than 10% formol–saline since hyaluronic acid is soluble in the latter[9]. In such fixed material the presence of intracellular and intraluminal alcian-blue-positive staining removed by pretreatment with hyaluronidase is almost diagnostic of mesothelioma.

Unusual Forms of Malignant Mesothelioma
Goldstein[10] described two cases of malignant mesothelioma which contained foci of calcification, cartilage formation and ossification together with malignant cartilaginous and fibrous stromal elements. We have also occasionally encountered foci of similar differentiation in otherwise typical malignant mesothelioma (Figure 21.12). This is not unexpected in view of the mesothelial cell's pluripotential capabilities of differentiation and has given rise to the concept of mesodermoma[11]. A rare variant of the papillary type of mesothelioma, we have encountered, exhibits sclerosis and mimics the so-called sclerosing haemangioma of lung (Figure 21.12).

References

1. Scharifker, D. and Kaneko, M. (1979) Localized fibrous 'mesothelioma' of pleura (submesothelial fibroma). *Cancer,* **43,** 627
2. Spencer, H. (1977). *Pathology of the lung.* (Oxford: Pergamon Press)
3. Wagner, J. C., Sleggs, C. A. and Marchand, P. (1960). Diffuse pleural mesothelioma and asbestos exposure in the North Western Cape Province. *Brit. J. Ind. Med.,* **17,** 160
4. McCaughey, W. T. E. (1965). Criteria for diagnosis of mesothelial tumours. *Ann. N.Y. Acad. Sci.,* **132,** 603
5. Churg, J., Rosen, S. H. and Moolten, S. (1965). Histological characteristics of mesothelioma associated with asbestos. *Am. N.Y. Acad. Sci.,* **132,** 614
6. Whitwell, F. and Rawcliffe, R. M. (1971). Diffuse malignant pleural mesothelioma and asbestos exposure. *Thorax,* **26,** 6
7. Hourihane, D. O. B. (1965). A biopsy series of mesotheliomata and attempts to identify asbestos within some of the tumour. *Am. N.Y. Acad. Sci.,* **132,** 647
8. Kannerstein, M. Churg, J. and Mayner, D. (1973). Histochemical studies in the diagnosis of mesothelioma. In *Biological Effects of Asbestos,* IARC Scientific Publications No.8, p.62. (Lyon: International Agency for Research in Cancer)
9. Wagner, J. C., Munday, D. E. and Harrington, J. S. (1962). Histochemical demonstration of hyaluronic acid in pleural mesotheliomas. *J. Pathol. Bacteriol.,* **84,** 73
10. Goldstein, B. (1979). Two malignant pleural mesotheliomas with unusual histological features. *Thorax,* **34,** 817.5Donna, A. and Provana, A. (1977). Considerations and proposals about mesotheliomas based on their morphological appearances (Note 1). *Pathologica,* **69,** 441

Index

(Italics refer to Figures)

Absidia spp. 34
acinic cell tumour 114
Actinomyces israeli 31
actinomycosis 31, *4.15*
adenocarcinoma 107, *16.4, 16.5, 16.17–16.19*
adenoid cystic carcinoma 111, *17.9*
adenomatoid malformation, congenital 14, *1.7*
adenovirus, and pneumonia 30
adrenal cortical tissues, heterotopic 11
agenesis 11
allergic granulomatosis and angiitis of Churg and Strauss
    (CSS) 78, *11.11*
aluminium pneumoconiosis 99, *15.1*
alveolar damage
    diffuse (DAD) 39, 42, *5.1–5.4*
    in influenza 27, *4.9*
    in mycoplasma pneumonia 30
    in systemic lupus erythematosus 63
alveolar microlithiasis, pulmonary 79, *12.6*
alveolar proteinosis 82, *12.12*
alveolitis, cryptogenic fibrosing (CFA) 42–3
amyloidosis, pulmonary 79, *12.1–12.4*
angiitis
    benign lymphocytic 122
    pulmonary 75
angioimmunoblastic lymphadenopathy 122,
    19.10–19.12
ankylosing spondylitis, pulmonary effects 66
anthraco-tuberculosis 51
antiproteolytic enzyme defects 22
a_1-antitrypsin deficiency, and emphysema 22
aplasia 11
arterioles 70
arteriovenous malformations, pulmonary 14
asbestos
    and interstitial pneumonias 43, *5.18*
    lung diseases induced by 91–2, 94–5, *14.1–14.11*,
        Plate *14.1*
asbestos bodies 91, *14.9–14.11*
asbestosis 92, 94–5, *14.1–14.11*
    grading guidelines 95
Ascaris, in eosinophilic pneumonia 62
aspergillosis 31, 34, *8.4, 8.6*
    mucoid impaction of bronchi 62
Aspergillus spp. 27, Plate *8.1*
    colonization following post-primary tuberculosis 50
    colonization in ankylosing spondylitis 66
    colonization of hyatid cyst 35
    in asthma 62
    in eosinophilic pneumonia 62
    A. fumigatus 31
asteroid bodies
    in sarcoidosis 54, *7.3*
    in Wegener's granulomatosis 75
asthma 59, 61–2
    Aspergillus infection 62
    'asthmatic plug' constituents 61, *8.3–8.5*

asthma – *continued*
    compared with chronic bronchitis 15
    histology 59, *8.1–8.2*
    mucoid impaction of bronchi 62, *8.5, 8.6*
    sputum examination 61–2, *8.3, 8.4*
atelectasis
    focal, in diffuse alveolar damage 39
    in bronchial asthma 59
    in systemic lupus erythematosus 63
    in Wilson–Mikity syndrome 14
    see also bronchiectasis, atelectatic
atherosclerosis, pulmonary 71
atrophy of lung, senile 22, *2.20*
azygos lobe 11

Bedsoniae, and pneumonia 30
berylliosis 99, *15.4*
    showing granulomata in lung 55
black fat tobacco, lipid pneumonia and 35
blastoma 118, *18.10, 18.11*
blood flow, pulmonary, decrease in, 74, *10.12*
bronchi
    adenoid cystic carcinoma 111, *17.9*
    displaced 11
    epithelial necrosis in influenza 27
    foreign body in *4.5*
    granulomatous reaction *8.9*
    hyatid cysts 35
    involvement in tuberculosis 50
    mucoid impaction 62, *8.5, 8.6*
    mucous plugs in asthma 59, *8.1*
    normal compared with chronic bronchitic *2.1*
    with diverticula 15, 18, *2.3–2.5*
bronchial tree, congenital abnormalities of 11
bronchiectasis 25–6
    and emphysema 22
    and lung carcinomas 103, *16.3*
    and organizing pneumonia *4.5*
    and rheumatoid arthritis 63
    atelectatic 26, *3.4*
    congenital 11, 26
        in Kartagener's syndrome 11
    'dry' *3.2*
    follicular 26, *3.1*
    in asthma 61, *8.6*
    in chronic bronchitis 15, *2.2*
    in cystic fibrosis 14, *1.11*
    saccular 26, *3.2, 3.3*
bronchiolectasis, in cystic fibrosis 14
bronchioles
    dust accumulation in 18
    earliest lesions in asbestosis 94
    epithelial necrosis in influenza 27
    inflammatory changes, in mycoplasma pneumonia 30
bronchiolitis 19, 22, *2.16*
    obliterans 39, 42, 43, 55, 62, *5.15*
    with EABA 55, *7.9*

bronchitis
    chronic 15, 18
        and emphysema 22
        and rheumatoid arthritis 63
        atrophic 18
        bronchial diverticulata 15, 18, *2.3*, *2.4*
        comparison with normal lung *2.1*
        inflammatory aspects 15
    monilial 34
    obliterative 63
    'plastic' 62
bronchocentric granulatosis 62, *8.11*
bronchogenic cysts 14, *1.5*, *1.6*
bronchopneumonia 27
    and *Streptococcus pneumoniae* 30
    gelatinous 34
    in cystic fibrosis 14
    Legionella pneumophila infection 31
    suppurative *4.13*
byssinosis 102, *15.11*

cadmium fume inhalation 102, *15.10*
calcification, dystrophic pulmonary 79, *12.8*
calcinosis, pulmonary 79, *12.7*
Candida albicans 34
    in eosinophilic pneumonia 62
candidiasis (moniliasis) 34
capillaries 70
    congestion in diffuse alveolar damage 39
Caplan lesions 87, 94, *13.12–13.15*
carcinoid tumourlets 111, *17.7*, *17.8*
carcinoid tumours 111, *17.1–17.6*
carcinomas 103–10, *16.1–16.24*, Plate 16.1
    adenosquamous 110, *16.24*
    and asbestosis 95
    and interstitial pneumonias 43, *5.8*, *5.10*
    associated with honeycomb lungs 66
    bronchio-alveolar 103, *16.6*
    clear cell 110, *16.22*, *16.23*
    histological typing 103
    large cell 107, 110, *16.20*, *16.21*
    lymphangitis carcinomatosa 103, *16.7*
    medullary, with amyloid stroma 126, *20.11*
    mucoepidermoid 111, 114, *17.10*
    oat cell 106–7, *16.10–16.15*
    obstructing lobar bronchus *4.6*
    peripheral growths 103, *16.4*, *16.5*
    possible misdiagnosis of Wegener's granulomatosis 75
    scar 110
    small cell 106–7, *16.10–16.15*
    spindle celled 106, *16.9*
    squamous cell 103, 106, *16.2*, *16.3*, *16.8*, *16.9*, *16.16*
carcinosarcoma 117–18, *18.8*, *18.9*
catarrh, and chronic bronchitis 15
chemodectoma, minute pulmonary 126, *20.9*
chondrosarcoma 126
Churg–Strauss syndrome 62, 78, *11.11*
cigarette smoking
    and chronic bronchitis 15
    and emphysema 22, 87, *2.15*, *2.18*
    and interstitial pneumonia 43
clear cell ('sugar') tumour, benign 114, *17.12*
coal workers, lung diseases of 18
    age comparisons 19, *2.7–2.14*
    see also pneumoconiosis
congenital disorders 11–14, *1.1–1.12*
corpora amylacea, pulmonary 79, *12.5*
Creola bodies *8.4*
cryptococcosis 34

Cryptococcus neoformans 34
cryptogenic fibrosing alveolitis (CFA) 42
    pathology 42–3
Curschmann's spirals 61
cyanosis, in diffuse alveolar damage 39
cylindroma 111, *17.9*
cystic fibrosis 14, *1.11*
    mucoid impaction of bronchi 62
cysts 11, *1.3*
    and neurofibromatosis *2.6*
    bronchogenic *1.5*, *1.6*
    congenital 14, *1.6*
        adenomatoid malformation 14
        cystic lymphangiectasis 14
    enterogenous 14, *1.10*
    hyatid disease 34
    in asbestosis 92
    see also pneumocysts
cytomegalovirus, and pneumocystis pneumonia 34

dental caries, and pneumonia *4.4*
desquamative interstitial pneumonia (DIP) 42
    distinguished from eosinophilic 62
    pathology 43, 45, *5.6*
Dietrle's silver impregnation technique 31
diffuse alveolar damage 39, 42, *5.1–5.4*
    and bronchiolitis obliterans 42
diverticula, bronchial, in chronic bronchitis 15, 18, *2.3*, *2.4*
drug-induced diseases 62
dust foci 18, *2.9–2.11*, *2.13*, *5.9*
    in coal worker's pneumoconiosis 86
    in non-miners 19
dusts, inhalation of 18, 19
    inert 99, 102, *15.9*
    see also occupational disorders
dyspnoea
    and interstitial pneumonias *5.15*, *5.21*, *9.10*, *9.11*
    in asbestosis 92
    in diffuse alveolar damage 39
dystrophic pulmonary calcification 79, *12.8*

Echinococcus granulosus 34
Eisenmenger syndrome 71
emphysema 18–19, 22
    and aluminium pneumoconiosis 99, *15.1*
    and interstitial pneumonias 43
    and lung carcinomas 103
    cadmium, chronic 22
    centrilobular 19, 22, *2.15–2.17*
        compared with focal 19
        tissue destruction 19, 22
    changes in nomenclature 23
    congenital lobar 14
    distribution 22
    focal 18–19, *2.7–2.14*
        compared with centrilobular 19
        related to age *2.8–2.10*, *2.12*
    investigative approaches 18
    panacinar (panlobular) 22, *2.2*, *2.18*
    relationship to pneumoconiosis 86, 87
    with EABA 55, *7.15*
empyema *4.3*
    and staphylococcal pneumonia 30
enterogenous cysts 14, *1.10*
eosinophilic granuloma 66
    comparison with histiocytosis X 67
epituberculosis 50
extrinsic allergic bronchiolo-alveolitis (EABA) 54–5, *7.8–7.15*

INDEX

Fallot's tetralogy 74, *10.12*
farmer's lung *see* occupational disorders: organic dust diseases
fibroma 126
    localized pleural 127, *21.1*
fibrosarcoma 126
fibrosis *see* interstitial fibrosis; progressive massive fibrosis; pulmonary massive fibrosis
fibrous histiocytoma 123, *20.6*
fibroxanthomatous pseudotumour 123, *20.1, 20.2*
finger clubbing 14
    and interstitial pneumonia *5.15, 5.21*
fuller's earth pneumoconiosis 97, *14.15*
fungal causes of disease
    in eosinophilic pneumonia 62
    showing granulomata in lung 55, 58

Ghon focus 47
giant cell carcinoma 110, *16.21*
giant cell interstitial pneumonia (GIP) 42–3, *5.22, 8.8*
giant cells
    in eosinophilic pneumonia 62, *8.8, 8.10*
    in necrotizing sarcoid granulomatosis 78, *11.10*
    in Wegener's granulomatosis 75, *11.7*
    reaction in amyloidosis 79
Goodpasture's syndrome 82, *12.11*
granular cell tumours (myoblastoma) 126
granulomatous conditions 53–8, *7.1–7.15*
    bronchocentric granulomatosis 62, *8.11*
    differential diagnosis 55, 58
    lymphomatoid granulomatosis (LYG) 122, *19.8*
    see also Wegener's granulomatosis (WG); necrotizing sarcoid granulomatosis (NSG)
grey hepatization *4.10*
    in lobar pneumonia 30, *4.1, 4.2*

haemangioma 123, *20.1, 20.2*
haemangiopericytoma 126
haematite pneumoconiosis 99, *15.5–15.7*
Haemophilus influenzae 15
    and bronchopneumonia 30
haemoptysis 14, *1.12*
    and lung carcinomas 103
haemorrhage
    diffuse intrapulmonary 82, *12.10, 12.11*
    in pneumonia *4.16*
        Pseudomonas aeruginosa 31
    intra-alveolar 26
haemosiderosis, pulmonary 71, *10.8*
    idiopathic 82, *12.10*
hamartoma 115, *18.2–18.5*
Hamazaki–Wesenberg bodies 54, *7.1*
Hamman–Rich syndrome 42
Hand–Schuller–Christian disease 66, 67
hard metal pneumoconiosis 99, *15.2, 15.3*
    showing granulomata in lung 55
helminth-borne pneumonias 34–5
    eosinophilic 62
herpes simplex, and pneumonia 30
heterotopic tissues 11
histiocytoma 123, *20.1, 20.2*
    fibrous 123, *20.6*
histiocytosis X 66, *9.8, 9.9*
    differentiation from eosinophilic pneumonia 62, *9.8, 9.9*
Histoplasma capsulatum 34
histoplasmosis 34
hyatid disease 34–5
hyperinflation
    in bronchial asthma 59
    in Wilson–Mikity syndrome 14

hypoplasia 11
hypoxia, chronic 71, 74

idiopathic chronic interstitial pneumonia (ICIP) 42
    alternative terms 42
    and systemic lupus erythematosus 63
    bronchoalveolar lavage 43
    compared with desquamative interstitial pneumonia 43
    pathology 42–3, *5.5, 5.7, 5.8, 5.11, 5.12, 5.14, 5.16–5.20*
idiopathic pulmonary haemosiderosis 82, *12.10*
influenza 27, *4.8*
infracardiac lobe 11
interstitial fibrosis 90, *13.19, 13.20*
    diffuse *9.10, 9.11*
        and rheumatoid arthritis 63, *9.3*
        and systemic sclerosis 66, *9.5*
    in aluminium pneumoconiosis 99, *15.1*
    in asbestosis 92, 94
    in coal workers 87, *13.16*
interstitium 42
    see also interstitial fibrosis; pneumonia, interstitial; pneumonitis, interstitial
intravascular broncho-alveolar tumour (IVSBAT) 123, *20.7, 20.8*
isocyanate vapour inhalation 102, *15.12*

kaolin pneumoconiosis 95, 97, *14.13, 14.14*
Kartegener's syndrome 11
Klebsiella pneumoniae 30, *4.12*

Legionella pneumophila pneumonia 31, *4.14*
    lobar 30
leiomyoma 126, *20.12*
leiomyosarcoma 126
Letterer–Siwe disease 66, 67
leukaemic infiltration 122, *19.11, 19.12*
lipoma 126
lobes
    congenital abnormalities 11
    emphysema, congenital 14
    sequestrated 11, *1.2, 1.3*
Löffler's syndrome 62
lupus erythematosus, systemic 63, 66, *9.4–9.6*
lymphadenopathy, angioimmunoblastic 122, *19.10–19.12*
lymphangiectasis, congenital cystic 14, *1.8–1.10*
lymphocytic angiitis, benign 122
lymphoid hyperplasia, benign 119, *19.7*
lymphoid interstitial pneumonia (LIP) 42, 119, *19.5, 19.6*
lymphoma 119, *19.1–19.4*
lymphomatoid granulomatosis (LYG) 122, *19.8*

malakoplakia of the lung 45
measles
    and atelactic bronchiectasis 26, *3.1*
    and pneumonia 27, *4.8*
melanoma, malignant 126
mercury vapour inhalation 102
mesothelioma
    localized fibrous 127, *21.1*
    malignant 127, 130
        mixed 130, *21.7–21.11*
        sarcomatous 127, 130, *21.5*
        tubulopapillary 127, *21.2–21.4*
        undifferentiated polygonal cell 130, *21.6*
        unusual forms 130, *21.12*
Microfilaria, in eosinophilic pneumonia 62
miliary lesions 34

miliary tuberculosis 50, *6.8, 6.10*
minute pulmonary chemodectoma 126, *20.9*
moniliasis 34
mucoepidermoid carcinoma 111, 114, *17.10*
mucoid impaction of bronchi 62
Mucor spp. 34
mucormycosis 34
mucous gland adenoma 114, *17.11*
mucous gland ducts 18, *2.4, 2.5*
    hyperplasia 15
mycetoma 34
    following silicosis with cavitary tuberculosis *6.12*
    nocardia colonization and 31
Mycobacterium bovis 47
Mycobacterium tuberculosis 47

nasal sinusitis, in Kartegener's syndrome 11
necrotizing sarcoid granulomatosis (NSG) 78, *11.9, 11.10*
neoplasms, showing granulomata in lung 55
neurilemmoma 126
neurofibroma 126, *2.6*
neurogenic sarcoma 126
nitrofurantoin, and desquamative interstitial pneumonia 43
nocardiosis 31

occupational disorders
    from coal and silica 83—90, *13.1—13.20*
    from metals, fumes and organic materials 99—102, *15.1—15.12*
    from silicates 91—7, *14.1—14.15*
    interstitial pneumonias 43
    organic dust diseases 54, *7.8—7.10, 7.12—7.15*
    showing granulomata in lung 55
    tuberculosis with pneumoconiosis 51, *6.12*
    see also pneumoconiosis
oedema
    in extrinsic allergic bronchiolo-alveolitis 55
    in *Klebsiella* pneumonia 30
    in lobar pneumonia 30
    intra-alveolar 39, *5.1*
oil granuloma, and exogenous lipid pneumonia 35
oncocytoma 114
ossification, pulmonary
    associated with mitral stenosis 79, *12.9*
    submucosal bone formation *1.4*
osteoplastica, tracheobronchopathia 11
osteosarcoma 126

papillary tumours, surface 126, *20.10*
paraquat, and diffuse alveolar damage *5.4*
phycomycosis (mucormycosis) 34
plasma cell granuloma 123, *20.3—20.5*
pleomorphic adenoma 114, 115, *18.1*
pleura
    lesions on *1.12*
    tumours of 127—30, *21.1—21.12*
pleural effusions, in asbestos workers 91
pleural fibroma, localized 127, *21.1*
pleural mesothelium, metaplasia 14, *1.11*
pleural plaques 91, 92, *14.1*
pleural thickening, following exposure to asbestos 92, *14.9*
pleurisy, and rheumatoid arthritis 63, *9.1, 21.11*
pneumococci, and bronchopneumonia 30
pneumoconiosis
    and angiitis 75
    conventional interpretation 83
    from aluminium 99, *15.1*
    from fuller's earth 97, *14.15*

pneumoconiosis — *continued*
    from graphite 87
    from haematite 99, *15.5—15.7*
    from kaolin (china clay) 95, 97, *14.13, 14.14*
    from silica 87, 90, *13.17, 13.18*
    from silicates 91—7, *14.1—14.15*
    from talc 95, *14.12*
    from tungsten carbide (hard metal) 99, *15.2, 15.3*
    in coal workers 83, 86—7
        Caplan lesions (rheumatoid pneumonia) 87, *13.12—13.15*
        lung assessment 83, 86, *13.1—13.11*
        pulmonary massive fibrosis (PMF) 86—7
        simple 86
        with tuberculosis 51, *5.9, 5.10, 5.16—5.18*
    with post-primary tuberculosis 51, *6.12*
Pneumocystis carinii 34
pneumocysts
    and cytomegalovirus infection 27
    dystrophic pulmonary calcification with 79, *12.8*
pneumonia
    bacterial forms 30—1
    classifications 27
        cytomegalovirus 27
    desquamative interstitial (DIP) 42—3, 45, 62, *5.6*
    eosinophilic 62, *8.7, 8.8*
    fungal forms 31, 34
    giant cell interstitial (GIP) 42, 43, *5.22, 8.8*
    Gram-negative organisms 31
    haemorrhagic *4.16*
    helminth-borne forms 34—5
    in immune compromised hosts 27
    interstitial 39—46
        classification 42
        in follicular bronchiectasis 26
        lymphoid (LIP) 42, 119, *19.5, 19.6*
        'of usual type' (UIP) 42
        with Wegener's granulomatosis *11.6*
    invasive 34
    Klebsiella 30
    Legionella pneumophila 31, *4.14*
    lipid 35
    lobar 30, *4.1, 4.2, 4.10, 4.11*
    mycoplasma 30
    pneumococcal 30
    pneumocystis 34
    staphylococcal 30
    viral forms 27, *5.14*
    see also bronchopneumonia
pneumonitis
    interstitial 55, *4.7, 4.9, 7.8—7.10, 8.7, 9.10, 9.11*
        with PM—DM 66
    obstructive 45, 103, *4.6, 16.2*
polyarteritis nodosa (PN) 78, *11.12*
polycythaemia 14
polymyositis—dermatomyositis (PM—DM) 66
progressive massive fibrosis (PMF) 51
protease mechanisms in emphysema 22
pseudolymphoma 119, *19.4*
Pseudomonas aeruginosa pneumonia 31, *4.13*
psittacosis 30
pulmonary arteries *10.1*
    dilatation lesions 70, *10.5*
    elastic 70, 71, *10.1*
    intimal proliferation *10.2, 10.3*
    medial hypertrophy 70, *10.2*
    muscular 70, *10.7, 10.11*
    necrotizing arteritis 70, *10.6*
    plexiform lesions 70, *10.4*
pulmonary hypertension
    and angiitis 75

INDEX

pulmonary hypertension — *continued*
   and fibrinoid necrosis *10.6*
   characteristic features 70
   classification of changes Plate *10.1*
   hypoxic 71, 74, *10.11*
   plexogenic 71, *10.3–10.5*
   thromboembolic 71, *10.7*
   vascular lesions 69–74, *10.1*
     classification 71, 74
     grading 70–1
   venous 71, *10.8–10.10*
pulmonary massive fibrosis (PMF) 86–7
pulmonary tumourlets 111, *17.7, 17.8*
pulmonary veins 70
   intimal fibrosis *10.8*
   lesions 71

red hepatization in lobar pneumonia 30
Rendu–Osler–Weber disease 14
respiratory distress syndrome *1.1*
   adult 39
   Wilson–Mikity syndrome 14
respiratory epithelium
   and submucosal bone formation *1.4*
   lining bronchogenic cyst *1.6*
respiratory insufficiency 39
rhabdomyosarcoma 126
rheumatoid arthritis
   and diffuse interstitial fibrosis 63, *9.3*
   and obliterative bronchitis 63
   and pulmonary disease 63, 75, *9.2*, Plate *9.1*
   necrobiotic nodules 63
rheumatoid disease
   similarities to bronchocentric granulomatosis 62, *8.9*
   with interstitial involvement 42
Rhizopus spp. 34
Rickettsiae and pneumonia 30

sarcoid granulomata 53, *7.1–7.3*
   see also necrotizing sarcoid granulomatosis (NSG)
sarcoidosis 53–4, *7.6*
   comparison with EABA 55
   role of biopsy 54
   similarities to necrotizing sarcoid granulomatosis 78
sarcoma, primary 126
Schaumann bodies 54, 55, *7.1, 7.6*
Schistoma in eosinophilic pneumonia 62
scleroderma see systemic sclerosis
sclerosing angioma 123, *20.1, 20.2*
senile lung 22, *2.20*
sequestrated lobe 11, *1.2, 1.3*
siderosis 99, *15.8*
silica see pneumoconiosis, from silica
silico-tuberculosis 51, *6.12*
silicosis 83
   acute 87
   nodular 90, *13.17, 13.18*
silo filler's disease 102
situs inversus, in Kartegener's syndrome 11
Sjögren's syndrome 66, 119, *9.7*
   associated pulmonary conditions 66
staphylococci
   and bronchopneumonia 30

staphylococci — *continued*
   and lobar pneumonia 30
Staphylococcus aureus 27, 30
streptococci
   and bronchopneumonia 30
   and lobar pneumonia 30
Streptococcus pneumoniae 30
striated muscle tissue, heterotopic 11
Strongyloides stercoralis 35
'sugar' tumour 114, *17.12*
syncytial virus, and pneumonia 30
systemic lupus erythematosus (SLE) 63, 66, *9.4–9.6*
systemic sclerosis (scleroderma) 66, *9.5*

talc pneumoconiosis 95, *14.12*
   showing granulomata in lung 55, 95
telangiectasis 14
teratoma 115, 117, *18.6, 18.7*
toluene diisocyanate (TDI) 102, *15.12*
Toxocara, in eosinophilic pneumonia 62
tracheal cartilage, and submucosal formation of bone *1.4*
tracheobronchopathia osteoplastica 11
tracheostomy stoma, infected *4.3*
transitional tumours 118
traumatic wet lung 39
tubercle
   differential diagnosis of histoplasmosis 34
   showing granulomata in lung 55
tuberculosis 47–51
   bacteriocidal treatment 47
   haematogenous spread 50
   histological appearances 47, *6.1–6.5*
   miliary 50, *6.8, 6.10*
   post-primary 50, *6.11*
   potential mycobacterial pathogens 47, *6.1*
   primary 47, Plate *6.1*
     complications 47, 50
     progressive 50, *6.10*
     'segmental lesion' (epituberculosis) 50, *6.9*
   tuberculous foci in atelectatic bronchiectasis 26
   with dust pneumoconiosis 51, *6.12*
tumours
   carcinoid and salivary-gland type 111–14, *17.1–17.12*
   of controversial diagnosis and histogenesis 115–18
   rare types 123–6, *20.1–20.12*
   see also carcinomas

varicella, and pneumonia 30
vasculitis
   eosinophilis 62
   showing granulomata in lung 55, *7.5*
veno-occlusive disease, pulmonary 71, *10.9, 10.10*
venules 70

Waldenström's macroglobulinaemia 122, *19.9*
Wegener's granulomatosis (WG) 75, 122, *11.1–11.8*
whooping cough, and atelectatic bronchiectasis 26
Wilson–Mikity syndrome 14

xanthofibroma 123, *20.1, 20.2*
xanthoma 123, *20.1, 20.2*

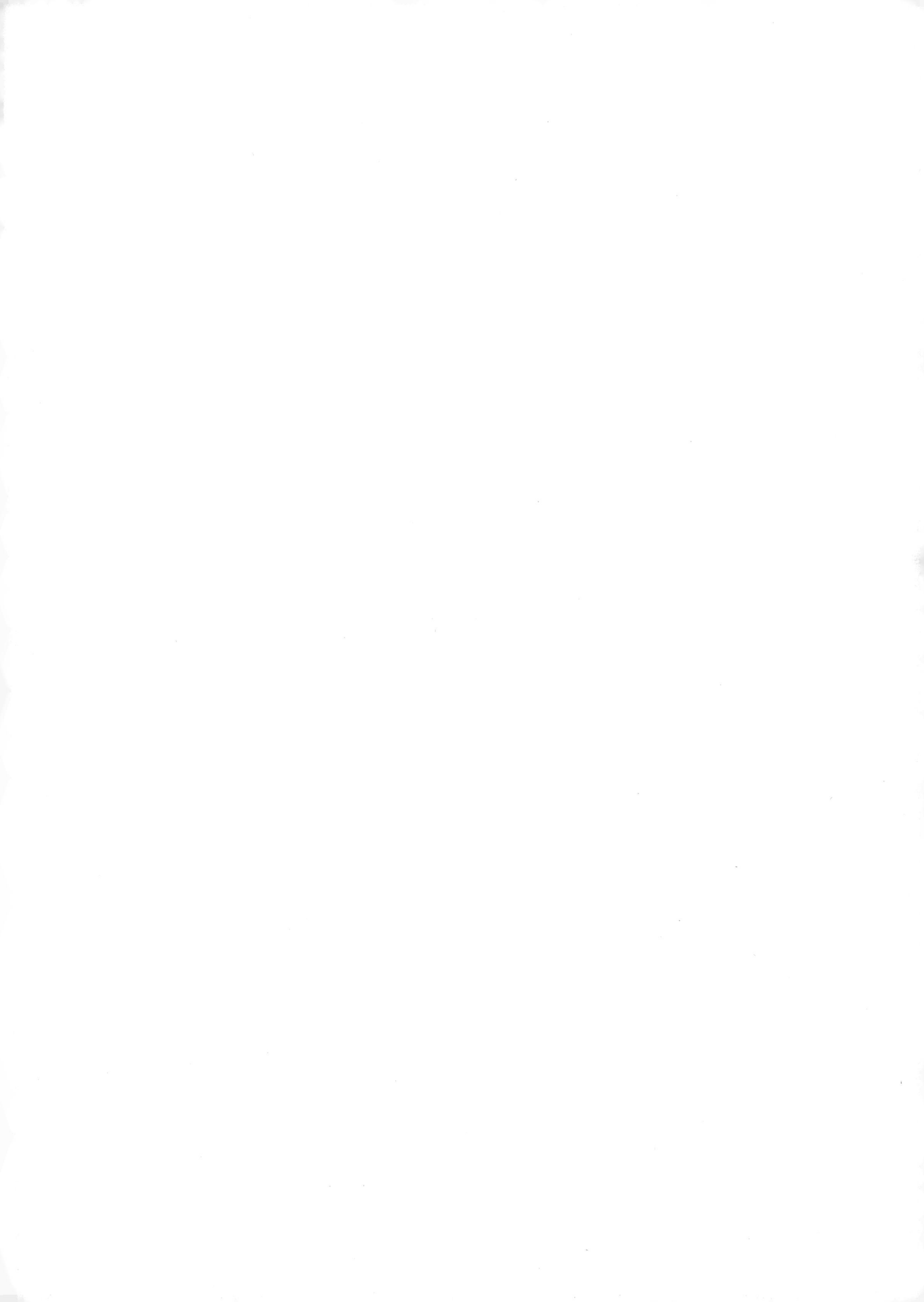